PSYCHIATRY BOARD REVIEW

PSYCHIATRY BOARD REVIEW

EDITED BY

Rajesh R. Tampi, MD, MS, DFAPA

PROFESSOR OF PSYCHIATRY, CASE WESTERN RESERVE UNIVERSITY SCHOOL OF MEDICINE
VICE CHAIRMAN FOR EDUCATION AND FACULTY DEVELOPMENT
RESIDENCY PROGRAM DIRECTOR
CHIEF OF GERIATRIC PSYCHIATRY
INTERIM DIRECTOR, PSYCHIATRY CONSULTATION LIAISON SERVICE
METROHEALTH, CLEVELAND, OHIO, USA
ASSOCIATE CLINICAL PROFESSOR OF PSYCHIATRY
YALE SCHOOL OF MEDICINE
NEW HAVEN, CT, USA

Kristina Zdanys, MD

ASSISTANT PROFESSOR OF PSYCHIATRY
GERIATRIC PSYCHIATRY FELLOWSHIP PROGRAM DIRECTOR
UCONN HEALTH
FARMINGTON, CT, USA

Mark Oldham, MD

ASSISTANT PROFESSOR OF PSYCHIATRY
YALE SCHOOL OF MEDICINE
ASSISTANT PROFESSOR OF PSYCHIATRY, YALE SCHOOL OF NURSING
MEDICAL DIRECTOR, BEHAVIORAL INTERVENTION TEAM
YALE-NEW HAVEN HOSPITAL
NEW HAVEN, CT, USA

OXFORD
UNIVERSITY PRESS

OXFORD
UNIVERSITY PRESS

Oxford University Press is a department of the University of Oxford. It furthers the University's objective of excellence in research, scholarship, and education by publishing worldwide. Oxford is a registered trade mark of Oxford University Press in the UK and certain other countries.

Published in the United States of America by Oxford University Press
198 Madison Avenue, New York, NY 10016, United States of America.

CIP data is on file at the Library of Congress
ISBN 978–0–19–026555–7

9 8 7 6 5 4 3 2 1

Printed by Webcom, Inc., Canada

TABLE OF CONTENTS

CONTRIBUTORS

Mohsina Ahmed, MD
Resident in Psychiatry
MetroHealth
Case Western Reserve University School of Medicine
Cleveland, OH, USA

Adefolake Akinsanya, MD
Resident in Psychiatry
MetroHealth
Case Western Reserve University School of Medicine
Cleveland, OH, USA

Lily Arora, MD
Clinical Assistant Professor
Rutgers-New Jersey Medical School
Newark, NJ, USA

Anil Bachu, MD
Resident in Psychiatry
MetroHealth
Case Western Reserve University School of Medicine
Cleveland, OH, USA

Silpa Balachandran, MD
Resident in Psychiatry
MetroHealth
Case Western Reserve University School of Medicine
Cleveland, OH, USA

Tatjana Barisic-Dujmovic, MD
Attending Psychiatrist
Rogers Memorial Hospital
Brown Deer, WI, USA

Isis Burgos-Chapman, MD, FAPA
Staff Adult and Geriatric Psychiatrist
Cornell Scott Hill Health Center
New Haven, CT, USA
Assistant Clinical Professor of Psychiatry
Yale School of Medicine
New Haven, CT, USA

Deepti Challagolla, MD
Attending Psychiatrist
Lighthouse Care Center of Conway
Conway, SC, USA

Jatinder Chawla, MBBS, MD
Staff psychiatrist
Manhattan Psychiatric Center
Manhattan, NY, USA

Suneela Cherlopalle, MD
Resident in Psychiatry
MetroHealth
Case Western Reserve University School of Medicine
Cleveland, OH, USA
Assistant Clinical Professor
Yale University School of Medicine
New Haven, CT, USA

Sarah de Asis, MD
Chairman
Department of Psychiatry
Day Kimball Hospital
Putnam, CT, USA
Assistant Clinical Professor
Yale University School of Medicine
New Haven, CT, USA

Nery Diaz, DO
Attending Psychiatrist
Audbon Clinic
Washington Heights Community Services
Instructor of Clinical Psychiatry
Columbia University New York State Psychiatric Institute
New York, New York, USA

Brian Frankel, MD
Fellow in Addiction Psychiatry
Yale School of Medicine
New Haven, CT, USA

Ambreen Ghori, MD
Resident in Psychiatry
MetroHealth
Case Western Reserve University School of Medicine
Cleveland, OH, USA

Aarti Gupta, MD
Principal Psychiatrist
Connecticut Valley Hospital
Middletown, CT, USA
Assistant Clinical Professor of Psychiatry
Yale School of Medicine
New Haven, CT, USA

Neha Gupta, MD
Fellow in Forensic Psychiatry
University of Pennsylvania School of Medicine
Philadelphia, PA, USA
Fellow in Child and Adolescent Psychiatry
University of Connecticut School of Medicine
Farmington, CT, USA

Swapnil Gupta, MBBS, MD
Assistant Professor
Department of Psychiatry
Yale School of Medicine
Attending Psychiatrist
Connecticut Mental Health Center
New Haven, CT, USA

Filza Hussain, MD
Consultant Psychiatrist
Mayo Clinic Health System
Eau Claire, WI, USA

Sarah Jillani, MD
Fellow Child and Adolescent Psychiatrist
Yale Child Study Center, Yale University
New Haven, CT, USA

Miyun Kang, MD
Department of Psychiatry
Yale School of Medicine
New Haven, CT, USA

Mahitha Kolli, MD
Resident in Psychiatry
MetroHealth
Case Western Reserve University School of Medicine
Cleveland, OH, USA

Mallika Lavakumar, MD
Attending Psychiatrist
Metrohealth
Assistant Professor of Psychiatry
Case Western Reserve University School of Medicine
Cleveland, OH, USA

Michael Maksimowski, MD, MA
Resident in Psychiatry
MetroHealth
Case Western Reserve University School of Medicine
Cleveland, OH, USA

Geetha Manikkara, MD
Research Assistant in Psychiatry
MetroHealth
Cleveland, OH, USA

Rabeea Mansoor, MD
Fellow in Child and Adolescent Psychiatry
Department of Psychiatry
Cleveland Clinic Foundation
Cleveland, OH, USA

Raman Marwaha, MD
Attending Psychiatrist
MetroHealth
Assistant Professor of Psychiatry
Case Western Reserve University School of Medicine
Cleveland, OH, USA

David Matuskey, MD
Associate Research Scientist in Radiology and Biomedical Imaging
Medical Director, Yale Positron Emission Tomography (PET) Center
Assistant Clinical Professor of Psychiatry
Yale School of Medicine
New Haven, CT, USA

Isabella Michna, MD
Fellow in Forensic Psychiatry
University of Colorado School of Medicine
Denver, CO, USA

Carlos E. Molina, MD
Resident in Psychiatry
MetroHealth
Case Western Reserve University School of Medicine
Cleveland, OH, USA

Mark Oldham, MD
Assistant Professor of Psychiatry, Yale School of Medicine
Assistant Professor of Psychiatry, Yale School of Nursing
Medical Director, Behavioral Intervention Team
Yale-New Haven Hospital
New Haven, CT, USA

Varma Penumetcha, MD
Fellow in Law and Psychiatry
Yale School of Medicine
New Haven, CT, USA

Rajiv Radhakrishnan, MBBS, MD
Department of Psychiatry
Yale School of Medicine
New Haven, CT, USA

Waqar Rizvi, MD
Fellow in Child and Adolescent Psychiatry
Yale Child Study Center, Yale University
New Haven, CT, USA

Kamalika Roy, MD
Fellow in Psychosomatic Medicine
University of Michigan
Ann Arbor, MI, USA

Ajay Shah, MD
Menninger Department of Psychiatry and Behavioral Sciences
Baylor College of Medicine
Houston, TX, USA

Esha Sharma, MBBS
Research Assistant
Psychiatric Genetic Epidemiology and Neurobiology Laboratory (PsychGENe Lab)
Department of Psychiatry and Behavioral Sciences
SUNY Upstate Medical University
Syracuse, NY, USA

Harvinder Singh, MD
Assistant Professor of Psychiatry
St. Luke's University Health Network
Bethlehem, PA, USA
Clinical Assistant Professor of Psychiatry (Adjunct)
Temple University School of Medicine
Philadelphia, PA, USA

Shirshendu Sinha, MBBS
Assistant Professor of Psychiatry
Mayo Clinic College of Medicine
Rochester, MN, USA
Senior Associate Consultant, Psychiatry
Mayo Clinic Health System
Mankato, MN, USA

Rajesh R. Tampi, MD, MS, DFAPA
Professor of Psychiatry
Case Western Reserve University School of Medicine
Vice Chairman for Education and Faculty Development
Residency Program Director
Chief of Geriatric Psychiatry
MetroHealth
Cleveland, OH, USA
Associate Clinical Professor of Psychiatry
Yale School of Medicine
New Haven, CT, USA

Tobias Wasser, MD
Assistant Professor of Psychiatry
Yale School of Medicine
New Haven, CT, USA

Rachel Wurmser, MD
Resident in Psychiatry
Yale School of Medicine
New Haven, CT, USA

Juan Young, MD
Resident in Psychiatry
MetroHealth
Case Western Reserve University School of Medicine
Cleveland, OH, USA

Kristina Zdanys, MD
Assistant Professor of Psychiatry
Geriatric Psychiatry Fellowship Program Director
UConn Health
Farmington, CT, USA

PART I

BASIC CONCEPTS IN PSYCHIATRY

Edited by Isis Burgos-Chapman

1.

DEVELOPMENT THROUGH THE LIFE CYCLE

Rachel Wurmser

1. A mother asks her daughter to babysit a younger sibling. The daughter asks her mother to add five dollars to her allowance in exchange for the babysitting work. What level is this child at in terms of Kohlberg's theory of moral development?

A. Conventional
B. Postconventional
C. Interpersonal accord and conformity
D. Social contract orientation
E. Preconventional

ANSWER: E

Lawrence Kohlberg's theory of moral development has six stages grouped within three levels. Stages generally cannot be skipped, and it is rare to regress in development. The first level is "preconventional" and includes stage 1 (punishment and obedience orientation) and stage 2 (instrumental relativist orientation e.g. self-interest orientation/exchange morality). At the preconventional level, the child is aware of rules and decision making is based on consequences. The child in this vignette is at the preconventional level within the instrumental relativist orientation stage because she asks, "What's in it for me?" The second level of moral development is "conventional" and includes stage 3 (interpersonal concordance) and stage 4 ("law and order" orientation). During the conventional level, morals and the social contract are internalized and valued. The last level is "postconventional" and includes stage 5 (social-contract legalistic orientation) and stage 6 (universal ethical principles orientation). At the postconventional level, morality is guided by self-chosen principles that the individual determines to be just.

REFERENCE

Sadock, B., Sadock, V., & Ruiz, P. (2015). *Kaplan and Sadock's synopsis of psychiatry: Behavioral sciences/clinical psychiatry* (11th ed., p. 1103). Philadelphia, PA: Wolters Kluwer.

Kohlberg, L. Stages and Aging in Moral Development. *The Gerontologist*. Winter 1973;13(4):497–502.

2. Kohut theorized that the difference between infantile narcissism and pathological narcissism is that pathological narcissism results from:

A. Early self-object failures
B. The core belief of being the center of the psychological universe
C. A life spent building self-esteem
D. The idealized parental imago
E. The grandiose–exhibitionistic self

ANSWER: A

Heinz Kohut was a psychoanalyst who developed self psychology. He asserted that psychopathology results from a lack of parental empathy during development. A self-object is a person or thing used by the child to complete the self and/or fulfill a function (such as maintaining self-structure) that the child will eventually learn to do on his own. The child is not aware that the person/object is separate from self. Pathological narcissism can result if self-object needs are not met.

REFERENCE

Sadock, B., Sadock, V., & Ruiz, P. (2015). *Kaplan and Sadock's synopsis of psychiatry: Behavioral sciences/clinical psychiatry* (11th ed., p. 181). Philadelphia, PA: Wolters Kluwer.

3. The second individuation process involves which of the following?

A. Infant becomes aware of difference between self and mother
B. Young child realizes that mobility signifies separateness between self and mother
C. Adolescent experiences the independence from parents to take responsibility for life choices
D. Pre-adult graduates from college and obtains first employment
E. Early adult marries and starts a new family

ANSWER: C

Margaret Mahler described the first individuation or "separation–individuation." This involves an infant becoming aware of the separation between self and mother and developing a sense of identity. Peter Blos developed the idea of "second individuation" as an adolescent separation from childhood and reworking of the parent–child bond. This involves experiencing the self as an individual, as well as the pursuit of love and responsibility for life choices.

REFERENCE

Gilmore, K. J., & Meersand, P. (2014). *Normal child and adolescent development: A psychodynamic primer* (p. 216). Arlington, VA: American Psychiatric Publishing.

4. According to Freud, a dependent person who is pessimistic, demanding, and envious of others is fixated at what stage of psychosexual development?

A. Oral stage
B. Anal stage
C. Urethral stage
D. Phallic stage
E. Genital stage

ANSWER: A

Psychosexual development progresses through the oral, anal, urethral, phallic, latency, and genital stages. The first stage is the oral stage, and one of the primary objectives is to establish a trusting relationship with sustaining objects. Traits associated with fixation at the oral stage include dependence, pessimism, narcissism, and envy.

REFERENCE

Sadock, B., Sadock, V., & Ruiz, P. (2015). *Kaplan and Sadock's synopsis of psychiatry: Behavioral sciences/clinical psychiatry* (11th ed., p. 157). Philadelphia, PA: Wolters Kluwer.

5. At what age should a child start to play simple pretend games, such as pretending to feed a doll?

A. 12 months
B. 18 months
C. 24 months
D. 36 months
E. 48 months

ANSWER: B

By 18 months, a child can engage in simple pretend play. By 2 years, children should be able to play simple make-believe games. By 3 years, make-believe games should be increasingly complex.

REFERENCE

Centers for Disease Control and Prevention (2009). Milestone moments. Retrieved from http://www.cdc.gov/ncbddd/actearly/pdf/parents_pdfs/milestonemomentseng508.pdf (accessed February 1, 2016)

6. At what age should a child be able to cooperate with other children and be more interested in playing with other children than by himself?

A. 18 months
B. 24 months
C. 36 months
D. 48 months
E. 60 months

ANSWER: D

By age 2, a child should be interested in the presence of other children. By age 3, a child should understand the concept of "mine" and "hers." A 3 year old child should also be able to show affection and concern for friends without prompting. At 4 years of age, a child should be able to cooperate with other children and be more interested in playing with other children than by himself.

REFERENCE

Centers for Disease Control and Prevention (2009). Milestone moments. Retrieved from http://www.cdc.gov/ncbddd/actearly/pdf/parents_pdfs/milestonemomentseng508.pdf (accessed February 1, 2016)

7. A child is able to understand that he can use water to make ice cubes and that if he leaves the ice cubes on the counter they will melt into water. At what stage of cognitive development is this child?

A. Sensorimotor
B. Preoperational
C. Concrete operational
D. Formal operational
E. Hypotheticodeductive

ANSWER: C

The child in this question understands the idea of reversibility. Both reversibility and conservation are achieved during the concrete operational stage. Jean Piaget made significant contributions to the subject of cognitive development. He described four stages that lead to the acquisition of adult thought and knowledge:

1. Sensorimotor stage (birth to 2 years)
2. Stage of preoperational thought (2–7 years)
3. Stage of concrete operations (7–11 years)
4. Stage of formal operations (11 years to end of adolescence)

Children progress through these stages at different rates, and the ages listed are an approximation.

REFERENCE

Sadock, B., Sadock, V., & Ruiz, P. (2015). *Kaplan and Sadock's synopsis of psychiatry: Behavioral sciences/clinical psychiatry* (11th ed., p. 93–97). Philadelphia, PA: Wolters Kluwer.

8. Piaget theorized that newborn babies turn their head toward something that touches the cheek as a result of:

A. An innate schema
B. Assimilation
C. Accommodation
D. Equilibration
E. Object constancy

ANSWER: A

This is a description of the rooting reflex. A schema is a unit of knowledge or framework that helps us organize or understand information. According to Piaget, innate schemas are the cognitive structures underlying neonatal reflexes. Assimilation and accommodation are forms of adaptation in the process of intellectual growth. Equilibration is the balance between accommodation and assimilation and helps drive development and learning. Object constancy is the understanding that an absent object continues to exist.

REFERENCE

Sadock, B., Sadock, V., & Ruiz, P. (2015). *Kaplan and Sadock's synopsis of psychiatry: Behavioral sciences/clinical psychiatry* (11th ed., p. 93). Philadelphia, PA: Wolters Kluwer.

9. A 3-year-old child carries a soiled blanket around with him at all times. His mother suggests that he not take the blanket to preschool, but he refuses to leave it at home. What is the blanket considered?

A. A blankie
B. A self-object
C. An attachment object
D. A solace object
E. A transitional object

ANSWER: E

A transitional object is an object (classically a blanket or stuffed animal) that provides psychological comfort. Donald Woods Winnicott established the idea of the transitional object as a soothing substitute for the mother as the child develops independence.

REFERENCE

Sadock, B., Sadock, V., & Ruiz, P. (2015). *Kaplan and Sadock's synopsis of psychiatry: Behavioral sciences/clinical psychiatry* (11th ed., p. 186). Philadelphia, PA: Wolters Kluwer.

10. According to Bowlby's work, what was crucial to a child's development and mental health?

A. Genetic predisposition
B. Parental care
C. Socioeconomic status
D. Quality of early education
E. Sibling relations

ANSWER: B

John Bowlby is considered to be the founder of attachment theory. He is known for his work on maternal care and deprivation and was commissioned by the World Health Organization to publish a report on the mental health of homeless children. He theorized that the parental relationship was crucial for a child's development and mental health. In cases of maternal deprivation or situations where the child is not proximate to the caregiver, the child may end up with anxiety, depression, neediness, or a reduced capacity for relationships.

REFERENCE

Sadock, B., Sadock, V., & Ruiz, P. (2015). *Kaplan and Sadock's synopsis of psychiatry: Behavioral sciences/clinical psychiatry* (11th ed., p. 176). Philadelphia, PA: Wolters Kluwer.

11. Considered to be the new developmental phase of the 21st century, this phase, marked by a tendency for early adults to delay achievements, has been coined:

A. Early adolescence
B. Late adolescence
C. Emerging adulthood
D. Early adulthood
E. Peter Pan-ification

ANSWER: C

Emerging adulthood is the phase following late adolescence that was officially named by James Arnett in 2000. Although there are conflicting age ranges for emerging adulthood, it is generally considered to occur in the 20s. It is still unclear whether this is a new developmental phase or a phenomenon due to current societal values. It is a period of wandering and uncertainty during which steady employment, marriage, parenthood, and financial independence are being delayed.

REFERENCE

Gilmore, K. J., & Meersand, P. (2014). *Normal child and adolescent development: A psychodynamic primer* (pp. 283–284). Arlington, VA: American Psychiatric Publishing.

12. In development, a period of solidification of competencies is called:

A. Plateau
B. Stage
C. Transition
D. Crisis
E. Rite of passage

ANSWER: B

A stage is a period of solidification of skills and abilities. A plateau is a period of stability. A transition is the link between stages. A crisis is an event or period usually marked by instability, difficulty, or change. A rite of passage is a social ritual such as graduation.

REFERENCE

Sadock, B., Sadock, V., & Ruiz, P. (2015). *Kaplan and Sadock's synopsis of psychiatry: Behavioral sciences/clinical psychiatry* (11th ed., p. 1326). Philadelphia, PA: Wolters Kluwer.

13. The developmental tasks of young adulthood include all of the following except:

A. Experience the third individuation
B. Develop age-appropriate play
C. Create a work identity
D. Establish new outlooks on time
E. Cope with the death of significant loved ones

ANSWER: E

The tasks of young adulthood include establishing a sense of self (third individuation) and work identity, creating adult friendships and a capacity for intimacy with a partner, becoming a parent, initiating a new relationship of equality with parents, engaging in age-appropriate play, and acquiring a new attitude with regard to time. Although it is possible to lose significant loved ones at any time in life, coping with the death of significant loved ones is considered to be a task of late adulthood.

REFERENCE

Sadock, B., Sadock, V., & Ruiz, P. (2015). *Kaplan and Sadock's synopsis of psychiatry: Behavioral sciences/clinical psychiatry* (11th ed., pp. 1326, 1335). Philadelphia, PA: Wolters Kluwer.

14. The theory of adult development called the stage-crisis view was developed by

A. Daniel Levinson
B. Erik Erikson
C. G. Stanley Hall
D. Elliott Jaques
E. Peter D. Kramer

ANSWER: A

The stage-crisis view was developed by Daniel Levinson and described in his work *The Seasons of a Man's Life*, published in 1978. He later wrote *The Seasons of a Woman's Life*. The Stage-Crisis View characterized adulthood as a series of different stages and transitions. His theory was based on research conducted with men and women aged 35 to 45.

REFERENCE

Levinson, DJ. The Conception of Adult Development. *American Psychologist*. 1986;41(1):3–13.
Sadock, B., Sadock, V., & Ruiz, P. (2015). *Kaplan and Sadock's synopsis of psychiatry: Behavioral sciences/clinical psychiatry* (11th ed., pp. 1331, 1339). Philadelphia, PA: Wolters Kluwer.

15. What term describes people in middle adulthood who provide care for their children and parents simultaneously?

A. Caregiver burnout
B. Sandwich generation
C. Baby boomers
D. Boomerang children
E. Burnout generation

ANSWER: B

The term *sandwich generation* describes the adult cohort caring for their children and aging parents concurrently. The term *boomerang children* is used to describe young adults who return home to live with their parents after leaving home for a period of time. The term *caregiver burnout* refers to the mental and physical exhaustion that may accompany being a caregiver.

REFERENCE

Sadock, B., Sadock, V., & Ruiz, P. (2015). *Kaplan and Sadock's synopsis of psychiatry: Behavioral sciences/clinical psychiatry* (11th ed., pp. 1326, 1331). Philadelphia, PA: Wolters Kluwer.
Miller, D. A. The 'Sandwich' Generation: Adult Children of the Aging. *Social Work*. 1981;26(5):419–423.

16. Which of the following is considered a normative crisis?

A. Rite of passage
B. Marriage
C. Graduation
D. Childbirth
E. Midlife crisis

ANSWER: E

Normative crises are periods of change that stretch a person's adaptive capabilities. A midlife crisis is a type of normative crisis. A midlife crisis is considered a critical point in a person's life associated with emotional instability involving alterations in major commitments (e.g., career or marriage). Marriage and graduation are considered rites of passage.

REFERENCE

Sadock, B., Sadock, V., & Ruiz, P. (2015). *Kaplan and Sadock's synopsis of psychiatry: Behavioral sciences/clinical psychiatry* (11th ed., pp. 1326, 1331). Philadelphia, PA: Wolters Kluwer.

17. Which of Erikson's stages is associated with ages 40 to 60?

A. Ego identity versus role confusion
B. Integrity versus despair
C. Generativity versus stagnation
D. Intimacy versus isolation
E. Industry versus inferiority

ANSWER: C

Erikson stages (Table 1.1):

Table 1.1

CONFLICT	VIRTUE	AGE IN YEARS (APPROXIMATION)
Trust vs. mistrust	Hope	Infancy 0–1.5
Autonomy vs. shame	Will	1.5-3
Initiative vs. guilt	Purpose	3–5
Industry vs. inferiority	Competency	5–12
Ego identity vs. role confusion	Fidelity	Adolescence 12–18
Intimacy vs. isolation	Love	Young adulthood 18–40
Generativity vs. stagnation	Care	Adulthood 40–60
Integrity vs. despair	Wisdom	>60

REFERENCE

Sadock, B., Sadock, V., & Ruiz, P. (2015). *Kaplan and Sadock's synopsis of psychiatry: Behavioral sciences/clinical psychiatry* (11th ed., p. 169). Philadelphia, PA: Wolters Kluwer.

18. Depression related to the last child's leaving home is more common:

A. When the children live close by after leaving the home
B. When the marriage was unhappy
C. When the marriage quality was good
D. In families where both parents work

ANSWER: B

Empty nest syndrome is described in this question. Depression can result when the last child departs home if the woman's primary role is mothering or if the parents are unhappily married but have chosen to remain in the marriage for the family.

REFERENCE

Sadock, B., Sadock, V., & Ruiz, P. (2015). *Kaplan and Sadock's synopsis of psychiatry: Behavioral sciences/clinical psychiatry* (11th ed., p. 1331). Philadelphia, PA: Wolters Kluwer.

19. Which of the following statements is true about adulthood?

A. Alcohol dependence, suicide, homicide, violence, and mental illness increase with unemployment.
B. Couples' friendships are easier to form and maintain.
C. The median age of first marriage has been decreasing since the 1950s.
D. The number of people never married has been decreasing since the 1950s.
E. Raising children helps promote sexual intimacy.

ANSWER: A

Unemployment has more than financial ramifications, with alcohol dependence, suicide, homicide, violence, and mental illness higher among the unemployed. Couples' friendships are considered more difficult to form and maintain because four people have to get along (as opposed to only two). The median age of first marriage has been increasing in men and women since the 1950s. The number of people never married also has been increasing since the 1950s. Raising children often interferes with sexual intimacy.

REFERENCE

Sadock, B., Sadock, V., & Ruiz, P. (2015). *Kaplan and Sadock's synopsis of psychiatry: Behavioral sciences/clinical psychiatry* (11th ed., pp. 1326–1331). Philadelphia, PA: Wolters Kluwer.

20. What characterizes the female climacterium?

A. Marriage
B. Childbirth
C. Pregnancy
D. Menopause
E. Death

ANSWER: D

Climacterium is a period of diminished biological function. For women, this is the menopausal period. For men, there is no clear corresponding period, though hormones decline in the 60s.

REFERENCE

Sadock, B., Sadock, V., & Ruiz, P. (2015). *Kaplan and Sadock's synopsis of psychiatry: Behavioral sciences/clinical psychiatry* (11th ed., p. 1331). Philadelphia, PA: Wolters Kluwer.

21. According to some longitudinal studies, individuals in the oldest age categories experience the following changes in basic personality traits:

A. Decrease in conscientiousness and openness
B. Increase in neuroticism, decrease in agreeableness
C. Increase in agreeableness, decrease in extroversion
D. Increase in agreeableness and extroversion
E. No appreciable change because personality becomes more rigid with age

ANSWER: C

There is evidence that the five basic personality traits are relatively stable over time. However, some studies have shown a modest decrease in extroversion and an increase in agreeableness.

REFERENCE

Sadock, B., Sadock, V., & Ruiz, P. (2015). *Kaplan and Sadock's synopsis of psychiatry: Behavioral sciences/clinical psychiatry* (11th ed., p. 1339). Philadelphia, PA: Wolters Kluwer.

22. Who theorized that improved control over the id and ego with advanced age gives rise to enhanced self-sufficiency?

A. Heinz Hartmann
B. Sigmund Freud
C. Erik Erikson
D. Bernice Neugarten
E. Daniel Levinson

ANSWER: B

Freud theorized that heightened control over the id and ego with advanced age leads to more autonomy. Heinz Hartmann was a founder of ego psychology. Erik Erikson is known for his theory of psychosocial development. Bernice Neugarten was a pioneer in the study of aging. Daniel Levinson developed the stage-crisis view of adult development.

REFERENCE

Sadock, B., Sadock, V., & Ruiz, P. (2015). *Kaplan and Sadock's synopsis of psychiatry: Behavioral sciences/clinical psychiatry* (11th d., p. 1339). Philadelphia, PA: Wolters Kluwer.

23. According to Levinson, what segment of development occurs between ages 60 and 65?

A. Middle adulthood stage
B. Late adulthood crisis
C. Late adulthood transition
D. Late adulthood stage
E. Pre-geriatric stage

ANSWER: C

Daniel Levinson developed the stage-crisis view of development, which involves different stages and transitions during adulthood, including pre-adulthood stage, early adult transition, early adulthood stages, midlife transition, middle adult stages, late adulthood transition, and late adulthood stage. Between ages 60 and 65 is the late adulthood transition, when the person experiences a decline in physical health and notices that friends are experiencing a similar decline or dying. Late adulthood stage is from 60 onward.

REFERENCE

Levinson, DJ. The Conception of Adult Development. *American Psychologist*. 1986;41(1):3–13.
Sadock, B., Sadock, V., & Ruiz, P. (2015). *Kaplan and Sadock's synopsis of psychiatry: Behavioral sciences/clinical psychiatry* (11th ed., p. 1139). Philadelphia, PA: Wolters Kluwer.

24. Which of Erikson's stages is associated with age older than 65?

A. Generativity versus stagnation
B. Integrity versus despair
C. Intimacy versus isolation
D. Industry versus inferiority
E. Ego identity versus role confusion

ANSWER: B

Erikson stages (Table 1.2):

REFERENCE

Sadock, B., Sadock, V., & Ruiz, P. (2015). *Kaplan and Sadock's synopsis of psychiatry: Behavioral sciences/clinical psychiatry* (11th ed., p. 169). Philadelphia, PA: Wolters Kluwer.

Table 1.2

CONFLICT	VIRTUE	AGE IN YEARS (APPROXIMATION)
Trust vs. mistrust	Hope	Infancy 0–1.5
Autonomy vs. shame	Will	1.5–3
Initiative vs. guilt	Purpose	3–5
Industry vs. inferiority	Competency	5–12
Ego identity vs. role confusion	Fidelity	Adolescence 12–18
Intimacy vs. isolation	Love	Young adulthood 18–40
Generativity vs. stagnation	Care	Adulthood 40–60
Integrity vs. despair	Wisdom	>60

25. All of the following are developmental tasks of late adulthood EXCEPT:

A. Maintenance of the body image
B. Maintenance of sexual activity
C. Acceptance of the failure of organs systems
D. Pursuit of wealth for retirement
E. Ridding oneself of an attachment to possessions

ANSWER: D

The pursuit of wealth is not a task of late adulthood. Developmental tasks of late adulthood include:

- Maintenance of the body image and physical integrity
- Performing a life review
- Maintenance of sexual activities
- Coping with the death of loved ones
- Acceptance of retirement
- Acceptance of the failure of organ systems
- Ridding oneself of the attachment to possessions
- Acceptance of relationships with grandchildren

REFERENCE

Sadock, B., Sadock, V., & Ruiz, P. (2015). *Kaplan and Sadock's synopsis of psychiatry: Behavioral sciences/clinical psychiatry* (11th ed., p. 1335). Philadelphia, PA: Wolters Kluwer.

26. In the United States, what percentage of persons older than 65 have severe dementia?

A. 1%
B. 2%
C. 5%
D. 10%
E. 15%

ANSWER: C

Five percent of persons in the United States over the age of 65 have severe dementia, and 15% of persons over the age of 65 have mild dementia. About 20% of persons over age 80 have severe dementia.

REFERENCE

Sadock, B., Sadock, V., & Ruiz, P. (2015). *Kaplan and Sadock's synopsis of psychiatry: Behavioral sciences/clinical psychiatry* (11th ed., p. 1346). Philadelphia, PA: Wolters Kluwer.

27. Which is NOT a risk factors for poor adjustment following the death of a loved one?

A. Male gender
B. Violent, stigmatized death
C. Depression soon after the death
D. Absence of grandchildren
E. Poor coping skills

ANSWER: D

Adjustment after the death of a loved one is variable among geriatric patients. Risk factors for poor adjustment include male gender, unexpected/violent/stigmatized death, symptoms of depression soon after the loss, low self-esteem, poor coping skills, and poor social support.

REFERENCE

Smoski, M. J., Jenal, S. T., & Thompson, L. W. (2009). Bereavement. In D. C. Steffens, D. G. Blazer, & M. E. Thakur (Eds.), *The American Psychiatric Publishing textbook of geriatric psychiatry*. Arlington, VA: American Psychiatric Publishing. http://psychiatryonline.org/doi/full/10.1176/appi.books.9781615370054.ds15. Accessed on February 1, 2016.

28. Which is TRUE about the psychosocial aspects of aging?

A. About 5% of older persons are living in nursing homes at any given time.

B. The amount of time spent in retirement has decreased since 1900.
C. The primary factor that determines geriatric sexual activity is proximity to potential partners in a nursing home.
D. Since the 1950s, the number of poor elderly persons has been increasing.
E. There is a significant decrease in social activity compared with prior social activity among healthy older adults.

ANSWER: A

About 5% of older people are living in nursing homes at any given time, and about 35% will require a long-term care facility at some point in their lives. The amount of time spent in retirement has increased since 1900 because the life span has increased. The main factors influencing sexual activity in older individuals are health, health of spouse, and past sexual activity. Since the 1950s, there has been a decline in poverty among the elderly. Healthy older adults typically experience a *slight* change in social activity compared with their prior level.

REFERENCE

Sadock, B., Sadock, V., & Ruiz, P. (2015). *Kaplan and Sadock's synopsis of psychiatry: Behavioral sciences/clinical psychiatry* (11th ed., p. 1339–1341). Philadelphia, PA: Wolters Kluwer.

29. Which of the following is NOT considered among the primary psychosocial factors contributing to the increased risk for suicide among older adults?

A. Loneliness
B. Access to potentially lethal medications
C. Advancing medical illness
D. Financial stressors
E. Depression

ANSWER: B

The elderly have a higher risk for suicide compared with the general population. Older adults cite loneliness, financial problems, medical illness, depression, and loss as reasons for suicidal ideation. Although access to potentially lethal medications such as opioids is common among older adults, access itself does not increase the risk of suicidal thoughts. Geriatric patients should be routinely evaluated for depression and suicidality.

REFERENCE

Sadock, B., Sadock, V., & Ruiz, P. (2015). *Kaplan and Sadock's synopsis of psychiatry: Behavioral sciences/clinical psychiatry* (11th ed., p. 1349). Philadelphia, PA: Wolters Kluwer.

30. According to Bernice Neugarten, the primary conflict of old age involves:

A. Financial concerns
B. Relinquishing authority and assessing accomplishments
C. Preoccupation with death and death anxiety
D. Preservation of self-esteem
E. Concerns about physical health

ANSWER: B

Bernice Neugarten dedicated much of her life's work to the subject of adult development and the psychology of aging. She believed that the primary conflict of old age involved relinquishing authority and assessing accomplishments. Kohut believed the major task of old age was preservation of self-esteem.

REFERENCE

Sadock, B., Sadock, V., & Ruiz, P. (2015). *Kaplan and Sadock's synopsis of psychiatry: Behavioral sciences/clinical psychiatry* (11th ed., p. 1339). Philadelphia, PA: Wolters Kluwer.

QUESTIONS AND ANSWERS

This chapter has accompanying questions and answers which are available to subscribers as part of the Oxford eLearning platform. To access the questions, follow the link below, or go to http://oxford-elearning.oup.com/books.

http://oxford-elearning.oup.com/books/test/67/10.1093/med/9780190265557.003.0001

2.

BEHAVIORAL AND SOCIAL SCIENCES

Adefolake Akinsanya

1. Which ethologist is best known for his study of imprinting?

A. Nikolaas Tinbergen
B. Konrad Lorenz
C. Karl Von Frisch
D. Richard Speck

ANSWER: B

The Austrian Konrad Lorenz is best known for his study of imprinting. Imprinting occurs during a susceptible period of early development when certain stimuli, such as interactions with the mother, cause a lasting behavioral pattern.

REFERENCE

Sadock, B. J., & Sadock, V. A. (2007). *Kaplan and Sadock's synopsis of psychiatry* (10th ed., p. 159). Philadelphia, PA: Lippincott Williams and Wilkins.

2. Which of the following correctly pairs developmental social isolation and its effects among nonhuman primates?

A. *Mother-only reared*: initial protest stage changing to despair 48 hours after separation
B. *Separation*: fails to leave mother and explore
C. *Total isolation*: self-orality, self-clasping, very fearful when placed with peers
D. *Partial isolation*: grasp others in clinging manner, easily frightened, reluctant to explore

ANSWER: C

Partial isolation results in vacant staring, self-mutilation, and stereotyped behavior. Total isolation leads to self-orality, self-clasping, and fearful behaviors among peers. Nonhuman primates reared only by their mother results in failure to leave mother and explore. These primates may be terrified when exposed to peers.

REFERENCE

Sadock, B. J., & Sadock, V. A. (2007). *Kaplan and Sadock's synopsis of psychiatry* (10th ed., p. 161). Philadelphia, PA: Lippincott Williams and Wilkins.

3. After repeated exposure to inescapable electric shock, the experimental dog eventually made no further attempts to avoid shocks and appeared helpless and apathetic. This is an example of:

A. Stress syndrome
B. Dominance
C. Learned helplessness
D. Temperament

ANSWER: C

Learned helplessness is an animal model of depression. In this example, the apparent giving up of the dog generalized to other situations, and eventually the dog developed helplessness and apathy. Because the cognitive, motivational, and affective deficits displayed by the dogs resembled symptoms common to human depressive disorder, learned helplessness, although controversial, was proposed as an animal model of human depression.

REFERENCE

Sadock, B. J., & Sadock, V. A. (2007). *Kaplan and Sadock's synopsis of psychiatry* (10th ed., p. 162). Philadelphia, PA: Lippincott Williams and Wilkins.

4. Who is widely known for his epigenetic model of human development, psychocultural biographies of Mahatma Gandhi and Martin Luther, and for the 1950 book *Childhood and Society*, in which he attempted to integrate individual psychosexual development with cultural influence?

A. Sigmund Freud
B. Carl Gustav Jung
C. Erik Erikson
D. Bronislaw Malinowski

ANSWER: C

Many aspects of Erik Erikson's theories were based on his experience with the Pine Ridge Indians in the Dakotas and the Yurok Indians in Oregon.

REFERENCE

Sadock, B. J., & Sadock, V. A. (2007). *Kaplan and Sadock's synopsis of psychiatry* (10th ed., p. 165). Philadelphia, PA: Lippincott Williams and Wilkins.

5. Brain fag occurs chiefly in which geographical region?

A. India
B. Caribbean
C. West Africa
D. Chinese
E. Iraq

ANSWER: C

Brain fag is a West African culture-bound syndrome experienced by high school or university students, characterized by difficulty concentrating, remembering, and thinking clearly. Somatic symptoms usually involve the head and neck. Students often describe their mind as being "fatigued." Amok, a dissociative episode characterized by a period of brooding followed by violent, aggressive or homicidal behaviors directed at humans or objects, is described among those from Puerto Rico, Papua New Guinea, and Malaysia. Koro describes an episode of sudden and intense anxiety over the fear that the penis (or, rarely, in women the vulva or nipples) will recede into the body and perhaps even cause death. It is reported in South and East Asia, China, and Thailand. Ataques de nervios is a common idiom of distress among Latinos in the United States and Latin America. It refers to a general state of vulnerability to stressful life experiences and encompasses a wide range of somatic and psychological symptoms (e.g., irritability, sleep difficulty, nervousness, easy tearfulness, inability to concentrate or function).

REFERENCE

Sadock, B. J., & Sadock, V. A. (2007). *Kaplan and Sadock's synopsis of psychiatry* (10th ed., p. 523). Philadelphia, PA: Lippincott Williams and Wilkins.

6. Amok is a culture-bound syndrome found among natives of which region?

A. West Africa
B. China
C. India
D. New Guinea

ANSWER: D

Amok, a dissociative episode characterized by a period of brooding followed by violent, aggressive, or homicidal behaviors directed at humans or objects, is described among those from Puerto Rico, Papua New Guinea, and Malaysia. Prevalent among men, it is precipitated by a perceived insult and accompanied by automatism, persecutory ideas, amnesia, and return to premorbid state following the episode.

REFERENCE

Sadock, B. J., & Sadock, V. A. (2007). *Kaplan and Sadock's synopsis of psychiatry* (10th ed., p. 523). Philadelphia, PA: Lippincott Williams and Wilkins.

7. Which term refers to a group of individuals who share a collective identity, ancestry, history, and beliefs?

A. Race
B. Ethnicity
C. Kinship
D. Cultural identity
E. People group

ANSWER: B

Race denotes human groupings that are biologically determined whereas ethnicity describes groups sharing a common identity, ancestry, history, and beliefs. Cultural identity describes the internalized self-definition resulting from a person's selective, developmentally mediated incorporation of values, beliefs, history, and customs from those available in one's native environment.

REFERENCE

Sadock, B. J., & Sadock, V. A. (2007). *Kaplan and Sadock's synopsis of psychiatry* (10th ed., p. 168). Philadelphia, PA: Lippincott Williams and Wilkins.

8. An immigrant who maintains his own cultural identity while participating in the host culture has done which of the following?

A. Marginated
B. Integrated
C. Assimilated
D. Acculturated
E. Separated

ANSWER: B

The broader process of learning culture through contact with family, friends, classmates, teachers, significant persons, and the media is termed *acculturation*. In this question, the immigrant has integrated. Assimilation occurs when a person adopts the host's culture entirely by shedding his own culture. The term *separation* describes maintenance of one's culture while rejecting the host culture. The term *marginalization* describes the rejection of both personal and host culture.

REFERENCE

Sadock, B. J., & Sadock, V. A. (2007). *Kaplan and Sadock's synopsis of psychiatry* (10th ed., p. 168). Philadelphia, PA: Lippincott Williams and Wilkins.

9. Which of the following tests involves asking a patient to make up a story when shown a picture?

A. Rorschach Test
B. Thematic Apperception Test
C. Holtzman Inkblot Technique
D. Minnesota Multiphasic Personality Inventory

ANSWER: D

The Thematic Apperception Test (TAT) was designed by Henry Murray and Christiana Morgan as part of a personality study conducted at the Harvard Psychology Clinic in 1943. The TAT consist of a series of 30 pictures and a blank card. The patient is shown 10 of these pictures and asked to make up a story about them. The patient is asked to describe what is going on in the picture and before the picture was taken, what the individual in the picture is thinking and feeling, and what is likely to happen in the future.

REFERENCE

Sadock, B. J., & Sadock, V. A. (2007). *Kaplan and Sadock's synopsis of psychiatry* (10th ed., p. 182). Philadelphia, PA: Lippincott Williams and Wilkins.

10. Which of the following is a projective personality assessment test?

A. Rorschach inkblot test
B. California Personality Inventory
C. Personality Assessment Inventory
D. Minnesota Multiphasic Personality Inventory

ANSWER: A

Projective personality assessment is defined by the use of unstructured, often ambiguous, test stimuli. A basic assumption is that when confronted with a vague stimulus and required to respond to it, persons naturally "project" their own personality onto this canvas. Examples are the Thematic Apperception Test, Rorschach (inkblot) test, sentence completion test, figure drawing, and make-a-picture story.

REFERENCE

Sadock, B. J., & Sadock, V. A. (2007). *Kaplan and Sadock's synopsis of psychiatry* (10th ed., pp. 180–182). Philadelphia, PA: Lippincott Williams and Wilkins.

11. Which of the following is an objective personality assessment test?

A. Rorschach test
B. Thematic Apperception Test
C. Holtzman inkblot technique
D. Minnesota Multiphasic Personality Inventory-2

ANSWER: D

Objective personality assessment involves structured, standardized measures, typically of a self-reported nature. Examples include Minnesota Multiphasic Personality Inventory-2, Personality Assessment Inventory, and California Personality Inventory.

REFERENCE

Sadock, B. J., & Sadock, V. A. (2007). *Kaplan and Sadock's synopsis of psychiatry* (10th ed., pp. 179–181). Philadelphia, PA: Lippincott Williams and Wilkins.

12. A 17-year-old male adolescent is being seen for developmental assessment. He was initially identified as having academic difficulties in second grade. Intelligence testing reveals an IQ of 60. What level of intellectual functioning does this suggest?

A. Borderline intellectual functioning
B. Mild intellectual disability
C. Moderate intellectual disability
D. Severe intellectual disability
E. Profound intellectual disability

ANSWER: B

IQ is normed, with an average score of 100 and a standard deviation of 15. Most individuals will fall into the range of 85 to 115. Borderline intellectual functioning spans from 70 to 79, mild intellectual disability (ID) from 55 to 69, moderate ID from 40 to 54, severe ID from 25 to 39, and profound ID 24 and below. Notably, a diagnosis of ID requires both impaired IQ and functional limitations.

REFERENCE

Sadock, B. J., & Sadock, V. A. (2007). *Kaplan and Sadock's synopsis of psychiatry* (10th ed., p. 179). Philadelphia, PA: Lippincott Williams and Wilkins.

13. Which of the following assesses abstract reasoning and flexibility in problem-solving?

A. Rorschach test
B. Thematic Apperception Test
C. Wisconsin Card Sorting Test
D. Draw-a-Person Test

ANSWER: C

The Wisconsin Card Sorting Test assesses abstract reasoning and flexibility in problem-solving. Cards with different colors, shapes, and numbers are presented to patients, who are then instructed to sort these cards into groups according to principles established by the examiner. The procedure is repeated several times to evaluate mental flexibility and pattern recognition.

REFERENCE

Sadock, B. J., & Sadock, V. A. (2007). *Kaplan and Sadock's synopsis of psychiatry* (10th ed., p. 184). Philadelphia, PA: Lippincott Williams and Wilkins.

14. According to Freud, the anal stage, which is characterized by a desire for independence from the parent, occurs over what ages?

A. First 18 months of life
B. 1 to 3 years of life
C. 3 to 5 years of life
D. 5 to 11 years of life

ANSWER: B

The oral stage is from birth to 18 months. The anal stage occurs from 1 to 3 years. The phallic stage extends from around age 3 to 5. The latency stage spans from 5 to 6 years to about 11 to 13 years of age. The last stage, the genital stage, begins at 11 to 13 years and stretches into adulthood.

REFERENCE

Sadock, B. J., & Sadock, V. A. (2007). *Kaplan and Sadock's synopsis of psychiatry* (10th ed., pp. 196–198) Philadelphia, PA: Lippincott Williams and Wilkins.

15. In Erikson's model of psychosocial stages, the development of trust versus mistrust occurs at what stage?

A. First 18 months of life

B. 3 to 5 years
C. 5 to 13 years
D. 13 to 21 years
E. 21 to 40 years

ANSWER: A

Erikson's epigenetic model describes eight stages of ego development across the life cycle. In the first 18 months of life, the infant's development of basic trust in the world stems from earliest experiences with his or her mother or primary caretaker. The stage-specific virtue is hope, and the central conflict to be mastered is trust over mistrust. Disruption during this stage leads to a failure of basic trust, theoretically leading to risk of psychosis, addiction, or depression later in life.

REFERENCE

Sadock, B. J., & Sadock, V. A. (2007). *Kaplan and Sadock's synopsis of psychiatry* (10th ed., p. 208). Philadelphia, PA: Lippincott Williams and Wilkins.

16. Who is generally considered the founder of attachment theory?

A. Kurt Goldstein
B. Erik Erikson
C. Karl Abraham
D. John Bowlby

ANSWER: D

John Bowlby is the founder of attachment theory. He formed ideas about attachment theory in the 1950s while he was consulting with the World Health Organization on the problems of homelessness in children. His theory of the mother–infant bond was biologically informed and drew extensively from ethology and evolutionary theory. A central tenet of attachment theory is that a core sense of safety is derived from a durable relationship with one's primary caregiver.

REFERENCE

Sadock, B. J., & Sadock, V. A. (2007). *Kaplan and Sadock's synopsis of psychiatry* (10th ed., p. 216). Philadelphia, PA: Lippincott Williams and Wilkins.

17. Freud's latency stage of psychosexual development corresponds with which of Erikson's psychosocial stages?

A. Autonomy versus shame
B. Initiative versus guilt
C. Integrity versus despair
D. Industry versus inferiority

ANSWER: D

The latency stage extends from about 5 to 6 years to about 11 to 13 years of age. Erikson's fourth stage, industry versus inferiority, occurs over this same age range. It is a period for developing important skills, exploring the environment, and becoming proficient in dealing with people and objects.

REFERENCE

Sadock, B. J., & Sadock, V. A. (2007). *Kaplan and Sadock's synopsis of psychiatry* (10th ed., p. 197–210). Philadelphia, PA: Lippincott Williams and Wilkins.

18. Which of the following is an immature defense mechanism?

A. Denial
B. Distortion
C. Displacement
D. Acting out
E. Suppression

ANSWER: D

Defense mechanisms are unconscious mental responses used by the ego to keep conflicts out of conscious awareness, thus decreasing anxiety and maintaining a person's sense of safety, equilibrium, and self-esteem. Immature defense mechanisms are manifestations of childlike disturbed behavior as seen in adolescents and some nonpsychotic patients. Examples include blocking, acting out, and introjection.

REFERENCES

Fadem, B. (2009). *Board review series behavioral science* (5th ed., p. 53). Philadelphia, PA: Lippincott Williams and Wilkins.

Sadock, B. J., & Sadock, V. A. (2007). *Kaplan and Sadock's synopsis of psychiatry* (10th ed., pp. 201–202). Philadelphia, PA: Lippincott Williams and Wilkins.

19. A 27-year-old man reports a latent desire of wanting to punch people in the face or punch walls; as a result, he pursues a career as a professional boxer. Which defense mechanism might he be using?

A. Intellectualization
B. Sublimation
C. Reaction formation
D. Rationalization

ANSWER: B

Sublimation is a mature form of defense mechanism through which individuals express a personally unacceptable feeling in a socially adaptive way.

REFERENCE

Fadem, B. (2009). *Board review series behavioral science* (5th ed., p. 54). Philadelphia, PA: Lippincott Williams and Wilkins.

20. A 35-year-old woman currently admitted to the inpatient psychiatric unit praises you as the "best doctor" and says you "completely understand my situation." She describes other caregivers as "terrible" and hopelessly unable to understand her. What defense mechanism accounts for these reports?

A. Acting out
B. Splitting
C. Reaction formation
D. Displacement
E. Projection

ANSWER: B

Splitting is an *unconscious* tendency to categorize people as either overly idealized or denigrated, often out of intolerance of ambiguity. This defense is common in borderline personality disorder. This term is often used indiscriminately by care providers to suggest that a patient is doing something consciously or maliciously as in, "Jessica has been splitting the staff," again as though this is a conscious action. This is *not* the nature of a defense mechanism, but splitting is likely occurring at an unconscious level in the patient's experience, and this is being played out or enacted in the staff. When staff have diametrically opposing responses to a patient—some with countertransferential hate and others with fantasies of rescue—this involves some degree of projective identification and collusion with the patient's unconscious defense of splitting.

REFERENCE

Fadem, B. (2009). *Board review series behavioral science* (5th ed., p. 54). Philadelphia, PA: Lippincott Williams and Wilkins.

QUESTIONS AND ANSWERS

This chapter has accompanying questions and answers which are available to subscribers as part of the Oxford eLearning platform. To access the questions, follow the link below, or go to http://oxford-elearning.oup.com/books.

http://oxford-elearning.oup.com/books/test/67/10.1093/med/9780190265557.003.0002

3.

EPIDEMIOLOGY AND PUBLIC POLICY

Carlos E. Molina

1. Which of the following describes positive predictive value?

A. The probability of having the disease when screening negative
B. The probability of having the disease when screening positive
C. The probability of not having the disease when screening positive
D. The probability of screening positive when not having the disease

ANSWER: B

Positive predictive value is the probability that someone with a positive screening test truly has the disease. Positive predictive value is the proportion of positive tests that are true positives. Unlike sensitivity and specificity, positive (and negative) predictive value is dependent on disease prevalence. Where disease prevalence is very low, even tests with relatively high specificity will have modest positive predictive value at best.

REFERENCE

Gordis, L. (1996). *Epidemiology* (5th ed.). Philadelphia, PA: Saunders Elsevier.

2. Which of these describes the mistake of missing a true difference between groups?

A. Type 1 error
B. Type 2 error
C. The alternative hypothesis
D. The null hypothesis
E. Selection bias

ANSWER: B

Type 2 error (or a "false negative") is failing to reject the null hypothesis when the null should, in fact, be rejected. Type 1 error (or a "false positive") is mistakenly rejecting the null hypothesis.

REFERENCE

Gordis, L. (1996). *Epidemiology* (5th ed.). Philadelphia, PA: Saunders Elsevier.

3. In a clinical trial, one group of patients diagnosed with depression receives an experimental SSRI, and another group receives a zplacebo. Six weeks later, both groups are scored using the Beck Depression Inventory. Which of the following tests is the most appropriate for comparing the mean of the scores of these two groups?

A. ANOVA
B. Chi-squareC. *t*-test
D. Pearson correlation
E. *z* score

ANSWER: C

A *t*-test is used to assess for differences between continuous variable outcomes between two groups. A chi-square test is used when comparing percentages (also known as proportions) across two or more groups. ANOVA assesses the variance across in means across two or more groups. Pearson correlation evaluates for a linear association between two continuous variables.

REFERENCE

Gordis, L. (1996). *Epidemiology* (5th ed.). Philadelphia, PA: Saunders Elsevier.

4. Which of the following categories of disorder has the highest 12-month prevalence among US adults?

A. Mood disorders
B. Anxiety disorders
C. Psychotic disorders
D. Substance use disorders
E. Impulse control disorders

ANSWER: B

Anxiety disorders are the most prevalent type of psychiatric disorder in US adults. As a result, patients who present for psychiatric evaluation should be systematically screened for the presence of anxiety disorders.

REFERENCE

The National Institute of Mental Health Epidemiologic Catchment Area Program and the National Comorbidity Survey, summary table. Retrieved from http://www.hcp.med.harvard.edu/ncs/ftp-dir/NCS-R_12-month_Prevalence_Estimates.pdf

5. Which of the following prevents or delays major neurocognitive disorder?

A. Genetic counseling
B. Pharmacological protective measures
C. Reducing exposure to environmental neurotoxins
D. Reducing risk in vulnerable groups showing prodromal signs of dementing process
E. Prevention of craniocerebral traumas earlier in life and control of vascular disease

ANSWER: E

The prevention of craniocerebral traumas earlier in life through highway speed limits, use of crash helmets and seatbelts, and drink-drive and vehicle licensing laws, prevents or delays onset of dementia. In addition, vascular disease is an evidence-based risk factor for dementia, and studies have suggested that controlling it by using antihypertensive medications or reducing cholesterol may prevent or delay the onset of dementia by more than 50%. Reducing exposure to neurotoxins (e.g., aluminum), pharmacological protective measures (e.g., estrogen replacement), antioxidants, vitamin E, and genetic counseling have all shown some promise, but evidence remains inconclusive.

REFERENCE

World Health Organization. 2004 Prevention of mental disorders effective interventions and policy options. Report. Prevention of mental disorders: effective interventions and policy options: summary report / a report of the World Health Organization Department of Mental Health and Substance Abuse in collaboration with the Prevention Research Centre of the Universities of Nijmegen and Maastricht. Retrieved from http://www.who.int/mental_health/evidence/en/prevention_of_mental_disorders_sr.pdf

6. Which of the following methods for suicide prevention has demonstrated the strongest effect?

A. Reducing access to the means to commit suicide
B. Hotlines
C. Crisis centers
D. School-based programs

ANSWER: A

Reducing access to the means of committing suicide prevents suicide. These strategies include safety measures on high buildings and bridges, restricted access to pesticides, detoxification of domestic gas and car exhaust, and control of availability of sedatives and analgesics. Hotlines, suicide education in school settings, and crisis centers have not been shown to have a similar effect on suicide prevention.

REFERENCE

World Health Organization 2004. Prevention of mental disorders effective interventions and policy options. Report. Prevention of mental disorders: effective interventions and policy options: summary report / a report of the World Health Organization Department of Mental Health and Substance Abuse in collaboration with the Prevention Research Centre of the Universities of Nijmegen and Maastricht. Retrieved from http://www.who.int/mental_health/evidence/en/prevention_of_mental_disorders_sr.pdf

7. Which of the following is/are TRUE concerning Assertive Community Treatment (ACT) services?

A. Offer social support in the community
B. Offer rehabilitation activities
C. Offer nursing care to patients
D. Decrease rates of rehospitalization
E. All of the above

ANSWER: E

The Assertive Community Treatment (ACT) program was developed by researchers in Madison, Wisconsin, in the 1970s for the delivery of services for persons with chronic mental illness. ACT programs consist of multidisciplinary teams with psychiatrists, nurses, social workers, and psychologists and assume the care of a designated number of adults with serious and persistent mental illness. ACT team members deliver services when and where needed by the patient *in the community*. The activities provided by this system include home delivery of medications, social skills training, monitoring of mental and physical health, and frequent contact with family members. The approach has a high staff-to-patient ratio (1:12) and reduces the risk of rehospitalization, particularly in persons with schizophrenia.

REFERENCE

Sadock, B. J., & Sadock, V. A. (2007). *Kaplan and Sadock's synopsis of psychiatry* (10th ed., p. 467). Philadelphia, PA: Lippincott Williams and Wilkins.

8. Which of the following statements regarding military psychiatry is true?

A. Confidentiality does not exist under the military code of conduct.
B. The principle "do no harm" may be superseded in military psychiatry settings.
C. Psychiatrists working for the military do not enter the military theater.
D. All of the above.
E. None of the above.

ANSWER: A

Confidentiality does not exist under the military code of conduct; hence, military psychiatrists face unique ethical problems. Mental health care providers must strike a balance between privacy that encourages persons to seek care with a responsibility of reporting to higher command regarding situations that pose various dangers. Psychiatrists are often deployed to war zones to provide immediate care to military personnel. The ethical principle of nonmaleficence applies.

REFERENCE

Sadock, B. J., & Sadock, V. A. (2007). *Kaplan and Sadock's synopsis of psychiatry* (10th ed., p. 683). Philadelphia, PA: Lippincott Williams and Wilkins.

9. Which of the following correctly describes principles of the wraparound approach?

A. Each child deserves individualized services.
B. Flexible funding allows for delivery of nontraditional services.
C. Interventions delivered for at-risk children are child and family centered.
D. The principal goal is to prevent hospitalization or residential placement.
E. All of the above.

ANSWER: E

The wraparound services approach is founded on the principle of individualization of services and proposes that an individualized service plan be wrapped around the child, including clinical, support, and nontraditional interventions. It is facilitated by the use of noncategorical and flexible funding of services and by these could enable a case manager and family to purchase whatever services the child and family needs. This level of service is distinct from inpatient or residential settings in that it supports a child at home.

REFERENCE

Sadock, B. J., & Sadock, V. A. (2007). *Kaplan and Sadock's synopsis of psychiatry* (10th ed., p. 1127). Philadelphia, PA: Lippincott Williams and Wilkins.

10. Which of the following terms describes the ability to generalize results of one study to other settings and/or populations?

A. Internal validity
B. External validity

C. Efficacy
D. Effectiveness
E. Fidelity

ANSWER: B

External validity refers to the ability to generalize the results of one study to other settings and/or populations beyond those included in the study. This is also called generalizability, relevance, or transferability. Internal validity is the degree to which research results are likely to be accurate and free of bias. Fidelity refers to the degree to which an intervention was administered as intended. Efficacy is whether a treatment works under ideal circumstances (e.g., randomized clinical trial) whereas effectiveness describes whether a treatment works in real-world practice.

REFERENCE

Miller, P. M. (2009). *Evidence based addiction treatment*. P. 1–18. New York, NY: Elsevier.

11. Which of the following study designs determines an individual's case status and risk factor exposure(s) at the same time?

A. Descriptive studies
B. Ecological studies
C. Cross-sectional studies
D. Case-control studies
E. Cohort studies

ANSWER: C

Cross-sectional studies examine individuals and determine their case status and risk factor exposures at the same time. Outcome rates between those with exposure can then be compared to those without. Descriptive studies describe the health status of a population or of a number of subjects. They can be useful for monitoring patients with rare conditions and in generating hypotheses for future study. In ecological studies, groups of individuals are studied as a whole, and the overall occurrence of disease is correlated with the aggregate level of exposure to a risk factor. In case-control studies, subjects are selected based on whether they have the outcome (case) or not (control), and their exposures are then determined by looking backward in time. In a cohort study, a group of healthy individuals is identified and followed over time to see who develops the outcomes of interest and who does not.

REFERENCE

Stern, T. A., Fava, M., Wilens, T.E, & Rosenbaum, J. F. (2015). *Massachusetts General Hospital comprehensive clinical psychiatry* (2nd ed.). China: Elsevier.

12. Which of the following is true about case-control studies?

A. Exposure status is determined at study enrollment.
B. They are not suitable for rare diseases.
C. They are not useful for distant and multiple exposures.
D. They are susceptible to selection bias.
E. None of the above.

ANSWER: D

Case-control studies are particularly susceptible to selection bias. These studies are population based, and participants should be representative of their respective populations. Case-control studies often recruit as part of a convenience sample, such as hospitalized patients who are solicited for study enrollment. These "cases" may then be compared with a similar convenience control of "willing volunteers." Disease status is determined before exposure status. Case-control studies, however, are suitable for rare disease or those for which the time between exposure and disease onset is relatively long.

REFERENCES

Gordis, L. (1996). *Epidemiology* (5th ed.). Philadelphia, PA: Saunders Elsevier.
Miller, P. M. (2009). *Evidence based addiction treatment*. P. 1–18. New York, NY: Elsevier.

13. Which of the following accurately describes Medicare?

A. Part A covers inpatient hospital stays, care in a skilled nursing facility, hospice care, and some health care.
B. Part B covers certain doctors' services, outpatient care, medical supplies, and preventive services.
C. Part C is a type of Medicare health plan offered by a private company that contracts with Medicare to provide you with all your Part A and Part B benefits.
D. Part D adds prescription drug coverage to Original Medicare, some Medicare Cost Plans,

some Medicare Private-Fee-for-Service Plans, and Medicare Medical Savings Account Plans.
E. All of the above.

ANSWER: E

Medicare Part A (Hospital Insurance) covers inpatient hospital stays, care in a skilled nursing facility, hospice care, and some home health care. Medicare Part B (Medical Insurance) covers certain doctors' services, outpatient care, medical supplies, and preventive services. Medicare Part C (Medicare Advantage Plans) is a type of Medicare health plan offered by a private company that contracts with Medicare to provide you with all your Part A and Part B benefits. Medicare Advantage Plans include Health Maintenance Organizations, Preferred Provider Organizations, Private Fee-for-Service Plans, Special Needs Plans, and Medicare Medical Savings Account Plans. Medicare Part D (prescription drug coverage) adds prescription drug coverage to Original Medicare, some Medicare Cost Plans, some Medicare Private-Fee-for-Service Plans, and Medicare Medical Savings Account Plans.

REFERENCE

Medicare.gov. The official government site for Medicare. Retrieved from https://www.medicare.gov

14. The federal insurance program for persons of all ages whose income and resources are insufficient to pay for health care is known as which of the following?

A. Medicare
B. Medicaid
C. Veterans Health Administration
D. Patient Protection and Affordable Care Act
E. Federal Employees Health Benefits Program

ANSWER: B

The Health Insurance Association of America describes Medicaid as a "government insurance program for persons of all ages whose income and resources are insufficient to pay for health care." The Patient Protection and Affordable Care Act, also known as Obamacare, is an expansion of Medicaid's eligibility that started in 2014 in which people with income up to 133% of the poverty line would qualify for coverage. The Veterans Health Administration and the Federal Employees Health Benefit Program are programs that provide medical assistance and health benefits to veterans and government employees, respectively.

REFERENCE

Medicare.gov. The official government site for Medicare. Retrieved from https://www.medicare.gov

The WHO World Mental Health Survey Consortium (2004). Prevalence, severity, and unmet need for treatment of mental disorders in the World Health Organization World Mental Health Surveys. *JAMA*, *291*, 2581–2590

15. Patients of which of the following ethnicities are more likely to be misdiagnosed as having Schizophrenia when their symptoms are more consistent with Bipolar Disorder or Major Depression with Psychotic Features?

A. German American
B. Caucasian
C. Native American
D. Italian American
E. African American

ANSWER: E

African American patients are frequently misdiagnosed as having Schizophrenia when instead they have Bipolar Disorder or Depression with Psychotic Features. They are also more likely to receive higher doses of antipsychotics, have higher rates of involuntary psychiatric hospitalizations, and have higher rates of seclusion and restraints.

REFERENCE

Sadock, B. J., & Sadock, V. A. (2007). *Kaplan and Sadock's synopsis of psychiatry* (10th ed., p. 467). Philadelphia, PA: Lippincott Williams and Wilkins.

16. Which of the following is correct regarding stigma related to mental illness?

A. Persons with chronic mental illness are viewed with fear.
B. Stigma has little effect on self-esteem.
C. Stigma affects individuals rather than their families.
D. Employment is unaffected by mental illness.
E. Patients with mental illness have an equivalent quality of life.

ANSWER: A

Persons with chronic mental illness are often viewed with fear, which can manifest as anger or worse. Views on those with mental illness lead to discrimination by others resulting in loss of self worth and confidence and unwillingness and thus a reluctance to participate in activities that may facilitate recovery.

REFERENCES

Sadock, B. J., & Sadock, V. A. (2007). *Kaplan and Sadock's synopsis of psychiatry* (10th ed., p. 683). Philadelphia, PA: Lippincott Williams and Wilkins.

Sadock, B. J., Sadock, V. A., & Ruiz, P. (2009). *Kaplan and Sadock's comprehensive textbook of psychiatry* (9th ed.). Philadelphia, PA: Lippincott Williams and Wilkins.

17. Which of the following is correct regarding antipsychiatry movements?

A. The development of diagnostic criteria was fueled in part by antipsychiatry advocates.
B. The Rosenhan experiment challenged objective validity in psychiatric diagnosis.
C. International differences in the rate of schizophrenia called diagnostic validity into question.
D. They led to limits on involuntary commitment and forcible treatment of patients.
E. All of the above are correct.

ANSWER: E

The development of diagnostic criteria started in the 1970s, partly in response to the challenge posed by antipsychiatry movements. The Rosenhan experiment, in which normal volunteers were diagnosed as having schizophrenia, created a furor and seemed to confirm the idea that psychiatric diagnosis had no objective validity. International research at this time also highlighted discrepancies in rates of diagnosis of schizophrenia between countries. Antipsychiatry ideas also influenced legislation. In England and Wales, the Mental Health Act of 1959 had given doctors more powers than any previous piece of legislation. This act was drafted and passed in an atmosphere of great optimism about the potential of psychiatry to solve all the problems posed by mental illness. However, antipsychiatry ideas suggested this optimism was misplaced and gave fuel to the civil rights movement's arguments that there should, at the very least, be more restrictions on the powers of doctors to admit and forcibly treat mental patients. The Mental Health Act of 1983 reflected these concerns. By narrowing definitions of certain categories of mental disorder, shortening periods of maximum detention, and placing restrictions on circumstances in which compulsory treatment can and cannot be given, it limited medical power and increased patients' rights.

REFERENCE

Black, D. W., & Andreasen, N. C. (2011). *Introductory textbook of psychiatry* (5th ed.). Arlington, VA: American Psychiatric Publishing.

18. Which of the following is a criminal issue that involves input from psychiatrists?

A. Involuntary hospitalization
B. Confidentiality
C. Competency to stand trial
D. Informed consent
E. Malpractice

ANSWER: C

Legal issues related to mental illness can be separated into two groups: civil and criminal. Civil law pertains to relationships between citizens, whereas criminal law centers on the individual's relationship to the state in the maintenance of social order. Civil issues relevant to psychiatry include confidentiality, informed consent, and involuntary treatment. Criminal issues that might involve input from psychiatrists include competence to stand a trial and criminal responsibility.

REFERENCE

Black, D. W., & Andreasen, N. C. (2011). *Introductory textbook of psychiatry* (5th ed.). Arlington, VA: American Psychiatric Publishing.

19. Which of the following rulings pertains to individuals who are not guilty by reason of insanity due to their mental illness making them unaware of the nature, the quality, and the consequences of their acts or if they were incapable of realizing that their acts were wrong?

A. Competency to stand trial
B. M'Naghten rule
C. Tarasoff I
D. Tarasoff II
E. Ted Bundy rule

ANSWER: B

This rule was named after Daniel M'Naghten, who for many years suffered from delusions, believing that he was persecuted by the Tory Party and its leader, Sir Robert Peel, the prime minister of Britain. In 1843 M'Naughten shot and killed Edward Drummond, who was Peel's private secretary. He was found not guilty on grounds of insanity. Competency to stand trial refers to a person's ability to understand the nature of the proceedings and to assist council regardless of the presence of mental illness. Tarasoff pertains to psychiatrists' legal responsibility to protect a third party and to break confidentiality by notifying the threatened person and the police. There is no eponymous legal rule named after the serial killer Ted Bundy.

REFERENCE

Black, D. W., & Andreasen, N. C. (2011). *Introductory textbook of psychiatry* (5th ed.). Arlington, VA: American Psychiatric Publishing.

20. Confidential information from a patient could be shared with which of the following without his or her permission?

A. Patient's insurance company
B. Patient's spouse
C. Patient's lawyer
D. Patient's supervisor
E. None of the above

ANSWER: E

Confidentiality is the ethical principle to hold secret all information given by patients. Confidentiality can be breached only to share information with other staff who may be treating the patient such as clinical supervisors and consultants.

REFERENCE

Sadock, B. J., & Sadock, V. A. (2007). *Kaplan and Sadock's synopsis of psychiatry* (10th ed., p. 1371). Philadelphia, PA: Lippincott Williams and Wilkins.

QUESTIONS AND ANSWERS

This chapter has accompanying questions and answers which are available to subscribers as part of the Oxford eLearning platform. To access the questions, follow the link below, or go to http://oxford-elearning.oup.com/books.

http://oxford-elearning.oup.com/books/test/67/10.1093/med/9780190265557.003.0003

4.

DIAGNOSTIC PROCEDURES

Ajay Shah, Varma Penumetcha, Rajesh R. Tampi, Mohsina Ahmed, Rabeea Mansoor, Raman Marwaha, and Juan Young

1. Which of the following is a semistructured interview?

A. Child and Adolescent Psychiatric Assessment (CAPA)
B. National Institute of Mental Health Interview Schedule for Child Version IV (NIMH DISC-IV)
C. Children Interview for Psychiatric Syndromes (ChIPS)
D. Diagnostic Interview for Children and Adolescents (DICA)

ANSWER: A

Semistructured interviews allow for interpretation of responses by the clinician, whereas structured interviews do not allow for interpretation. Of the above examples, the Child and Adolescent Psychiatric Assessment (CAPA) is the semistructured interview. It assesses symptoms across multiple psychiatric disorders and has been updated for use with *DSM-5*.

BIBLIOGRAPHY

Sadock, B.J., & Ruiz, P. (2015). Assessment, examination and psychological testing. In *Kaplan and Sadock's synopsis of psychiatry: Behavioral sciences, clinical psychiatry* (11th ed., p. 1110) (J.A.Sadock, Ed.). Philadelphia, PA: Wolters Kluwer.

2. Which of the following is an open-ended question?

A. Are you having suicidal thoughts?
B. Are you feeling depressed?
C. Have you had voices for the past week?
D. What brought you to the hospital?

ANSWER: D

Open-ended questions usually call for a narrative from the patients and elicit more information. In contrast, closed-ended questions elicit limited, often direct yes/no responses.

BIBLIOGRAPHY

Sadock, B.J, & Ruiz, P. (2015). Assessment, examination and psychological testing. In *Kaplan and Sadock's synopsis of psychiatry: Behavioral sciences, clinical psychiatry* (11th ed., p. 1109). (J.A.Sadock, Ed.). Philadelphia, PA : Wolters Kluwer.

3. Which of the following types of information elicited during a psychiatric interview is not protected under doctor–patient confidentiality?

A. Presence of a sexually transmitted disease
B. Ownership of a firearm
C. Intent to harm an identifiable person
D. History of spousal abuse

ANSWER: C

If a patient reports intent to harm an identifiable person, this information is not protected by doctor–patient confidentiality. Spousal abuse is not considered reportable. Presence of firearm in itself does not necessitate an obligation to report unless there is an intention to use it to harm a third party. Although patients are encouraged to report sexually transmitted diseases to their spouses, this does not necessitate breaking confidentiality. It is important to remember that states vary in their duty-to-warn statutes.

BIBLIOGRAPHY

Johnson, R., Persad, G., & Sisti, D. (2014). The Tarasoff rule: The implications of interstate variation and gaps in professional training. *Journal of the American Academy of Psychiatry and the Law Online, 42*, 469–477.

4. In which version of the *DSM* was the multiaxial system of diagnosing first introduced?

A. DSM-II
B. DSM-III
C. DSM-IV
D. DSM-IV-TR

ANSWER: B

The American Psychiatric Association introduced the multiaxial system of diagnosis in *DSM-III*, and this system persisted through *DSM-IV-TR*. *DSM-5* has done away with this pentaxial system. One reason to move away from this system is that the distinction between "axis I" psychiatric conditions and "axis III" medical conditions is artificial and arguably even stigmatizing.

BIBLIOGRAPHY

American Psychiatric Association. (2013). Introduction: The multiaxial system (2013). In *Diagnostic and statistical manual of mental disorders* (5th ed., p. 16). Arlington, VA: American Psychiatric Publishing.

5. A psychiatrist feels attracted to his patient, and later in the day he realizes that the patient reminds him of the girlfriend he took to prom. This is an example of what?

A. Transference
B. Countertransference
C. Denial
D. Blocking
E. Sublimation

ANSWER: B

Countertransference describes the unconscious response toward a patient based on previous relationships. Transference occurs when a patients' unconsciously displaces their feelings for significant people in their life onto the treating physician. Recognition of countertransference is critical to prevent unintended responses toward patients. For example, a physician may choose to not charge a patient for a missed appointment or may give preference in scheduling based on a countertransferential response.

BIBLIOGRAPHY

Sadock, B.J, & Ruiz, P. (2015). Psychiatric interview, history and mental status Examination. In *Kaplan and Sadock's synopsis of psychiatry: Behavioral sciences, clinical psychiatry* (11th ed., p. 194). (J.A.Sadock, Ed.). Philadelphia, PA : Wolters Kluwer.

6. You experience attraction to your patient during initial evaluation to the point that you have difficulty focusing on the interview. What is the next appropriate step in this situation?

A. Transfer the patient immediately.
B. Tell the patient that you are attracted to her.
C. Ignore this feeling because it will pass away with time.
D. Discuss this issue with a colleague or a supervisor.
E. Discharge the patient so that you can ask her out on a date.

ANSWER: D

Although transferring the patient may ultimately be appropriate, it is essential to identify and discuss this issue with a colleague or a supervisor because you are having difficulty responding objectively in this situation. Telling patients about countertransference, particularly early in the course of care, is not advisable unless there is a firm therapeutic alliance and introducing this information is intended for the patient's benefit rather than for the benefit of the physician.

BIBLIOGRAPHY

Sadock, B.J, & Ruiz, P. (2015). Psychiatric interview, history and mental status examination. In *Kaplan and Sadock's synopsis of psychiatry: Behavioral sciences, clinical psychiatry* (11th ed., p. 194). (J.A.Sadock, Ed.). Philadelphia, PA: Wolters Kluwer.

7. Who introduced the biopsychosocial model?

A. Robert Spitzer
B. Phillipe Pinel
C. George Engel
D. Aaron Beck

ANSWER: C

George Engel introduced the biopsychosocial model, which maintains that biological, psychological, and social factors each contribute to the patient and their overall well-being.

BIBLIOGRAPHY

Borrell-Carrió, F., Suchman, A. L., & Epstein, R. M. (2004). The biopsychosocial model 25 years later: Principles, practice, and scientific inquiry. *Annals of Family Medicine, 2*, 576–582. http://doi.org/10.1370/afm.245

8. Which of the following is most important to ask about during the initial interview to assess suicidal risk?

A. History of prior suicide attempts
B. History of suicide attempts in the family
C. History of substance use disorder
D. History of having guns at home

ANSWER: A

Whereas all these options inform risk of suicide, history of previous suicide attempts has the highest predictive value for future attempts. Additionally, current suicidal ideation, intent, and plan are essential for the assessment of acuity of risk.

BIBLIOGRAPHY

Sadock, B.J, & Ruiz, P. (2015). Psychiatric interview, history and mental status examination. In *Kaplan and Sadock's synopsis of psychiatry: Behavioral sciences, clinical psychiatry* (11th ed., p. 198). (J.A. Sadock, Ed.). Philadelphia, PA: Wolters Kluwer.

9. Which of the following is an example of thought content?

A. Auditory hallucinations
B. Visual hallucinations
C. Circumstantiality
D. Delusions
E. Knight's move thinking

ANSWER: D

Delusions, ruminations, and obsessions are types of thought content, as is the presence of suicidal or homicidal thoughts. Both auditory and visual hallucinations are perceptual disturbances. Circumstantiality describes a thought process in which the original topic is reached in a roundabout way as opposed to reaching it in a linear and goal-directed fashion. Knight's move thinking is a nonstandard synonym for loosening of associations.

BIBLIOGRAPHY

Sadock, B.J, & Ruiz, P. (2015). Psychiatric interview, history and mental status examination. In *Kaplan and Sadock's synopsis of psychiatry: Behavioral sciences, clinical psychiatry* (11th ed., p. 201). (J.A.Sadock, Ed.). Philadelphia, PA Wolters Kluwer.

10. What domain is assessed by asking the patient to explain the similarity between an orange and an apple?

A. Insight
B. Judgment
C. Orientation
D. Concentration
E. Abstract reasoning

ANSWER: E

Abstract reasoning is the ability to shift back and forth between general concepts and specific examples. Asking about similarities tests a patient's ability to use abstraction. Examples of a concrete sense of abstraction include "They are round" or "They both have seeds." The appropriate answer, "They are both fruit," requires that the patient grasp the abstract prototype of a fruit and correctly identify that both of these items fit into this abstract category.

BIBLIOGRAPHY

Sadock, B.J, & Ruiz, P. (2015). Psychiatric interview, history and mental status examination. In *Kaplan and Sadock's synopsis of psychiatry: Behavioral sciences, clinical psychiatry* (11th ed., p. 203). (J.A.Sadock, Ed.). Philadelphia, PA Wolters Kluwer.

11. A 25-year-old patient with schizophrenia and tobacco use disorder comes to the clinic for routine follow-up. During the appointment, the patient says he cut down from 12 cigarettes a day to 10 a day. When the psychiatrist asks, "What led you to cut down on your smoking?," the patient refers to his chronic cough. "So smoking has been hurting your health," the doctor

responds. This line of conversation is consistent with which of the following techniques?

A. Confrontation
B. Harm reduction
C. Facilitating interview
D. Motivational interviewing
E. Transference interpretation

ANSWER: D

The interviewer is exploring ambivalence in relation to smoking. Enhancing and capitalizing on ambivalence is the core feature of motivational interviewing, which is widely recommended for substance use disorders.

BIBLIOGRAPHY

Sadock, B.J, & Ruiz, P. (2015). Psychiatric interview, history and mental status examination. In *Kaplan and Sadock's synopsis of psychiatry: Behavioral sciences, clinical psychiatry* (11th ed., p. 208). (J.A.Sadock, Ed.). Philadelphia, PA: Wolters Kluwer.

12. Which of the following statements is FALSE regarding the examination of a patient using an interpreter?

A. The interpreter should paraphrase what the patient said.
B. A family member can be used as an interpreter.
C. The interviewer should face the interpreter.
D. The interviewer should refer to the patient in the third person.
E. All the above.

ANSWER: E

As much as possible, it is essential that interpreters provide a verbatim translation of what the patient has said. Using a family member as an interpreter makes it difficult for the patient to discuss sensitive issues such as suicidal thoughts or sexual fantasies, and the family member might fail to convey an accurate picture of the patient. The interviewer should face the patient and use first/second person (e.g., "How can we help today?" as opposed to turning to the interpreter and saying, "Can you ask him what brought him to the hospital?").

BIBLIOGRAPHY

Sadock, B., & Ruiz, P. (2015). Psychiatric interview, history and mental status examination. In *Kaplan and Sadock's synopsis of psychiatry: Behavioral sciences, clinical psychiatry* (11th ed., internat. ed., p. 209). Philadelphia, PA [u.a.]: Wolters Kluwer.

13. An 18-year-old woman is brought to the emergency department by her parents, who found a note in her bedroom stating that she just took a bottle of Tylenol to end her "worthless" life. You notice that her lab results show that her acetaminophen levels are significantly elevated. When you interview the patient, she reports that she wrote the letter to get her parents' attention and did not intend to overdose to end her life. You cite the lab results and say that it's impossible to have this high level without a serious overdose. What interviewing technique is being used?

A. Clarification
B. Reflection
C. Confrontation
D. Facilitation

ANSWER: C

This is an example of confrontation, where the patient is provided with information (that she may or may not be aware of) that contradicts what she has been saying.

BIBLIOGRAPHY

Sadock, B., & Ruiz, P. (2015). Psychiatric interview, history and mental status examination. In *Kaplan and Sadock's synopsis of psychiatry: Behavioral sciences, clinical psychiatry* (11th ed., internat. ed., p. 211). Philadelphia, PA [u.a.]: Wolters Kluwer.

14. Which of the following is a self-administered disability assessment scale?

A. World Health Organization Disability Assessment Scale, 2.0
B. Yale-Brown Obsessive Compulsive Scale
C. Structured Clinical Interview for the *DSM*
D. Mini-International Neuropsychiatric Interview
E. Hamilton Anxiety Rating Scale

ANSWER: A

The World Health Organization Disability Assessment Scale (WHODAS), currently in its second iteration, is a self-administered scale for functional disability. It measures impairment in the following domains: understanding and communicating, getting around, self-care, getting along with people, life activities, and participation in society. The Yale-Brown Obsessive Compulsive Scale (YBOCS) is part of a semistructured interview to evaluate severity of obsessive–compulsive disorder (OCD). The Structured Clinical Interview for *DSM* (SCID) and the Mini-International Neuropsychiatric Interview (MINI) are common structured psychiatric diagnostic instruments. The Hamilton Anxiety Rating Scale (HAM-A) is a clinician-rated scale that assesses for anxiety.

BIBLIOGRAPHY

Sadock, B., & Ruiz, P. (2015). Psychiatric rating scales. In *Kaplan and Sadock's synopsis of psychiatry: Behavioral sciences, clinical psychiatry* (11th ed., internat. ed., pp. 219–232). Philadelphia, PA: Wolters Kluwer.

15. Which of the following scales assesses for psychotic disorder?

A. Brief Psychiatric Rating Scale
B. Positive and Negative Syndrome Scale
C. Scale for the Assessment of Positive Symptoms
D. Scale for the Assessment of Negative Symptoms
E. All of the above

ANSWER: E

All of the above scales are designed to be used with psychotic patients. The Brief Psychiatric Rating Scale, which requires an experienced rater to administer, was the earliest of those scales developed to assess psychotic inpatients. The Positive and Negative Syndrome Scale (PANSS) is a semistructured scale that assesses both positive and negative symptoms of schizophrenia. The Scale for the Assessment of Positive Symptoms (SAPS) and the Scale for the Assessment of Negative Symptoms (SANS) assess positive and negative symptoms of psychosis, respectively.

BIBLIOGRAPHY

Sadock, B., & Ruiz, P. (2015). Psychiatric rating scales. In *Kaplan and Sadock's synopsis of psychiatry: Behavioral sciences, clinical psychiatry* (11th ed., internat. ed., pp. 222–226). Philadelphia, PA: Wolters Kluwer.

16. Which of the following is a clinician-administered scale?

A. Hamilton Rating Scale for Depression
B. Beck Depression Inventory
C. Geriatric Depression Scale
D. Patient Health Questionnaire
E. Both A and B

ANSWER: A

The Hamilton Rating Scale for Depression (HAM-D) is a clinician-administered scale that evaluates depression severity. This scale has two versions, one with 17 questionnaire items and the other with 24 items. This scale can be used by both physician and trained laypersons. The other scales are self-administered.

BIBLIOGRAPHY

Sadock, B., & Ruiz, P. (2015). Psychiatric rating scales. In *Kaplan and Sadock's synopsis of psychiatry: Behavioral sciences, clinical psychiatry* (11th ed., internat. ed., pp. 222–227). Philadelphia, PA: Wolters Kluwer.

17. Which of the following instruments consists of the three subscales of problem behaviors, academic functioning, and adaptive behaviors and is designed to be completed by parents, teachers, and children?

A. Diagnostic Interview Schedule for Children (DISC)
B. Autistic Diagnostic Interview- Revised (ADI-R)
C. Corners Ratings Scale
D. Child Behavior Checklist (CBCL)

ANSWER: D

The Child Behavior Checklist (CBCL) has two versions. One of them has to be completed by parents of children between 4 and 18 years of age. Another version is available for children between the ages of 2 and 3 years. The scale includes problematic behaviors and academic and social strengths. Three subscales are available, including problem behaviors, academic functioning, and adaptive behaviors.

BIBLIOGRAPHY

Sadock, B., & Ruiz, P. (2015). Psychiatric rating scales. In *Kaplan and Sadock's synopsis of psychiatry: Behavioral sciences, clinical psychiatry* (11th ed., internat. ed., pp. 235). Philadelphia, PA: Wolters Kluwer.

18. Which of the following scales assesses for physical sequelae of neuroleptics?

A. Brief Psychiatric Rating Scale
B. Positive and Negative Syndrome Scale
C. Scale for the Assessment of Positive Symptoms
D. Abnormal Involuntary Movement Scale

ANSWER: D

The Abnormal Involuntary Movement Scale (AIMS) is a brief rating scale that detects abnormal movements (in particular, tardive dyskinesia) caused by antipsychotics. It uses a 5-point rating scale to detect and monitor movement disorders in seven body areas: the face, lips, jaw, tongue, upper extremities, lower extremities, and tongue.

BIBLIOGRAPHY

AIMS Abnormal Involuntary Movement Scale. (n.d.). Retrieved November 1, 2015, from http://www.psychiatrictimes.com/clinical-scales-movement-disorders/clinical-scales-movement-disorders/aims-abnormal-involuntary-movement-scale

19. A patient is examined in the emergency department following a suicide attempt. After the patient declines to provide additional information, the psychiatrist says, "If you do not give me a consent, I will have to admit you involuntarily." Which ethical principle has been violated?

A. Beneficence
B. Nonmaleficence
C. Autonomy
D. None

ANSWER: C

In this scenario, it is coercive to tell the patient that he/she will be admitted involuntarily if informed consent is not provided. This action challenges the ethical principle of Autonomy.

BIBLIOGRAPHY

Sadock, B., & Ruiz, P. (2015). Ethics in psychiatry. In *Kaplan and Sadock's synopsis of psychiatry: Behavioral sciences, clinical psychiatry* (11th ed., internat. ed., p. 1392). Philadelphia, PA [u.a.]: Wolters Kluwer.

20. Which of the following projective tests used in children uses a combination of animal figures and human figures to elicit a story based on psychodynamic theory?

A. Rorschach inkblot test
B. Children's apperception test
C. Adolescent apperception cards
D. Sentence and story completion tests

ANSWER: B

The children's apperception test uses animal and human figures in different social situations and elicits stories from children. Scoring and interpretation are based on various elements of the children's stories because they disclose interpersonal dynamics and unconscious or otherwise preverbal content.

BIBLIOGRAPHY

Sadock, B., & Ruiz, P. (2015). Personality assessment: Adults and children. In *Kaplan and Sadock's synopsis of psychiatry: Behavioral sciences, clinical psychiatry* (11th ed., internet. ed., p. 252). Philadelphia, PA [u.a.]: Wolters Kluwer.

21. Why are structured patient interviews not suitable for routine psychiatric assessment?

A. They are less time-consuming.
B. They are mainly designed for research.
C. They help establish rapport with patients.
D. Limited training is required.
E. The interviewer can be creative with questions.

ANSWER: B

Psychiatrists do not use structured interviews in real clinical settings mainly for the following reasons: (A) Structured interviews are designed as research tools to be used in research settings and are not designed for psychiatrists to use in real clinical settings; (B) structured interviews are time-consuming; and (C) the rules of structured interviews make it difficult for the psychiatrist to establish rapport with the patient.

REFERENCE

Aboraya, A. (2009). Use of structured interviews by psychiatrists in real clinical settings. *Psychiatry (Edgmont) 6*(6), 24–28.

22. A psychiatrist asks his 40-year-old patient, "Have you had trouble sleeping lately?" The patient replies, "I usually sleep in my bed, but now I am sleeping on the sofa." This response reveals which of the following disorders of thought?

A. Circumstantiality
B. Flight of ideas
C. Loose associations
D. Tangentiality
E. None of the above

ANSWER: D

Tengentiality occurs when a patient gives a reply that is appropriate to the topic without actually answering the question. Circumstantiality is including irrelevant details that impede getting to the point. Flight of ideas is a succession of multiple associations in which thoughts move abruptly from idea to idea. Ideas are unrelated in loose associations.

REFERENCE:

Sadock, B. J., Sadock, V. A, & Ruiz, P. (2007). Clinical examination of the psychiatric patient. In *Kaplan and Sadock's synopsis of psychiatry* (10th ed., pp. 227–272). Philadelphia, PA: Lippincott Williams and Wilkins.

23. A 54-year-old woman is brought to the emergency department by her partner with thoughts of "not wanting to be here." She was recently diagnosed with diabetes and has been nonadherent with diabetes medications and the recommended diet. She reports having had depression for "a while," citing the loss of her job 2 months prior and her sister's death a month ago. On interview, she is "sad," and she mentions loss of appetite, feeling tired all day, low energy, and hopelessness about her future. Which of the following is the most important risk factor for suicide in this patient?

A. Age
B. Loss of job
C. Loss of sister
D. Hopelessness
E. Uncontrolled diabetes

ANSWER: D

The most important risk factors for suicide are previous suicide attempt, feelings of hopelessness, impulsive aggression, and borderline personality disorder.

REFERENCE

Soloff, P. H., Lynch, K. G., Kelly, T. M., & Malone, K. M. (2000). Characteristics of suicide attempts of patients with major depressive episode and borderline personality disorder: A comparative study. *American Journal of Psychiatry, 157*, 601–608.

24. A speech disorder characterized by repetition of syllables, words, or phrases is best described as which of the following?

A. Palilalia
B. Echolalia
C. Echopraxia
D. Coprolalia
E. Monotonous speech

ANSWER: A

Palilalia is a speech disorder characterized by repetition of one's own words, phrases, or sentences and is commonly seen in autistic patients. Echolalia is meaningless repetition of another person's spoken words; it is found in autism spectrum disorder or catatonia. Echopraxia is meaningless repetition or imitation of the movements of others and may also be seen in catatonia. Coprolalia is the use of obscene language.

REFERENCE

Karmali, I., Greer, D., Nuzzolo-Gomez, R., & Ross, D. E. (2005). Reducing palilalia by presenting tact corrections to young children with autism. *Analysis of Verbal Behavior, 21*, 145–153.

25. Which of the following cognitive functions is tested when patients draw intersecting pentagons?

A. Language
B. Memory
C. Attention
D. Visual motor ability
E. Thought process

ANSWER: D

The task of drawing intersecting pentagons tests for visual motor ability.

REFERENCE

Fountoulakis, K. N., Siamouli, M., Panagiotidis, P. T., et al. (2001). The standardised copy of pentagons test. *Annals of General Psychiatry, 10*(1), 13.

26. Loose associations are an abnormality of which of the following?

A. Memory
B. Thought process
C. Attention
D. Language
E. Thought content

ANSWER: B

Loose associations are an abnormality of thought process on a mental status examination.

REFERENCE

McIntyre, K. M., Norton, J. R., & McIntyre, J. S. (2009). Psychiatric interview, history, and mental status examination. In B. J. Sadock, V. A. Sadock, & P. Ruiz (Eds.), *Kaplan and Sadock's comprehensive textbook of psychiatry* (9th ed., pp. 896–897). Philadelphia, PA: Lippincott Williams and Wilkins.

27. Which of the following is an example of a facilitating intervention in a psychiatric interview?

A. Reflection
B. Clarifying
C. Leading
D. Probing
E. Transitions

ANSWER: A

Reflection is an example of a facilitating intervention in a psychiatric interview, whereas clarifying, leading, probing, and transitions are examples of expanding interventions.

REFERENCE

McIntyre, K. M., Norton, J. R., & McIntyre, J. S. (2009). Psychiatric interview, history, and mental status examination. In B. J. Sadock, V. A. Sadock, & P. Ruiz (Eds.), *Kaplan and Sadock's comprehensive textbook of psychiatry* (9th ed., pp. 899–901). Philadelphia, PA: Lippincott Williams and Wilkins.

28. Which of the following terms describes a profound disruption of self-awareness characterized by feelings of disembodiment and subjective emotional numbing?

A. Delusion
B. Hallucination
C. Overvalued idea
D. Depersonalization
E. Derealization

ANSWER: D

Depersonalization is the correct term to describe a profound disruption of self-awareness characterized by feelings of disembodiment and subjective emotional numbing.

REFERENCE

Sierra, M., & David, A. S. (2011). Depersonalization: A selective impairment of self-awareness. *Conscious Cogn., 20*, 99–108.

29. Which of the following is appropriate when using an interpreter for a psychiatric interview?

A. Family members are acceptable as interpreters for psychiatric evaluation.
B. Interpreters should provide verbatim translations of all that is being said by patients.
C. The psychiatrist should address the interpreter directly during the interview.
D. Contact with the interview should be limited to the face-to-face psychiatric evaluation.
E. All of the above.

ANSWER: B

Always use a non–family member professional interpreter for a psychiatric interview. Family members may be reluctant to discuss sensitive personal and family issues. Furthermore, the patient may be less likely to disclose sensitive information, or the family member doing the interpreting may censor what the patient says. The interpreter should always provide a verbatim translation of everything the patient says. The psychiatrist should directly address the patient, not the interpreter, to facilitate therapeutic contact. It is important to meet with the interpreter before and after the interview to clarify goals for the interview and also receive helpful insights regarding norms from the patient's own culture.

REFERENCE

McIntyre, K. M., Norton, J. R., & McIntyre, J. S. (2009). Psychiatric interview, history, and mental status examination. In B. J. Sadock,

V. A. Sadock, & P. Ruiz (Eds.), *Kaplan and Sadock's comprehensive textbook of psychiatry* (9th ed., p. 903). Philadelphia, PA: Lippincott Williams and Wilkins.

30. Which one of the following is not an abnormality of thought content?

A. Delusions
B. Obsessions
C. Homicidal ideation
D. Illusions
E. Paranoia

ANSWER: D

Illusions are an abnormality of perception and not of thought content.

REFERENCE

McIntyre, K. M., Norton, J. R., & McIntyre, J. S. (2009). Psychiatric interview, history, and mental status examination. In B. J. Sadock, V. A. Sadock, & P. Ruiz (Eds.), *Kaplan and Sadock's comprehensive textbook of psychiatry* (9th ed., pp. 896–897). Philadelphia, PA: Lippincott Williams and Wilkins.

31. Which of the following is FALSE regarding a no-suicide contract?

A. Almost 80% of mental health professionals report that they use such contracts
B. A no-suicide contract is used more frequently with high-risk patients.
C. A no-suicide contract may provide a crisis plan for the patient.
D. Use of no-suicide contract may be disruptive to a therapeutic relationship.
E. A no-suicide contract offers protection for the clinician from malpractice claims.

ANSWER: E

The no-suicide contract (often documented in notes as "the patient contracts for safety") is not legally binding and does not protection from malpractice claims for the clinician. Available data indicate that almost 80% of mental health professionals report using these contracts. Safety contracts are used most frequently with highest risk patients. No-suicide contracts may provide some guidance for what to do in an emergency, but their use may be disruptive to a therapeutic relationship.

REFERENCE

Matarazzo, B. B., Homaifar, B. Y., & Wortzel, H. S. (2014). Therapeutic risk management of the suicidal patient: Safety planning. *Journal of Psychiatric Practice, 20*, 220–224.

32. Which of the following is not covered in the CAGE questionnaire for alcohol use disorder?

A. Anterograde amnesia after alcohol use
B. Annoyance that others criticize one's drinking
C. Guilt about current drinking
D. Attempts to reduce drinking
E. Drinking in the morning to feel better

ANSWER: A

The CAGE questionnaire does not cover anterograde amnesia.

REFERENCE

McIntyre, K. M., Norton, J. R., & McIntyre, J. S. (2009). Psychiatric interview, history, and mental status examination. In B. J. Sadock, V. A. Sadock, & P. Ruiz (Eds.), *Kaplan and Sadock's comprehensive textbook of psychiatry* (9th ed., p. 894). Philadelphia, PA: Lippincott Williams and Wilkins.

33. Which of the following is not tested on the Mini Mental State Examination?

A. Orientation
B. Attention
C. Concentration
D. Executive functioning
E. Visual motor ability

ANSWER: D

The Mini Mental State Examination does not assess for executive functioning, which is often an early feature of neurocognitive disorders such as vascular neurocognitive disorder.

REFERENCE

Spencer, R. J., Wendell, C. R., Giggey, P. P., et al. (2013). Psychometric limitations of the Mini-Mental State Examination among nondemented older adults: An evaluation of neurocognitive and magnetic resonance imaging correlates. *Exp Aging Res., 394*, 382–397.

34. Which of the following is NOT part of the assessment of an agitated patient?

A. Safety for the patient and psychiatrist is a priority.
B. The room should be arranged so that the patient and interviewer can exit if necessary.
C. The patient should be approached in a calm, direct manner.
D. Making promises to elicit cooperation should be employed.
E. Security should be available in case of an emergency.

ANSWER: D

Making promises to elicit cooperation should be avoided because it may escalate the agitation. The other choices describe essential aspects of the assessment of an agitated patient.

REFERENCE

McIntyre, K. M., Norton, J. R., & McIntyre, J. S. (2009). Psychiatric interview, history, and mental status examination. In B. J. Sadock, V. A. Sadock, & P. Ruiz (Eds.), *Kaplan and Sadock's comprehensive textbook of psychiatry* (9th ed., p. 906). Philadelphia, PA: Lippincott Williams and Wilkins.

35. A 72-year-old Chinese man with chronic schizophrenia presented to the emergency department with suicidal ideation after a suicide attempt in which he cut his wrists. The patient is seen with his son, who is his primary caregiver. The son reports that the patient "ran out" of his medication 2 months ago and has become increasingly paranoid of the son and other family members. The patient has also had command auditory hallucinations telling him to kill himself and other family members. The patient speaks only Mandarin, but the patient's son speaks both English and Mandarin. After obtaining more collateral information, the son offers to interpret during the psychiatric interview. Which of the following is the most appropriate next step?

A. Accept the son's proposal to translate due to the acute nature of the situation.
B. Wait for a professional interpreter
C. Request a nearby staff member who is fluent in Mandarin to interpret.
D. Ask the legal department whether the son can interpret in accordance with HIPAA.
E. Have the son ask the patient whether he would give permission for his son to interpret for evaluation.

ANSWER: B

Interpretation by family should be avoided because patients may be reluctant to speak in front of family members. In this case, the patient may be actively paranoid of his son and may not provide a forthcoming history if the son acts as the interpreter. Additionally, family members may be hesitant to portray the patient's presentation accurately due to the intimate nature of their relationship. The best choice is always to use a professional interpreter when conducting a psychiatric interview to obtain the most accurate history and allow for the most objectivity.

REFERENCE

Sadock, B. J., Sadock, V. A., & Ruiz, P. (2014). In *Kaplan and Sadock's synopsis of psychiatry: Behavioral sciences/clinical psychiatry* (11th ed.). Philadelphia, PA: Lippincott Williams and Wilkins.

36. Which of the following is true concerning the use of the Mini Mental State Examination to evaluate capacity in older patients?

A. High sensitivity but low specificity when scores are below 20.
B. Low sensitivity but high specificity when scores are below 20.
C. Both high sensitivity and specificity when scores are below 20.
D. Both low sensitivity and specificity when scores are below 20.
E. The Mini Mental State Examination is useful in evaluating capacity only when scores are 20 or above.

ANSWER: B

The Mini Mental State Examination (MMSE) has poor sensitivity when screening for incapacity in groups with dementia, acquired brain injury, or psychiatric disorders. In contrast, the MMSE has high specificity when evaluating for capacity in these diagnostic groups. In fact, MMSE use had a specificity of 91% if the score cutoff was 22 or lower. Even higher specificity was found when the cutoff was below 20.

REFERENCE

Pachet, A., Astner, K., & Brown, L. (2010). Clinical utility of the Mini-Mental Status Examination when assessing decision-making capacity. *Journal of Geriatric Psychiatry and Neurology, 23*, 3–8.

37. A 24-year-old Caucasian man was brought by police to the emergency department for disorderly conduct and making threats against his neighbors. When first evaluated, the patient presented with psychomotor agitation, irritability, and paranoid statements about his neighbors trying to break into his home and steal from him. The patient is guarded, is suspicious of all medical staff, and becomes verbally combative when evaluated by staff. Which of the following is the most appropriate next step?

A. Administer intramuscular haloperidol and lorazepam for acute psychotic decompensation and agitation.
B. Seclude the patient to prevent harm to others.
C. Conduct the interview in a closed, isolated room to establish rapport with the patient and lessen the patient's paranoia.
D. Prescribe divalproex for mood stabilization and discharge the patient.
E. Evaluate the patient for possible delirium.

ANSWER: E

In an agitated patient, the first question that should be resolved is whether or not the patient has delirium. Patients who are agitated, disoriented, and disorganized may present similar to psychotic patients, but care should be taken to determine if causes of delirium (e.g., illicit substance use, alcohol withdrawal, electrolyte imbalances, or other medical illnesses) may actually be contributing to a patient's current aggressive behavior.

REFERENCE

Stowell, K. R., Florence, P., Harman, H. J., & Glick, R. L (2012). Psychiatric evaluation of the agitated patient: Consensus statement of the American Association for Emergency Psychiatry Project Beta psychiatric evaluation workgroup. *West J Emerg Med., 13*, 11–16.

38. Which of the following is true about screening for major depressive disorder using full-length questionnaires?

A. The PHQ-9 has the most data in screening for depression.
B. The HADS-D questionnaire performs the best in determining depression severity.
C. The PHQ-2 performs as well in identifying depression as does the full-length PHQ-9.
D. There is little to no difference between the performances of PHQ-9, HADS-D, and BDI in screening for recurrence of major depression.
E. The BDI questionnaire is the most commonly used questionnaire in screening for major depressive disorder.

ANSWER: D

All three screening questionnaires performed equally in accurately defining major depressive disorder recurrence as compared with a semistructured psychiatric interview. PHQ-2 performed as well as the PHQ-9 scale only if two items from the PHQ-9 scale were added to the PHQ-2 questionnaire.

REFERENCE

Thapar, A., Hammerton, G., Collishaw, S., Potter, R., Rice, F., Harold G., et al. (2014). Detecting recurrent major depressive disorder within primary care rapidly and reliably using short questionnaire measures. *British Journal of General Practice, 64*, e31–e37.

39. Which of the following is correct regarding standardized neurocognitive tests?

A. The Mini Mental State Examination (MMSE) includes cube and clock drawing to assess visuospatial skills.
B. The Montreal Cognitive Assessment includes an abbreviated trail-making test to assess spatial attention and working memory.
C. The Confusion Assessment Method can detect delirium in less than a minute.
D. The MMSE assesses for frontal-subcortical executive functions.
E. The Continuous Performance Test, third edition, can be used to evaluate word-finding difficulty.

ANSWER: B

The Montreal Cognitive Assessment (often simply "MoCA") is used to evaluate frontal executive dysfunction in patients with declining cognitive ability. It does this by testing visuoconstructive abilities, language, and memory. Notably, the Confusion Assessment Method (CAM) is a fast, reliable screen for delirium, but its use has been validated *only* when it is used in conjunction with a formal assessment of cognition such as the MMSE or other evaluation for memory, attention, and clarity of thought.

REFERENCE

Finney, G. R., Minagar, A., & Heilman, K. M. (2016). Assessment of mental status. *Neurologic Clinics, 34,* 1–16. doi:10.1016/j.ncl.2015.08.001

40. Which of the following cognitive domains is being tested in the part of the Mini Mental State Examination (MMSE) that asks the person to spell the word *world* backward?

A. Registration
B. Attention
C. Executive functioning
D. Orientation
E. Abstraction

ANSWER: B

The MMSE is a 30-point test for assessment of cognitive function, including orientation, registration, attention, memory, language, and visuomotor integrity. The MMSE tests attention by having the patient spell the word *world* backward or perform serial 7s (i.e., have the patient count backward from 100 by 7s).

REFERENCE

Beresin, E. (2010). The psychiatric interview. In T. Stern (Ed.), *MGH handbook of general hospital psychiatry* (6th ed., pp. 25–38). Saunders.

41. Which of the following is not a perceptual disturbance?

A. Hallucination
B. Illusion
C. Delusion
D. Depersonalization
E. Derealization

ANSWER: C

Perceptual disturbances include hallucinations, illusions, depersonalization, and derealization. Delusions are included in disturbances of thought content and are fixed, false beliefs out of keeping with a patient's cultural background.

REFERENCE

Sadock, B. J., & Sadock, V. A. (2007). *Kaplan and Sadock's synopsis of psychiatry* (10th ed., pp. 233–234). Philadelphia, PA: Lippincott Williams and Wilkins.

42. Which of the following neuropsychological deficits is associated with a right hemisphere brain damage?

A. Finger agnosia
B. Right–left disorientation
C. Aphasia
D. Anosognosia

ANSWER: D

In general, the dominant hemisphere (left side in the majority of people) is responsible for contralateral awareness, whereas the nondominant hemisphere (right brain) exhibits global awareness. This explains why patients with right-brain syndromes typically have hemineglect and often demonstrate anosognosia. Finger agnosia, right–left disorientation, and aphasia are the deficits found in patients with left-sided injury.

BIBLIOGRAPHY

Sadock, B.J, & Ruiz, P. (2015). Clinical neuropsychology and intellectual assessment of adults. In *Kaplan and Sadock's synopsis of psychiatry: Behavioral sciences, clinical psychiatry* (11th ed.,p. 236). (J.A.Sadock, Ed.). Philadelphia, PA: Wolters Kluwer.

43. Which of the following clusters of symptoms is associated with Gerstmann's syndrome?

A. Finger agnosia, dyscalculia, dysgraphia, right–left disorientation
B. Dysgraphia, hemineglect, right–left disorientation, finger agnosia
C. Limb apraxia, agnosia, dyscalculia, right–left disorientation
D. Constructional apraxia, finger agnosia, dyscalculia, hemineglect

ANSWER: A

Patients presenting with Gerstmann's syndrome have a damage classically involving the angular gyrus of the parietal lobe. It is commonly caused by a stroke in this region of the brain.

BIBLIOGRAPHY

NINDS Gerstmann's syndrome information page. (n.d.). Retrieved October 30, 2015, from http://www.ninds.nih.gov/disorders/gerstmanns/gerstmanns.htm

44. A 55-year-old man was brought to the emergency department by family for garbled speech. Upon clinical examination, you find the patient is unable to understand what you are asking him. However, the patient is able to speak fluently, albeit with paraphasia and neologisms. CT scan of head reveals a hemmorhagic stroke. Which region in the brain is most likely affected because of the stroke?

A. Superior temporal gyrus
B. Inferior frontal gyrus
C. Arcuate fasciculus
D. Prefrontal cortex

ANSWER: A

The patient presents with Wernicke's aphasia characterized by receptive aphasia (difficulty with comprehension) with fluent speech associated with neologisms and paraphasia. Wernicke's aphasia is seen in damage to the superior temporal gyrus in the dominant hemisphere. Broca's aphasia, also called an expressive aphasia, is associated with damage of the left posterior inferior frontal gyrus. Damage to the arcuate fasciculus is associated with conduction aphasia.

BIBLIOGRAPHY

Sadock, B.J., & Ruiz, P. (2015). Clinical neuropsychology and intellectual assessment of adults. In *Kaplan and Sadock's synopsis of psychiatry: Behavioral sciences, clinical psychiatry* (11th ed., p. 237). (J.A.Sadock, Ed.). Philadelphia, PA: Wolters Kluwer

45. Which of the following tests was originally designed to localize a brain lesion?

A. Mini Mental State Examination
B. Halstead-Reitan Neuropsychological Test Battery
C. Montreal Cognitive Assessment
D. Clock drawing test

ANSWER: B

The Mini Mental State Examination, the Montreal Cognitive Assessment, and the Clock drawing test assess cognitive function. However, the Halstead-Reitan Neuropsychological Test Battery was developed to localize brain lesions.

BIBLIOGRAPHY

Reitan, R. M., & Wolfson, D. (2009). The Halstead–Reitan Neuropsychological Test Battery for Adults—Theoretical, methodological, and validational bases. In *Neuropsychological assessment of neuropsychiatric and neuromedical disorders* (3rd ed., pp. 3–24). New York, NY: Oxford University Press, Inc.

46. Which of the following scales is a self-report patient questionnaire?

A. Beck Depression Inventory
B. Hamilton Depression Rating Scale
C. Trail making test
D. Wisconsin Card Sorting Test

ANSWER: A

The Beck Depression Inventory is a self-report questionnaire that is sensitive for screening for depression in adults. The Hamilton Depression Rating Scale, though, is an observer-rated scale. The trail making test is not a questionnaire; it requires a person to draw a line connecting numbers (or numbers/letters) in series and evaluates executive functioning. The Wisconsin Card Sorting Test also assesses executive function.

BIBLIOGRAPHY

Sadock, B.J., & Ruiz, P. (2015). Clinical neuropsychology and intellectual assessment of adults. In *Kaplan and Sadock's synopsis of psychiatry: Behavioral sciences, clinical psychiatry* (11th ed., p. 242). (J.A.Sadock, Ed.). Philadelphia, PA : Wolters Kluwer.

47. Which of the following tests was developed to assess abstract reasoning and the ability to shift cognitive strategies in response to environmental changes?

A. Finger tapping test
B. Clock drawing test

C. Token test
D. Wisconsin Card Sorting Test

ANSWER: D

The Wisconsin Card Sorting Test is a neuropsychological assessment in which where the subject is presented with a series of cards and is instructed to determine the pattern by a sequence of trial and error. It tests executive function, and scores are reported as percentages and percentiles of categories achieved, trials, and errors. The clock drawing test is used to detect a range of cognitive impairment, particularly in dementia or other acquired cognitive disorders. The finger tapping test is used to assess motor speed and lateralization, whereas the token test is used to test auditory comprehension in patients affected with disorders affecting language.

BIBLIOGRAPHY

Agrell, B., & Dehlin, O. (1998). The clock-drawing test. *Age and Ageing, 27,* 399–404.
Mountain, M. A., & Snow, W. G. (1993). Wisconsin Card Sorting Test as a measure of frontal pathology: A review. *The Clinical Neuropsychologist, 7*(1), 108–118.

48. Which of the following is an objective personality test?

A. Rorschach test
B. Minnesota Multiphasic Personality Inventory
C. Thematic Apperception Test
D. Figure-drawing test

ANSWER: B

The MMPI is a true/false format self-report questionnaire, which requires comprehension at an eighth-grade level. Individual results are compared to a normative sample. Subjective (or projective) tests like the Rorschach inkblot, Thematic Apperception Test, and figure drawing test require an experienced evaluator to administer and to interpret the test results.

BIBLIOGRAPHY

Sadock, B.J., & Ruiz, P. (2015). Personality assessment: Adults and children. In *Kaplan and Sadock's synopsis of psychiatry: Behavioral sciences, clinical psychiatry* (11th ed., p. 247). (J.A.Sadock, Ed.). Philadelphia, PA: Wolters Kluwer.

49. A patient is presented with a picture of two people of different ages standing next to each other and is asked to tell a story about the picture. What test is being administered?

A. Thematic Apperception Test
B. Figure drawing test
C. Sentence completion test
D. Rorschach test

ANSWER: A

The Thematic Apperception Test was developed by Henry Murray and Christiana Morgan at Harvard Psychological Clinic. As described in this question stem, a patient is asked to tell a story based on a picture, and the patient's response will reflect elements of his or her personal needs, thoughts, desires, and view of the future. In the Rorschach (inkblot) test, a patient is presented with 10 ambiguous symmetrical inkblots and asked to identify the figures. Patients are then asked to explain their responses to the examiner. In the sentence completion test, the patient is presented with a series of incomplete sentences and asked to complete each sentence with the first response that comes to mind. All of the above options are examples of projective personality tests.

BIBLIOGRAPHY

Sadock, B.J., & Ruiz, P. (2015). Personality assessment: Adults and children. In *Kaplan and Sadock's synopsis of psychiatry: Behavioral sciences, clinical psychiatry* (11th ed.,p. 249). (J.A.Sadock, Ed.). Philadelphia, PA : Wolters Kluwer.

50. A psychiatrist sits next to a patient, shows the patient a series of symmetrical designs on cards, and asks the patient to "free associate" what is seen on the card. What test is being administered?

A. Rorschach test
B. Thematic Apperception Test
C. Figure drawing test
D. Sentence completion test

ANSWER: A

The Thematic Apperception Test was developed by Henry Murray and Christiana Morgan at Harvard Psychological Clinic. As described in this question stem, a patient is asked to tell a story based on a picture, and the patient's response will reflect elements of his or her personal needs, thoughts, desires, and view of the future. In the Rorschach (inkblot) test, a patient is presented with 10 ambiguous symmetrical inkblots and asked to identify the figures. Patients are then asked to explain their responses to the examiner. In the sentence completion test the patient is presented with a series of incomplete sentences and asked to complete each sentence with the first response that comes to mind. All of the above options are examples of projective personality tests.

BIBLIOGRAPHY

Sadock, B.J., & Ruiz, P. (2015). Personality assessment: Adults and children. In *Kaplan and Sadock's synopsis of psychiatry: Behavioral sciences, clinical psychiatry* (11th ed.,p. 249). (J.A.Sadock, Ed.). Philadelphia, PA: Wolters Kluwer.

51. A psychology student is developing a scale to screen for borderline personality disorder. She prepares a series of questions and forwards it to personality experts at her university to see whether her individual questions measure the characteristic features of borderline personality disorder. Which of the following test characteristics is the student trying to improve?

A. Factor validity
B. Criteria validity
C. Face validity
D. Predictive validity

ANSWER: C

The student is trying to improve the face validity of the test. Face validity refers to the content of the questions and whether they measure what they are intended to measure. In this regard, personality experts at the student's university would provide feedback on whether her questions accurately capture elements of borderline personality disorder.

BIBLIOGRAPHY

Sadock, B.J., & Ruiz, P. (2015). Personality assessment: Adults and children. In *Kaplan and Sadock's synopsis of psychiatry: Behavioral sciences, clinical psychiatry* (11th ed., p. 247). (J.A.Sadock, Ed.) Philadelphia, PA: Wolters Kluwer.

52. Which of the following tests has weak interrater reliability?

A. Personality Inventory of Children
B. Children's Personality Questionnaire
C. High School Personality Questionnaire
D. Thematic Apperception Test

ANSWER: D

Interrater reliability is the ability of a test to produce consistent results when administered by different raters. Projective tests such as the Thematic Apperception Test have lower interrater reliability given the subjectivity involved in rating. By comparison, objective personality tests have much more limited responses and are compared with a normative sample.

BIBLIOGRAPHY

Gwet, K. L. (2014). *Handbook of inter-rater reliability: The definitive guide to measuring the extent of agreement among raters.* (3rd edition).Gaithersburg, MD: Advanced Analytics, LLC.

53. When you ask a patient to repeat the five words "face, velvet, church, daisy, red" and ask him or her to recall the words after 5 minutes, what type of memory are you testing?

A. Recent memory
B. Retrograde memory
C. Remote memory
D. Episodic memory
E. Recent past memory

ANSWER: A

This is an example of recent memory. An example of recent past memory would be recalling current events or what a person had for breakfast. An example of remote or long-term memory would be when a person recalls when he or she was married or the first car he or she owned.

BIBLIOGRAPHY

MoCA Montreal—Cognitive Assessment. (n.d.). Retrieved November 1, 2015, from http://www.mocatest.org/
Sadock, B.J, & Ruiz, P. (2015). Geriatric psychiatry. In *Kaplan and Sadock's synopsis of psychiatry: Behavioral sciences, clinical psychiatry* (11th ed., p. 1344). (J.A.Sadock, Ed.) Philadelphia, PA: Wolters Kluwer.

54. At what age do intelligence quotient scores in children stabilize?

A. 2 to 3 years
B. 4 to 5 years
C. 5 to 7 years
D. 10 to 12 years

ANSWER: C

The intelligence quotient (or IQ) is a measure of intellectual functioning at a particular age. IQ scores tend to stabilize from 5 to 7 years of age. Children tested after this age tend to have stable IQ scores if they are tested within a short period of time.

BIBLIOGRAPHY

Sadock, B.J., & Ruiz, P. (2015). Neurological and psychological assessment of children. In *Kaplan and Sadock's synopsis of psychiatry: Behavioral sciences, clinical psychiatry* (11th ed.,p. 258). (J.A.Sadock, Ed.). Philadelphia, PA: Wolters Kluwer.

55. A 13-year-old boy is performing poorly in school and has difficulty with nonverbal cues. What scale would you use to measure his functional ability?

A. Vineland Adaptive Behavior Rating Scale
B. Beck Youth Inventory
C. Child Behavior Checklist
D. Symptom Checklist-90

ANSWER: A

Adaptive behavior is the ability of a person to work successfully in a community. IQ tests assess cognition and intellect, but functional intelligence requires additional assessment. The Vineland Adaptive Behavior Rating Scale, standardized for use from birth to 18 years, measures adaptive functioning in four domains: communication, daily living skills, socialization, and gross motor skills.

BIBLIOGRAPHY

Sadock, B.J, & Ruiz, P. (2015). Intellectual disability. In *Kaplan and Sadock's synopsis of psychiatry: Behavioral sciences, clinical psychiatry* (11th ed., p. 1119). (J.A.Sadock, Ed.). Philadelphia, PA: Wolters Kluwer.

56. In addition to clinical evaluation of a child to assess for symptoms of attention deficit hyperactivity disorder (ADHD), which of the following is required to establish the diagnosis?

A. Interviewing the parents to assess the child's presentation at home is sufficient to establish the diagnosis.
B. Interviewing a teacher at school about the child's behavior should be sufficient.
C. The clinical interview in itself is sufficient to establish the diagnosis.
D. Information should be obtained from both parents and teachers to establish the diagnosis.

ANSWER: D

Behavior assessments of children across multiple settings in addition to the clinical interview are essential for the diagnosis of the ADHD. Clinical examination by itself is insufficient to make a diagnosis.

BIBLIOGRAPHY

Sadock, B.J., & Ruiz, P. (2015). Personality assessment: Adults and children. In *Kaplan and Sadock's synopsis of psychiatry: Behavioral sciences, clinical psychiatry* (11th ed., p. 255). (J.A.Sadock, Ed.). Philadelphia, PA: Wolters Kluwer.

57. Which of the following is a disadvantage of using the Mini Mental State Examination for screening of cognitive deficits?

A. It overestimates cognitive deficits in patients with less education.
B. It underestimates cognitive deficits in well-educated patients.
C. It does not assess executive functioning.
D. All the above.

ANSWER: D

The MMSE is a 30-point questionnaire used as a screening tool to detect and monitor cognitive function. MMSE lacks sensitivity to distinguish between individuals with mild cognitive impairment and normal cognitive function. MMSE lacks measures to assess for executive cognitive function.

BIBLIOGRAPHY

Sadock, B.J., & Ruiz, P. (2015). Clinical neuropsychology and intellectual assessment of adults. In *Kaplan and Sadock's synopsis of psychiatry: Behavioral sciences, clinical psychiatry* (11th ed., p. 241). (J.A.Sadock, Ed.) Philadelphia, PA: Wolters Kluwer.

58. Which of the following tests measures visuospatial and constructional ability?

A. Finger tapping test B. Grip strength
C. Clock drawing test
D. Reverse digit span test

ANSWER: C

The clock drawing test is a simple screening tool in which a subject is asked to draw a clock face. It is reliable for assessing cognitive impairment. Among the cognitive domains assessed are visuospatial and constructional ability.

BIBLIOGRAPHY

Eknoyan, D., Hurley, R. A., & Taber, K. H. (2014). The clock drawing task: Common errors and functional neuroanatomy. *Journal of Neuropsychiatry and Clinical Neurosciences, 24*(3), 260–265

59. Which of the following indices of the Minnesota Multiphasic Personality Inventory (MMPI) indicates malingering to feign illness?

A. L scale
B. D scale
C. Pa scale
D. Sc scale

ANSWER: A

The Lie Scale is one of the validity scales used in the MMPI; a high score on this scale suggests that the subject could be providing untruthful responses. The other three options, the D (Depression) scale, Pa (Paranoia) scale, and Sc (Schizophrenia) scale, assess for symptoms of each respective domain.

REFERENCE

Interpretation of the MMPI Scales. (n.d.). Retrieved November 1, 2015, from http://schatz.sju.edu/intro/1001lowfi/personality/mmpi/mmpi_interpretation.html

60. Which of the following tests is used to detect malingering?

A. The Rey 15-item memory test
B. 16 Personality Factor Questionnaire
C. California Personality Inventory
D. Jackson Personality Inventory

ANSWER: A

The Rey 15-item memory test is frequently used to detect malingering. It shows high specificity with low sensitivity, excluding patients with depression, to detect malingering.

REFERENCE

Reznek, L. (2005). The Rey 15-item memory test for malingering: A meta-analysis. *Brain Injury, 19*, 539–543.

61. Which of the following self report scales assesses a broad range of psychiatric symptoms?

A. Patient Health Questionnaire-9
B. Mood Disorder Questionnaire
C. Symptom Checklist-90-R
D. Liebowitz Social Anxiety Scale

ANSWER: C

The Symptom Checklist is a self-report questionnaire for use in those 13 years and older. It assesses a variety of psychological domains as opposed to, for instance, the PHQ-9 (which evaluates for depression), the MDQ (for bipolar disorder), or the LSA scale (for social anxiety).

REFERENCE

Leonard. R Derogatis Retrieved November 1, 2015 Clinical psychology. (n.d.). from http://www.pearsonclinical.com/psychology/products/100000645/symptom-checklist-90-revised-scl90r.html? Pid=PAg514

62. Patients of which of the following backgrounds should be screened for the HLA-B*1502 allele before initiating carbamazepine to prevent potentially fatal dermatological reactions?

A. Native American
B. Chinese
C. Caucasian
D. African American
E. Hispanic

ANSWER: B

Stevens–Johnson syndrome (SJS)/toxic epidermal necrolysis (TEN) occurs in roughly 1 to 6 per 10,000 persons of mainly Caucasian descent treated with carbamazepine. This risk is thought to be 10 times higher in persons of Chinese ancestry, primarily due to the increased prevalence of the HLA-B*1502 allele. Carbamazepine carries a black box warning for serious dermatologic reactions, including SJS/TEN, in individuals testing positive for HLA-B*1502. If an individual is found to be HLA-B*1502 positive, he or she should not be treated with carbamazepine unless the benefits clearly outweigh the risks.

REFERENCES

Ketter, T. A., Wang, P.W., Post, R. M. (2009). Carbamazepine and oxcarbazepine. In A. F. Schatzberg & C. B. Meneroff (Eds.), *The American Psychiatric Publishing textbook of psychopharmacology* (4th ed.). Washington, DC: American Psychiatric Publishing. doi:10.1176/appi.books.9781585623860. Retrieved from http://psychiatryonline.org/doi/full/10.1176/appi.books.9781585623860.as37#x18567.8330986

US Food and Drug Administration Alert. (December 12, 2007). Information for Healthcare Professionals: Dangerous or even fatal skin reactions—Carbamazepine (marketed as Carbatrol, Equetro, Tegretol, and generics). Retrieved from http://www.fda.gov/Drugs/DrugSafety/PostmarketDrugSafetyInformationforPatientsandProviders/ucm124718.htm

Tegretol (carbamazepine) [prescribing information]. East Hanover, NJ: Novartis Pharmaceuticals. September 2015. Retrieved from https://www.pharma.us.novartis.com/product/pi/pdf/tegretol.pdf

63. A 53-year-old woman with bipolar I disorder in remission on lithium for several years now presents with worsening depression, fatigue, abdominal pain, weight loss, and bone pain. Which of the following laboratory tests is most likely to reveal the underlying cause of her symptoms?

A. BUN/Cr
B. Creatine kinase
C. TSH
D. Serum B12
E. Ca++

ANSWER: E

This patient is experiencing signs and symptoms of hypercalcemia. The common mnemonic for remembering the symptoms of hypercalcemia is "stones, bones, groans, thrones, and psychiatric overtones." Prolonged lithium therapy can result in hyperparathyroidism, which in turn causes hypercalcemia. Patients treated with lithium should be regularly monitored for hypercalcemia. Although hypothyroidism can cause depression and fatigue, it is less likely to cause weight loss and bone pain, thus making Ca++ a better choice than TSH.

REFERENCE

Saunders, B. D., Saunders, E. F., & Gauger, P. G. (2009). Lithium therapy and hyperparathyroidism: An evidence-based assessment. *World Journal of Surgery, 33*, 2314–2323.

64. A 46-year-old man presents with an uncomfortable sensation in the legs that occurs mainly at night. He has a constant urge to move his legs, which is worsened with rest and improved with activity. Which of the following laboratory tests may aid in the diagnosis?

A. Mean corpuscular volume (MCV)
B. Serum glucose
C. Ca++
D. Serum ferritin
E. Mg++

ANSWER: D

Restless legs syndrome (RLS), which was upgraded to an independent disorder in *DSM-5*, is a sleep–wake disorder characterized by an uncomfortable sensation, typically in the legs, that worsens with rest, improves with activity, and occurs mainly in the late evening to at nighttime. Iron deficiency can present with symptoms indistinguishable from those of RLS. Iron is an important cofactor in the synthesis of dopamine, which has been implicated in the pathophysiology of RLS. Serum ferritin is a measure of iron body stores, and iron replacement is recommended in patients with serum ferritin lower than 50 ng/ml.

REFERENCES

Reite, M., & Weissberg, M. (2014). Sleep–wake disorders. In R. E. Hales, S. C. Yudofsky, & L. W. Roberts (Eds.), *The American Psychiatric Publishing textbook of psychiatry* (6th ed.). Arlington, VA, American Psychiatric Publishing. doi:10.1176/appi.books.9781585625031. Retrieved from http://psychiatryonline.org/doi/full/10.1176/appi.books.9781585625031.rh19#x63142.8237922

Sadock, B. J., & Sadock, V. A. (2007). *Kaplan and Sadock's synopsis of psychiatry* (10th ed., pp. 765, 997). Philadelphia, PA: Lippincott Williams and Wilkins.

65. Central deficiency of which of the following neurotransmitters is thought to underlie narcolepsy?

A. Norepinephrine
B. Dopamine
C. Hypocretin
D. Acetylcholine
E. Serotonin

ANSWER: C

Hypocretin, also known as orexin, is released from the hypothalamus and regulates wakefulness and arousal. Hypocretin-1 deficiency, measured via cerebrospinal fluid (CSF), is now a part of *DSM-5* diagnostic criteria for narcolepsy. Hypocretin deficiency is considered to be less than 110 pg/ml in CSF. Interestingly, in the United States, CSF evaluation for hypocretin is available exclusively for research purposes at the time of this writing.

REFERENCES

American Psychiatric Association. (2013). *Diagnostic and statistical manual of mental disorders* (5th ed., pp. 372–378). Arlington, VA: American Psychiatric Publishing.

Bourgin, P., Zeitzer, J. M., & Mignot, E. (2008). Review: CSF hypocretin-1 assessment in sleep and neurological disorders. *Lancet Neurology, 7*, 649–662.

Sadock, B. J., & Sadock, V. A. (2007). *Kaplan and Sadock's synopsis of psychiatry* (10th ed., pp. 759–761). Philadelphia, PA: Lippincott Williams and Wilkins.

66. A patient being treated with olanzapine for schizophrenia is concerned about metabolic side effects and asks how frequently her lipid profile will be checked. What frequency do guidelines recommend?

A. Baseline, 3 months, and annually
B. Baseline and annually
C. 3 months and annually
D. Annually
E. Baseline and every 6 months afterward

ANSWER: A

In 2004, the American Diabetes Association and the American Psychiatric Association released a consensus statement on metabolic monitoring. The statement recommends that patients being treated with atypical antipsychotics have their fasting lipid panel checked at baseline, 3 months after initiation, and annually thereafter.

REFERENCE

American Diabetes Association, American Psychiatric Association, American Association of Clinical Endocrinologists, & North American Association for the Study of Obesity. (2004). Consensus Development Conference on Antipsychotic Drugs and Obesity and Diabetes. *Diabetes Care, 27*, 596–601. Retrieved from http://care.diabetesjournals.org/content/27/2/596.long

Sadock, B. J., & Sadock, V. A. (2007). *Kaplan and Sadock's synopsis of psychiatry* (10th ed., pp. 743–744). Philadelphia, PA: Lippincott Williams and Wilkins.

67. A 20-year-old man with schizophrenia has been treated with risperidone for several months. He presents for follow-up stating he has noticed swelling and tenderness in the area of his chest. Upon exam, glandular breast tissue is palpable. Which of the following would be most helpful in determining the cause of this patient's symptoms?

A. TSH level
B. Prolactin level
C. Dopamine level
D. Cortisol level
E. Aldosterone level

ANSWER: B

Antipsychotics, which are D2 antagonists, can lead to an increase in prolactin in the tuberoinfundibular pathway because dopamine serves as prolactin inhibiting hormone. Symptoms of hyperprolactinemia often occur early in the course of treatment and include gynecomastia, galactorrhea, sexual dysfunction, and menstrual cycle changes such as amenorrhea. Per American Psychiatric Association practice guidelines, monitoring of these symptoms should be done at each visit; however, prolactin should be measured only if the patient is symptomatic as in this example. Risperidone carries a higher risk of hyperprolactinemia than do other antipsychotic medications. Dopamine level would not be the correct choice as prolactin level is more specific to the symptoms the patient is exhibiting.

REFERENCES

Janicak, P. G. (2014). Pharmacological treatment of psychosis. In G. O. Gabbard (Ed.), *Gabbard's treatment of psychiatric disorders* (5th ed.). Arlington, VA: American Psychiatric Publishing. doi:10.1176/appi.books.9781585625048. Retrieved from http://psychiatryonline.org/doi/full/10.1176/appi.books.9781585625048.gg11#x86291.8326682

Lehman, A. F., Lieberman, J. A., Dixon, L. B., McGlashan, T. H., Miller, A. L., Perkins, D. O.,Kreyenbuhl, J,; American Psychiatric Association; Steering Committee on Practice Guidelines (2004). Practice guideline for the treatment of patients with schizophrenia, second edition. American Psychiatric Association Steering Committee on Practice Guidelines. *American Journal of Psychiatry, 161*(2 suppl.):1–56.

Risperdal (risperidone) [prescribing information]. Titusville, NJ: Janssen Pharmaceuticals. April 2014. Retrieved from http://www.janssen.com/us/sites/www_janssen_com_usa/files/products-documents/risperdal.pdf

68. Which of the following laboratory tests is most helpful in determining long-term heavy drinking in a patient with alcohol dependence (*DSM-IV-TR*)/alcohol use disorder (*DSM-5*)?

A. Blood alcohol level (BAL) or breathalyzer
B. Ethyl glucuronide
C. Aspartate Aminotransferase (AST):Alanine Aminotransferase (ALT) ratio
D. Gamma glutamyl transferase (GGT)
E. Carbohydrate-deficient transferrin (CDT)

ANSWER: E

At-risk drinking is defined as having greater than 4 drinks per day or greater than 14 drinks per week in men. In women and the elderly, it is defined as having greater than 3 drinks per day or greater than 7 drinks per week. Of the choices listed, CDT is the best option because it is the most specific for alcohol use compared with the others. Patients who drink alcohol have lower levels of sialic acid on circulating transferrin; this is measured by the CDT test, which assesses alcohol use over the past 2 to 4 weeks. BAL provides a measure of active or very recent alcohol intake. Ethyl glucuronide is a metabolite of alcohol found in urine for up to 80 hours after alcohol intake. AST and ALT can be affected by a variety of liver pathologies, and GGT can be affected by obesity, hypertension, and certain cardiovascular or biliary disorders.

REFERENCES

Gough, G., Heathers, L., Puckett, D., Westerhold, C., Ren, X., Yu, Z., Crabb, D. W., Liangpunsakul, S. (2015). The utility of commonly used laboratory tests to screen for excessive alcohol use in clinical practice. *Alcoholism: Clinical and Experimental Research, 39*, 1493–1500.

National Institute on Alcohol Abuse and Alcoholism. (2007). *Helping patients who drink too much: A clinician's guide* (Updated 2005 edition). Bethesda, MD: National Institutes of Health.

National Institute on Alcohol Abuse and Alcoholism. Allen, J. P., Sillanaukee, P., Strid, N., Litten, R. Z. (2004). *Biomarkers of heavy drinking*. Bethesda, MD: National Institutes of Health. Retrieved from http://pubs.niaaa.nih.gov/publications/AssessingAlcohol/biomarkers.htm

69. Which of the following medications requires intact kidney function?

A. Valproic acid
B. Acamprosate
C. Naltrexone
D. Disulfiram
E. Chlordiazepoxide

ANSWER: B

Acamprosate is eliminated via the kidneys without hepatic involvement. Other psychotropics that have exclusive renal clearance include lithium, gabapentin, and pregabalin. The benzodiazepines oxazepam, temazepam, and lorazepam are metabolized via glucuronidation, which occurs both intrahepatically and systemically. The other choices listed undergo hepatic metabolism.

REFERENCE

Prescribing information for these medications can be found at www.dailymed.nlm.nih.gov.

70. What is the appropriate monitoring of absolute neutrophil count in a Caucasian patient being initiated on clozapine?

A. Monthly for 6 months, followed by every 2 months afterward
B. Weekly for 6 months, followed by monthly for 6 months, followed by every 3 months afterward
C. Every 2 weeks for 6 months, followed by every month for 6 months, followed by every 3 months afterward

D. Weekly for 6 months, followed by every 2 weeks for 6 months, followed by every 3 months afterward
E. Weekly for 6 months, followed by every 2 weeks for 6 months, followed by monthly afterward

ANSWER: E

Patients being initiated on clozapine should have their absolute neutrophil count (ANC) monitored weekly for 6 months, followed by every 2 weeks for 6 months, followed by monthly thereafter. As of October 12, 2015, the Food and Drug Administration (FDA) has updated guidelines to now include only ANC in the monitoring of patients on clozapine and no longer requires both ANC and WBC counts. These new guidelines include slightly separate criteria for patients with benign ethnic neutropenia (BEN). Along with updated monitoring guidelines, clozapine is now available only through a centralized program called the Clozapine Risk Evaluation and Mitigation Strategy (REMS) program, which replaces the previous 6 clozapine registries.

REFERENCES

Clozapine REMS. https://www.clozapinerems.com/CpmgClozapineUI/home.u
Clozaril (clozapine) [prescribing information]. East Hanover, NJ: Novartis Pharmaceuticals. September 2015.
US Food and Drug Administration Drug Safety Communication (September 15, 2015). FDA modifies monitoring for neutropenia associated with schizophrenia medicine clozapine; approves new shared REMS program for all clozapine medicines. Retrieved from http://www.fda.gov/Drugs/DrugSafety/ucm461853.htm

71. Which abnormality may be seen in a patient with self-induced vomiting?

A. Hypochloremic, hypokalemic metabolic alkalosis
B. Hypochloremic, hypernatremic metabolic alkalosis
C. Hyperchloremic, hypernatremic metabolic acidosis
D. Hyperchloremic, hyponatremic metabolic acidosis
E. Hypochloremic, hypokalemic metabolic acidosis

ANSWER: A

Purging may be seen in anorexia or bulimia nervosa. It is important to pay attention to the type of compensatory behavior described in the question. Choice A is the correct choice for a patient with vomiting. Vomiting leads to loss of gastric chloride, leaving comparatively higher levels of bicarbonate, thus leading to a metabolic alkalosis. Choice D may be seen in a patient with acute diarrhea secondary to laxative abuse. Electrolytes such as potassium, calcium, phosphorus, and magnesium are all generally low regardless of the compensatory behavior.

REFERENCES

Mitchel, J. E., & Wonderlich, S. A. (2014). Feeding and eating disorders. In R. E. Hales, S. C. Yudofsky, & L. W. Roberts (Eds.), *The American Psychiatric Publishing textbook of psychiatry* (6th ed.). Arlington, VA: American Psychiatric Publishing. doi:10.1176/appi.books.9781585625031. Retrieved from http://psychiatryonline.org/doi/full/10.1176/appi.books.9781585625031.rh17
Stern, T. A., Fricchione, G. L., Cassem, N. H., Jellinek, M., & Rosenbaum, J. F. (Eds.). *Massachusetts General Hospital handbook of general hospital psychiatry* (6th ed., p. 6). Philadelphia, PA: Saunders Elsevier.

72. A 21-year-old woman with anorexia nervosa is hospitalized for weight restoration after losing 40 pounds over the past 3 months. Which of the following lab abnormalities would be important to monitor during nutrition replacement?

A. Hypophosphatemia and hypomagnesemia
B. Hypophosphatemia and hyperkalemia
C. Hypermagnesemia and hyperkalemia
D. Hypermagnesemia and hypokalemia
E. Hyperphophatemia and hypokalemia

ANSWER: A

Refeeding syndrome can occur when the nutritional state of a starved person is restored too rapidly. It occurs within the first few days of re-nutrition secondary to insulin release, which activates protein, fat, and glycogen synthesis. These pathways require electrolytes such as phosphorus, magnesium, and potassium, leading to their rapid depletion. More important, these electrolyte disturbances can lead to arrhythmias, which are the most common cause of death in refeeding syndrome. Management includes replenishing phosphate and more gradual re-nourishment.

REFERENCES

American Psychiatric Association. (2013). *Diagnostic and statistical manual of mental disorders* (5th ed., pp. 345–350). Arlington, VA: American Psychiatric Publishing.
Mehanna, H. M., Moledina, J., & Travis, J. (2008). Refeeding syndrome: What it is, and how to prevent and treat it. *British Medical Journal, 336*, 1495–1498.
Mitchel, J. E., & Wonderlich, S. A. (2014). Feeding and eating disorders. In R. E. Hales, S. C. Yudofsky, & L. W. Roberts (Eds.), *The*

American Psychiatric Publishing textbook of psychiatry (6th ed.). Arlington, VA: American Psychiatric Publishing. doi:10.1176/appi.books.9781585625031. Retrieved from http://psychiatryonline.org/doi/full/10.1176/appi.books.9781585625031.rh17

73. A patient with opioid dependence (*DSM-IV-TR*)/opioid use disorder (*DSM-5*) presents to the emergency room seeking opiate detox. He states that his last use was just a couple of hours ago. Physical exam and labs, including a standard urine toxicology, are negative. Which of the following was the patient most likely taking?

A. Heroin
B. Codeine
C. Morphine
D. Thebaine
E. Oxycodone

ANSWER: E

Many standard urine tests detect only naturally occurring opiates that are derived from the opium poppy. Semisynthetic or synthetic opioids such as oxycodone, hydromorphone, hydrocodone, methadone, fentanyl, and buprenorphine are often not detected by standard urine drug testing and require more specific tests. Several "expanded opioid panels" exist, but specific testing varies by site.

REFERENCES

Center for Substance Abuse Treatment. (2006). Detoxification and substance abuse treatment (pp. 50–51). Treatment Improvement Protocol (TIP) Series 45. DHHS Publication No. (SMA) 06-4131. Rockville, MD: Substance Abuse and Mental Health Services Administration.
Substance Abuse and Mental Health Services Administration. (2012). Clinical drug testing in primary care (pp. 58–60). Technical Assistance Publication (TAP) 32. HHS Publication No. (SMA) 12-4668. Rockville, MD: Substance Abuse and Mental Health Services Administration.

74. Which of the following electrolytes should be monitored in patients taking oxcarbazepine?

A. Sodium
B. Potassium
C. Calcium
D. Magnesium
E. Chloride

ANSWER: A

Clinically significant hyponatremia (Na+ < 125 mmol/L) generally occurs within the first 3 months of treatment with oxcarbazepine. Up to 5% of patients treated with oxcarbazepine develop hyponatremia, and it is more commonly seen than with carbamazepine. Symptoms of hyponatremia can include nausea, headache, fatigue, delirium, seizures, and coma.

REFERENCES

Sadock, B J., & Sadock, V A. (2007). *Kaplan and Sadock's synopsis of psychiatry* (10th ed., p. 1033). Philadelphia, PA: Lippincott Williams and Wilkins.
Trileptal (oxcarbazepine) [prescribing information]. East Hanover, NJ: Novartis Pharmaceuticals. March 2013.

75. In which of the following clinical scenarios would an electrocardiogram be recommended prior to initiating dextroamphetamine?

A. No previous stimulant exposure
B. Family history of sudden death
C. Age < 12 years
D. Concomitant use of fluoxetine
E. Comorbid diagnosis of autism

ANSWER: B

There is currently no indication for routine screening with an EKG prior to initiating stimulant medications in healthy children or adults. EKG screening may be useful in patients with cardiovascular disease, chest pain, palpitations, syncope, or a family history of sudden cardiac death.

REFERENCES

Perrin, J. M., Friedman, R. A., Knilans, T. K.; Black Box Working Group; Section on Cardiology and Cardiac Surgery (2008). Cardiovascular monitoring and stimulant drugs for attention-deficit/hyperactivity disorder. *Pediatrics, 122*, 451–453.
Pliszka, S; AACAP Work Group on Quality Issues. (2007). Practice parameter for the assessment and treatment of children and adolescents with attention-deficit/hyperactivity disorder. *Journal of the American Academy of Child and Adolescent Psychiatry, 46*,894–921.
Vetter, V. L., Elia, J., Erickson, C., Berger, S., Blum, N., Uzark, K., Webb, C. L.. (2008). Cardiovascular monitoring of children and

adolescents with heart disease receiving medications for attention deficit/hyperactivity disorder [corrected]: A scientific statement from the American Heart Association Council on Cardiovascular Disease in the Young Congenital Cardiac Defects Committee and the Council on Cardiovascular Nursing. *Circulation, 18*, 2407–2423.

76. A 24-year-old woman with bipolar I disorder presents to your office as a new patient. She is currently off medication but reports being treated effectively with valproic acid in the past. Which of the following tests is the most important to check prior to reinitiating this medication?

A. Lipase
B. BUN/Cr
C. TSH
D. Pregnancy test
E. Liver enzymes

ANSWER: D

Valproic acid carries a risk of teratogenicity in pregnant women, specifically neural tube defects (NTDs). Lipase and liver enzymes are measures of pancreatic and hepatic function, respectively. Valproic acid can affect both the pancreas and the liver, but ruling out pregnancy to avoid the risk of NTDs prior to initiating treatment is the first step in women of childbearing age. BUN/Cr and TSH monitoring are indicated for patients on lithium.

REFERENCE

Sadock, B. J., & Sadock, V. A. (2007). *Kaplan and Sadock's synopsis of psychiatry* (10th ed., pp. 1113–1116). Philadelphia, PA: Lippincott Williams and Wilkins.

77. A 49-year-old man with bipolar I disorder is being treated with twice-daily dosing of immediate-release lithium. You are considering a dose increase but would like to check a lithium level prior to doing so. How many hours following a dose of lithium should a level be checked?

A. 4 hours
B. 6 hours
C. 8 hours
D. 10 hours
E. 12 hours

ANSWER: E

Checking blood levels for lithium is important secondary to its narrow therapeutic index. Blood levels should be checked at a steady state, which is 5 half-lives. For lithium, this is about 5 days. Blood levels are checked by measuring the trough, which is the lowest point of the medication prior to the next dose. For twice-daily dosing, that is 12 hours after first dose. Of note, single daily dosing is often preferred for improved adherence, comparable efficacy, and possible reduction in nephrotoxicity.

REFERENCES

Carter, L., Zolezzi, M., & Lewczyk, A. (2013). An updated review of the optimal lithium dosage regimen for renal protection. *Canadian Journal of Psychiatry, 58*, 595.
Sadock, B. J., & Sadock, V. A. (2007). *Kaplan and Sadock's synopsis of psychiatry* (10th ed., pp. 1056–1063). Philadelphia, PA: Lippincott Williams and Wilkins.

78. A 52-year-old woman on valproic acid presents with nausea, delirium, and tremor. Which of the following is the most likely cause?

A. Elevated ammonia
B. Decreased sodium
C. Elevated AST and ALT
D. Decreased calcium
E. Decreased glucose

ANSWER: A

Although rare, treatment with valproic acid can lead to hyperammonemia. This can occur *with or without abnormality in liver enzymes.* The rate of symptomatic hyperammonemia secondary to valproic acid use is unknown; however, when symptoms do occur, they can include nausea, fatigue, mental status changes, and tremor. In a study of 123 patients treated with valproic acid, half had elevated ammonia levels but remained asymptomatic compared with 21.7% of patients who were not on valproic acid. Valproic acid is not commonly associated with decreased sodium, calcium, or glucose.

REFERENCE

Schatzberg A.F., DeBattista C (2015). Mood Stabilizers. *Manual of Clinical Psychopharmacology* (8th ed.). Arlington, VA: American

Psychiatric Publishing. doi:10.1176/appi.books.9781615370047. Retrieved from http://psychiatryonline.org/doi/10.1176/appi.books.9781615370047.AS05

Raja, M., & Azzoni, A. (2002). Valproate-induced hyperammonaemia. *Journal of Clinical Psychopharmacology, 22*, 631–633.

79. A previously healthy 84-year-old man presents to the emergency room from his home via ambulance. On exam he is calm and cooperative but smells of urine. His wife reports that he has had nighttime incontinence and bouts of confusion, agitation, and visual hallucinations for 3 days. Which of the following should be the first step?

A. Give haloperidol.
B. Order urinalysis.
C. Apply restraints
D. Start donepezil.
E. File for conservatorship.

ANSWER: B

This patient is displaying symptoms of delirium (impairment in awareness and attention, thought disorganization, agitation, and visual hallucinations). The first step is to first check a urinalysis to rule out an infection that could be causing his symptoms. Putting the patient in restraints or giving haloperidol is inappropriate at this time because he is calm and cooperative in the emergency department, and these should be considered only if less assertive behavioral measures such as redirection and de-escalation fail. Starting donepezil is not appropriate because the patient is experiencing symptoms of delirium, not dementia. Filing for conservatorship is also unnecessary because the patient was seemingly healthy 3 days ago and is now experiencing a sudden change in his mental status.

REFERENCE

Sadock, B. J., & Sadock, V. A. (2007). *Kaplan and Sadock's synopsis of psychiatry* (10th ed., pp. 326–327). Philadelphia, PA: Lippincott Williams and Wilkins.

80. Activity of which of the following medications is least affected by changes in liver function?

A. Naltrexone
B. Disulfiram
C. Temazepam
D. Chlordiazepoxide
E. Valproic acid

ANSWER: C

Of the medications listed, temazepam is safest in patients with hepatic impairment. The mnemonic "outside the liver" is helpful in remembering the benzodiazepines that have extrahepatic metabolism: oxazepam, temazepam, and lorazepam. Valproic acid, naltrexone, and disulfiram can impact liver function.

REFERENCES

Ferrando, S. J., Owen J.A., Levenson J.L. (2014). Psychopharmacology. In R. E. Hales, S. C. Yudofsky, & L. W. Roberts (Eds.), *The American Psychiatric Publishing textbook of psychiatry* (6th ed.). Arlington, VA: American Psychiatric Publishing. doi:10.1176/appi.books.9781585625031. Retrieved from http://psychiatryonline.org/doi/full/10.1176/appi.books.9781585625031.rh27

Schatzberg A.F., DeBattista C. (2015). Pharmacotherapy for substance use disorders. *Manual of Clinical Psychopharmacology* (8th ed.). Arlington, VA, American Psychiatric Publishing. doi:10.1176/appi.books.9781615370047. Retrieved from http://psychiatryonline.org/doi/full/10.1176/appi.books.9781615370047.AS11

81. Which of the following is important to monitor in patients taking topiramate?

A. Bicarbonate
B. Glucose
C. Creatine kinase
D. Platelets
E. Absolute neutrophil count

ANSWER: A

Topiramate inhibits carbonic anhydrase, which can cause kidney stones. Because it is a carbonic anhydrase inhibitor, bicarbonate levels are decreased, and thus periodic monitoring of bicarbonate is recommended.

REFERENCES

McElroy, S. L., & Keck, P. E. (2009). Topiramate. In A. F. Schatzberg & C. B Nemeroff (Eds.), *The American Psychiatric*

Publishing textbook of psychopharmacology (4th ed.). Washington, DC: American Psychiatric Publishing. doi:10.1176/appi.books.9781585623860. Retrieved from http://psychiatryonline.org/doi/full/10.1176/appi.books.9781585623860.as40
Schatzberg A.F., DeBattista C (2015). Mood stabilizers. *Manual of clinical psychopharmacology* (8th ed.). Arlington, VA: American Psychiatric Publishing. doi:10.1176/appi.books.9781615370047. Retrieved from http://psychiatryonline.org/doi/10.1176/appi.books.9781615370047.AS05

QUESTIONS AND ANSWERS

This chapter has accompanying questions and answers which are available to subscribers as part of the Oxford eLearning platform. To access the questions, follow the link below, or go to http://oxford-elearning.oup.com/books.

http://oxford-learning.oup.com/books/test/67/10.1093/med/9780190265557.003.0004

5.

CLINICAL ASPECTS OF PSYCHIATRIC DISORDERS

Neha Gupta, Ajay Shah, Kamalika Roy, Varma Penumetcha, and Mark Oldham

SECTION A

Disorders usually first diagnosed in infancy, childhood, or adolescence (*DSM-IV*)/disruptive, impulse control, and conduct disorders (*DSM-5*); neurodevelopmental disorders (*DSM-5*); elimination disorders (*DSM-5*)

1. Which of the following disease processes is the most common genetic cause of intellectual disability?

A. Fetal alcohol syndrome
B. Down syndrome
C. Fragile X syndrome
D. Edward syndrome
E. Autism spectrum disorder

ANSWER: B

Intellectual disability is a disorder that requires deficits in both intellectual functioning (i.e., reasoning, problem-solving, abstract thinking, etc.) and adaptive functioning (i.e., social participation and responsibility, independent living, etc.). IQ is no longer used as a measure of severity of intellectual disability because adaptive functioning better correlates with the level of assistance a patient will need. Down syndrome, the most common genetic cause of intellectual disability, is most often caused by an error in cell division called nondisjunction (not heritable), leading to three copies of chromosome 21 rather than two. Down syndrome has an incidence of 1:1,000. Fetal alcohol syndrome is thought to be the most common *preventable* cause of intellectual disability. Fragile X (an X-linked dominant disorder due to a CGG trinucleotide repeat in the *FMR1* gene) has an incidence of 1:4,000 males and 1:8,000 females and is the most common *inherited* cause of intellectual disability. Edward syndrome is significantly rarer than these others, and autism spectrum disorder is not a cause of intellectual disability, though it may be associated with it.

REFERENCE

American Psychiatric Association. (2013). *Diagnostic and statistical manual of mental disorders* (5th ed., pp. 33–41). Arlington, VA: American Psychiatric Publishing.

Toth, K., de Lacy, N., and King, B. (2016). Intellectual disability. In M. K. Dulcan (Ed.), *Dulcan's textbook of child and adolescent psychiatry* (2nd ed.). Arlington, VA: American Psychiatric Publishing. doi:10.1176/appi.books.9781615370306. Retrieved from http://psychiatryonline.org/doi/full/10.1176/appi.books.9781615370306.md07

2. A 5-year-old boy is brought to your office by his parents, who say that he has been not speaking at school for the last several months. The parents are concerned because this has impacted the patient's academic performance. They are perplexed by these symptoms because when the patient is at home with them, he is quite talkative. Which of the following is the most likely diagnosis?

A. Selective mutism
B. Avoidant personality disorder
C. Post-traumatic stress disorder
D. Autism spectrum disorder
E. Language disorder

ANSWER: A

This patient is displaying refusal to speak while at school but willingness to do so while at home. Children with selective mutism will often speak around their immediate family, but when in social situations such as school or even with extended family, they will not speak. Selective mutism generally occurs before the age of 5 and requires that the child not speak in situations in which there is an expectation to do so. Personality disorders are generally not diagnosed until adolescence, and there is no indication of trauma in this patient. Patients with autism spectrum disorder or language disorder would show skill deficits in all situations rather than select ones as in this patient.

REFERENCE

American Psychiatric Association. (2013). *Diagnostic and statistical manual of mental disorders* (5th ed., pp. 189, 195–197). Arlington, VA: American Psychiatric Publishing.

3. A 10-year-old boy is brought to the clinic by his parents with complaints of eye blinking and clearing of throat. Symptoms have been present for the past 14 months. Which disorder does he most likely have?

A. Tourette's disorder
B. Persistent (chronic) motor tic disorder
C. Provisional tic disorder
D. Other specified tic disorder
E. Stereotypic movement disorder

ANSWER: A

The diagnosis of Tourette's disorder requires the presence of both motor and vocal tics for at least 1 year. Persistent (chronic) motor or vocal tic disorder is diagnosed when the patient has either motor or vocal tics, but not both. In provisional tic disorder, both motor and vocal tics may be present, but the patient has been experiencing symptoms for less than 1 year. Other specified tic disorder is diagnosed when symptoms of a tic disorder are present and impairing, but full criteria are not met (i.e., onset of symptoms after the age of 18). Stereotypic movement disorder is characterized by a fixed pattern of movement, which, unlike tics, can be variable in severity and affect different muscle groups.

REFERENCE

American Psychiatric Association. (2013). *Diagnostic and statistical manual of mental disorders* (5th ed., pp. 77–85). Arlington, VA: American Psychiatric Publishing.

4. A 9-year-old girl with normal body weight and no history of developmental delay is brought for outpatient evaluation by her parents. They state that the patient has been eating mostly chalk for the past 1 month. What is the most appropriate diagnosis?

A. Rumination disorder
B. Anorexia nervosa
C. Avoidant/restrictive food intake disorder (ARFID)
D. Intellectual disability disorder
E. Pica

ANSWER: E

Pica, previously categorized as a "disorder of infancy or early childhood," has been recategorized as a "feeding and eating disorder" in *DSM-5* because the disorder can begin at any age, although childhood onset is most common. A diagnosis of pica requires that the patient be eating nonnutritive, nonfood substances for at least 1 month and that this is not accounted for by the patient's developmental level. It is also important to rule out this type of behavior as being socially acceptable within the patient's culture. Rumination disorder involves the regurgitation of food following meals, and anorexia nervosa requires a low body weight as part of its criteria. ARFID, which is new in *DSM-5*, is characterized by restriction of food intake as in anorexia, but patients with ARFID do not have fear of gaining weight or misperceptions about body image as seen in anorexia. Although pica may be seen in patients with intellectual disability, this patient has no history of developmental delay.

REFERENCES

American Psychiatric Association. (2013). *Diagnostic and statistical manual of mental disorders* (5th ed., pp. 329–354). Arlington, VA: American Psychiatric Publishing.
Sadock, B. J., & Sadock, V. A. (Eds.). (2007). *Kaplan and Sadock's synopsis of psychiatry* (10th ed., pp. 1228–1233). Philadelphia, PA: Lippincott Williams and Wilkins.

5. In *DSM-5*, how is autism spectrum disorder (ASD) differentiated from social (pragmatic) communication disorder (SCD)?

A. Patients with SCD do not have repetitive or restrictive behaviors, interests, or activities.
B. Patients with ASD do not have repetitive or restrictive behaviors, interests, or activities.
C. SCD is initially diagnosed in adulthood, whereas ASD is initially diagnosed in children.
D. ASD presents with impaired nonverbal communication (e.g., interpreting body language), whereas SCD does not.
E. ASD impairs function, whereas SCD does not.

ANSWER: A

Both ASD and SCD present with language difficulties in social or learning situations. They both involve difficulty in communicating emotions or problem-solving with language, but the key difference is the lack of restrictive or repetitive interests, behaviors, or activities in SCD. Both ASD and SCD begin in childhood, and both require functional impairment to be diagnosed.

REFERENCE

American Psychiatric Association. (2013). *Diagnostic and statistical manual of mental disorders* (5th ed., pp. 47–59). Arlington, VA: American Psychiatric Publishing.

6. Which of the following is the most common reason that children in school receive special education?

A. Emotional dysregulation
B. Intellectual disability
C. Autism spectrum disorder
D. Learning disorder
E. Attention-deficit/hyperactivity disorder

ANSWER: D

According to the US Department of Education, in 2012–2013 children received special education most commonly for a specific learning disability such as in math, reading, or writing. Specific learning disability was the cause for 35% of patients in special education. Autism accounted for 8%, intellectual disability accounted for 7%, emotional disturbance accounted for 6%, and ADHD under the classification of "other health impairment" accounted for 12% of patients in special education.

REFERENCE

Cortiella, C., & Horowitz, S. H. (2014). *The state of learning disabilities: Facts, trends and emerging issues.* New York: National Center for Learning Disabilities. Retrieved from https://www.ncld.org/wp-content/uploads/2014/11/2014-State-of-LD.pdf

Kena, G., Musu-Gillette, L., Robinson, J., Wang, X., Rathbun, A., Zhang, J., Wilkinson-Flicker, S., ... Dunlop Velez, E. (2015). *The condition of education 2015* (NCES 2015-144). Washington, DC: US Department of Education, National Center for Education Statistics. Retrieved from http://nces.ed.gov/pubsearch

7. In *DSM-5*, which of the following diagnoses is now included as an obsessive–compulsive related disorder?

A. Pyromania
B. Kleptomania
C. Trichotillomania
D. Intermittent explosive disorder
E. Gambling disorder

ANSWER: C

In *DSM-5*, a new chapter on disruptive, impulse control, and conduct disorders includes oppositional defiant disorder (ODD), conduct disorder (CD), intermittent explosive disorder (IED), pyromania, and kleptomania. This is a change from *DSM-IV-TR*, in which IED, pyromania, and kleptomania were included under "impulse control disorders not elsewhere classified," and ODD and CD under "disorders first diagnosed in infancy, childhood, or adolescence." Trichotillomania (or skin-picking disorder) was previously included under "impulse control disorders not elsewhere classified" but has been recategorized to the obsessive–compulsive and related disorders label in *DSM-5*.

REFERENCE

American Psychiatric Association. (2013). Highlights of changes from *DSM-IV-TR* to *DSM-5*. In *Diagnostic and statistical manual of mental disorders* (5th ed., pp. 7, 15–16). Arlington, VA: American Psychiatric Publishing. Also available at http://www.dsm5.org/Documents/changes%20from%20dsm-iv-tr%20to%20dsm-5.pdf

8. Presence of which of the following is associated with progression of oppositional defiant disorder to conduct disorder?

A. Healthy older sibling
B. Early age of onset
C. Lack of family history
D. Higher socioeconomic status
E. Close attachment to a parental figure

ANSWER: B

Children with early age of onset for oppositional defiant disorder were three times more likely to develop conduct disorder. Approximately 30% of children with early-onset oppositional defiant disorder go on to develop conduct disorder. The other choices are relatively protective and account for positive support.

REFERENCE

Steiner, H., & Remsing, L. (2007). Work Group on Quality Issues: Practice parameter for the assessment and treatment of children and adolescents with oppositional defiant disorder. *Journal of the American Academy of Child and Adolescent Psychiatry,* 46, 126–141.

9. A 5-year-old boy is brought to the clinic by his parents with complaints of bedwetting for the past 3 months. The boy's bedwetting episodes occur about 3 times per week, and his parents are concerned about whether these symptoms will persist into adulthood. What is the best answer to their question?

A. Most patients with bedwetting will experience remission of symptoms as they age.
B. Once diagnosed, most patients with bedwetting will continue to have symptoms of similar severity into adulthood.
C. Symptoms will improve only if the patient is treated with pharmacological interventions.
D. Symptoms will initially improve and then worsen with age.

ANSWER: A

Enuresis is the repeated voiding of urine in inappropriate situations such as on the bed or clothing. A developmental age of at least 5 is required to make the diagnosis. The prevalence is thought to be 5% to 10% in 5-year-olds, and this number decreases with age. The yearly spontaneous remission rate has been reported to be anywhere from 5% to 16%, with only 1% of patients retaining a diagnosis of enuresis into adulthood. Use of a bed alarm (i.e., behavioral management) is first-line treatment.

REFERENCES

American Psychiatric Association: (2013). *Diagnostic and statistical manual of mental disorders* (5th ed., pp. 355–357). Arlington, VA: American Psychiatric Publishing.

Fritz, G., Rockney, R., Bernet, W., Arnold, V., Beitchman, J., Benson, R., *et al.* (2004). Practice parameter for the assessment and treatment of children and adolescents with enuresis. *Journal of the American Academy of Child and Adolescent Psychiatry,* 43, 1540–1550.

10. A 9-year-old boy with a family history of attention deficit hyperactivity disorder (ADHD) and substance use disorder is brought to the clinic by his mother for evaluation of inattention, hyperactivity, and poor academic performance. After making a diagnosis of ADHD in the patient, you recommend treatment with a stimulant. The mother is concerned about the family history of substance use and asks you how treatment with a stimulant will impact the risk of developing a substance use disorder in the patient. Which of the following is the best response?

A. It is likely to *increase* the likelihood of developing a substance use disorder.
B. It is likely to *decrease* the likelihood of developing a substance use disorder.
C. It should have *no impact* on the likelihood of developing a substance use disorder.
D. It will increase the likelihood of developing only cocaine use disorder.

ANSWER: B

A diagnosis of ADHD is itself a risk factor for the development of substance use; however, treatment for ADHD with a stimulant is considered to decrease the future likelihood of developing a substance use disorder.

REFERENCES

Groenman, A. P., Oosterlaan, J., Rommelse, N., Franke, B., Roeyers, H., Oades, R., et al. (2013) Substance use disorders in adolescents with attention deficit hyperactivity disorder: A 4-year follow-up study. *Addiction,* 108, 1503–1511.

Wilens, T. E., Adamson, J., Monuteaux, M. C., Faraone, S., Schillinger, M., Westerberg, D., & Biederman, J. (2008). Effect of prior stimulant treatment for attention-deficit/hyperactivity disorder on subsequent risk for cigarette smoking and alcohol and drug use disorders in adolescents. *Archives of Pediatrics and Adolescent Medicine,* 162, 916–921.

SECTION B: SUBSTANCE-RELATED DISORDERS

1. A 34-year-old woman with unknown history presents to the emergency room confused and agitated. The local police found her in the park while they were on patrol. The police report that the patient had difficulty identifying herself, could not stand in one place, was unable to walk in a straight line, and had slow responses to the questions they asked her. What is the best initial course of treatment?

A. Folic acid
B. Haloperidol
C. IV normal saline
D. Olanzapine
E. Thiamine

ANSWER: E

Administration of thiamine (100 mg IV) should occur immediately for all suspected cases of alcohol intoxication. Wernicke–Korsakoff syndrome is a medical emergency and may develop in alcohol-dependent patients secondary to thiamine deficiency. Wernicke's encephalopathy develops suddenly, and although it is classically described as the triad of ophthalmoplegia, ataxia, and altered mental status, these three *rarely* will be found in the same patient. Korsakoff's syndrome (or psychosis; also known as confabulatory psychosis or alcohol-induced persisting amnestic disorder) develops over days to weeks. Features include confabulation, diminished spontaneous verbal output, limited understanding of the degree of one's memory loss, and poor insight into one's illness.

REFERENCE

Fava, M., Rosenbaum, J., Stern, T., & Wilens, T. (Eds.). (2016). *Massachusetts General Hospital comprehensive clinical psychiatry* (2nd ed., pp. 274–276). New York, NY: Elsevier.

2. What is the most effective form of psychotherapy to treat individuals with a gambling disorder?

A. Dialectic behavioral therapy
B. Psychodynamic psychotherapy
C. Cognitive behavioral therapy
D. Group therapy
E. Interpersonal therapy

ANSWER: C

Cognitive restructuring involves addressing false beliefs about gambling, including the illusion of control and of memory biases where the gambler remembers only the winnings. Training is focused on problem-solving and social skills to reduce the distress that triggers the need to gamble. The gambler can self-monitor by journaling in a workbook.

REFERENCE

Fava, M., Rosenbaum, J., Stern, T., & Wilens, T. (Eds.). (2016). *Massachusetts General Hospital comprehensive clinical psychiatry* (2nd ed., pp. 250–252). New York, NY: Elsevier.

3. Which of the following is not a sign or symptom of caffeine withdrawal?

A. Difficulty concentrating
B. Flu-like symptoms
C. Headache
D. Tachycardia
E. Dysphoric mood

ANSWER: D

Tachycardia is a symptom of caffeine intoxication. Caffeine withdrawal presents with headache, marked fatigue or drowsiness, dysphoric mood, depressed mood, or irritability, difficulty concentrating, and flu-like symptoms (nausea, vomiting, or muscle pain/stiffness).

REFERENCE

American Psychiatric Association. (2013). *Diagnostic and statistical manual of mental disorders* (5th ed.). Arlington, VA: American Psychiatric Publishing.

4. A 32-year-old woman is found unresponsive is and taken to the emergency room. She awakens to naloxone. Standard urine toxicology is negative for opiates but positive for benzodiazepines. What is the likely explanation for the patient's response to naloxone?

A. It was most likely a false negative drug screen.
B. Naloxone exerts cross-reactive antagonism for benzodiazepines.
C. She used a synthetic or semisynthetic opioid.
D. The patient is malingering.

ANSWER: C

Several synthetic and semisynthetic opioids are not detected on routine urine toxicology screening. For instance, fentanyl, buprenorphine, and methadone require assays for these substances in particular given structural differences relative to naturally occurring opioids (i.e., opiates), including morphine and codeine. Of note, all agents that activate mu receptors are known as opioids (literally, "resembling opiates"), and agonists that are structurally related to compounds derived from opium poppy are opiates proper. The *DSM-5* uses the more encompassing term *opioid*, as in "opioid use disorder" and "opioid withdrawal."

REFERENCE

Tenore, P. L. (2010). Advanced urine toxicology testing. *Journal of Addictive Disorders, 29*, 436–448.

5. What is the most common long-term risk of classic hallucinogen use?

A. Chronic suicidality
B. Hypomania
C. Auditory hallucinations
D. Visual hallucinations
E. Flashbacks

ANSWER: E

The most common long-term risk of classic hallucinogen use is hallucinogen persisting perception disorder (HPPD), also referred to as flashbacks. A flashback includes reinforcement of the perceptual, emotional, or somatic effects of a previous hallucinogen experience. For the psychiatric diagnostic criteria for HPPD to be met, perceptual disturbances must last beyond the normal duration of drug effects and must be clinically distressing or impairing.

REFERENCE

Galanter, M. Kleber, H. D., & Brady, K. T. (Eds.). (2015). *The American Psychiatric Publishing textbook of substance abuse treatment* (5th ed., Chapter 15). Washington, DC: American Psychiatric Association Publishing.

6. How long can a urine drug screen test stay positive for delta-9-tetrahydrocannabinol in a heavy cannabis user?

A. 12 to 24 hours
B. 1 to 2 days
C. 4 to 6 days
D. 1 to 2 weeks
E. 2 to 4 weeks

ANSWER: E

A positive urine test for delta-9-tetrahydrocannabinol (THC) is limited for diagnosis because it signifies past use but cannot be used to diagnose acute intoxication. Cannabinoids are highly lipophilic and can remain in body fluids for weeks after cessation of *heavy* use. Occasional use, though, rarely leads to positive urine screens for more than a few days after last use.

REFERENCE

Bailey, J. A., DuPont, R. L., & Teitelbaum, S. A (2014). *Cannabis use disorder: Clinical features and diagnosis.* In UpToDate, Waltham, MA.

7. A 58-year-old man with tobacco use disorder was recently diagnosed with peripheral vascular disease by his primary care physician. He now wishes to quit smoking cigarettes. Which of the following FDA-approved medications for smoking cessation is best avoided in this patient?

A. Varenicline
B. Nicotine inhaler
C. Nicotine nasal spray
D. Buproprion
E. Nicotine patch

ANSWER: A

Varenicline is approved by the FDA for smoking cessation; however, the FDA has issued black box warnings for psychiatric and cardiac symptoms. Psychiatric symptoms include agitation, dysthymia, and suicidal ideations. Cardiac symptoms include angina pectoris, nonfatal myocardial infarction, need for coronary revascularization, and new diagnosis of peripheral vascular disease. Ongoing studies continue to explore the nature of potential cardiac risk with varenicline.

REFERENCE

Galanter, M. Kleber, H. D., & Brady, K. T. (Eds). (2015). *The American Psychiatric Publishing textbook of substance abuse treatment* (5th ed., Chapter 16). Washington, DC: American Psychiatric Association Publishing.

8. How long after the last drink does alcohol withdrawal delirium typically present?

A. 10 to 12 hours
B. 12 to 24 hours
C. 1 to 2 days
D. 2 to 4 days
E. 6 to 8 days

ANSWER: D

Alcohol withdrawal delirium (or "delirium tremens") is the most serious withdrawal syndrome associated with alcohol withdrawal. Symptoms usually begin 2 to 4 days after the last drink. The average length of an episode of alcohol withdrawal delirium is less than 1 week; however, there have been reports of its lasting for several weeks.

REFERENCE

Galanter, M. Kleber, H. D., & Brady, K. T. (Eds). (2015). *The American Psychiatric Publishing textbook of substance abuse treatment* (5th ed., Chapter 11). Washington, DC: American Psychiatric Publishing.

SECTION C: SCHIZOPHRENIA AND OTHER PSYCHOTIC DISORDERS (*DSM-IV*)/ SCHIZOPHRENIA SPECTRUM AND OTHER PSYCHOTIC DISORDERS (*DSM-5*)

1. Which of the following is NOT a poor prognostic factor in schizophrenia?

A. Autistic behavior
B. Abnormal dexamethasone suppression test
C. Focal neurological signs
D. Aggressive behavior
E. Acute onset

ANSWER: E

Withdrawn autistic behavior, focal neurological signs, insidious onset, younger age of onset, history of aggressive behavior and aggressiveness, and nonsuppression of dexamethasone suppression test are associated with poor prognosis in schizophrenia. Conversely, later age of onset, presence of clear precipitant, acute onset, comorbid mood symptoms, family history of mood disorders, and positive symptoms are considered to have better prognosis. Only 20% to 30% of individuals with schizophrenia are able to lead a relatively "normal" life. Roughly half of patients with schizophrenia remain significantly impaired.

REFERENCE

Sadock, B., & Sadock, V. (2015). Schizophrenia. In *Synopsis of psychiatry* (11th ed., pp. 305–318). Philadelphia, PA: Wolters Kluwer.

2. Which of the following is TRUE for nicotine use in schizophrenia?

A. Half of those with schizophrenia are nicotine dependent.
B. Nicotine worsens negative symptoms.
C. Tobacco use increases the blood level of haloperidol.
D. Tobacco use increases the blood level of risperidone.
E. Nicotine reduces auditory hallucinations.

ANSWER: E

Up to 90% of patients with schizophrenia may be dependent on nicotine. A specific polymorphism in a nicotine receptor has been shown to be linked with an increased risk of schizophrenia. Nicotine administration is shown to improve some cognitive symptoms and some positive symptoms as well, through its effect on nicotine receptors in the brain that reduce the perception of outside stimuli. Tobacco use reduces the blood level of haloperidol and has no or minimal significant effect on the blood level of risperidone. (*Note*: The polycyclic aromatic compounds in tobacco, not nicotine itself, induce CYP1A2. This is important because when patients who smoke are placed on nicotine replacement in the hospital, several medication levels can change and then change again upon discharge when tobacco use resumes.) Haloperidol, olanzapine, and clozapine are metabolized by CYP1A2. Risperidone is mainly metabolized by CYP2D6, and the level is not significantly affected by smoking.

REFERENCES

Lucas, C., & Martin, J. (2013). Smoking and drug interactions. *Australian Prescriber, 36*, 102–104.
Sadock, B., & Sadock, V. (2015). Schizophrenia. In *Synopsis of psychiatry* (11th ed., pp. 305–318). Wolters Kluwer.

3. Which one of the following is TRUE about suicide in schizophrenia?

A. Roughly 1% of those with schizophrenia commit suicide.
B. Comorbid depression does not influence suicide risk.
C. Younger men with higher aspirations have a lower suicide risk.
D. Having fewer negative symptoms may decrease suicide risk.
E. Suicide is often sudden and unexpected in patients with schizophrenia.

ANSWER: E

Almost 20% to 50% patients with schizophrenia attempt suicide. According to *DSM-5*, at least 5% to 6% may die by suicide. Nearly 80% of patients with schizophrenia will have a lifetime major depressive episode, and the presence of depression is a strong risk factor for suicide in schizophrenia. Younger men with higher expectations paradoxically have a *higher* risk of suicide. Fewer negative symptoms and better abstract thinking are also associated with *higher* risk. Suicide is often sudden and unexpected in schizophrenia. Two thirds of the patients who commit suicide may have seen an otherwise-unsuspecting clinician within 72 hours of the act. Clozapine *decreases* risk of suicide in patients with schizophrenia.

REFERENCE

Sadock, B., & Sadock, V. (2015). Schizophrenia. In *Synopsis of psychiatry* (11th ed., pp. 305–318). Wolters Kluwer.

4. According to *DSM-5*, which of the following is sufficient on its own to satisfy criterion A for schizophrenia?

A. Two voices having a conversation with each other
B. Auditory hallucination providing a real-time commentary
C. A belief that an alien resides in one's big toe
D. Mental automatisms
E. None of the above

ANSWER: E

In *DSM-IV-TR*, choices A through C would have been sufficient to satisfy criterion A. These are among Schneider's first-rank symptoms of schizophrenia. Mental automatisms are another first-rank symptom. *DSM-5* removed the eminence of such symptoms from schizophrenia diagnosis because the nature of the delusion (i.e., whether it is bizarre) or the content of auditory hallucination is not specific for schizophrenia. Any two of the following symptoms have to be present for criterion A: delusions, hallucinations, disorganized speech, grossly disorganized or catatonic behavior, and negative symptoms.

REFERENCE

American Psychiatric Association. (2013). *Diagnostic and statistical manual of mental disorders* (5th ed., p. 99). Arlington, VA: American Psychiatric Publishing.

5. What percentage of those with attenuated psychosis syndrome (APS) progress to a formal psychotic disorder the year following APS diagnosis?

A. 75%
B. 50%
C. 35%
D. 15%
E. 2%

ANSWER: D

Attenuated psychosis syndrome is diagnosed when at least one of the three psychotic symptoms (hallucination, delusion, disorganized speech) is present in an attenuated form for at least 1 week in the last month. These symptoms are transient and accompanied by largely maintained insight. Difficulty in concentration, anxiety, social withdrawal, and disrupted sleep–wake cycle are commonly associated with the syndrome. The symptoms usually start in late adolescence to early adulthood. In help-seeking populations, 18% may progress to meet criteria for psychotic disorder in 1 year. Some of them may transition to mood disorders. Presence of negative symptoms and cognitive impairment are poor prognostic factors for later development of a psychotic disorder.

REFERENCE

American Psychiatric Association. (2013). *Diagnostic and statistical manual of mental disorders* (5th ed., p. 785). Arlington, VA: American Psychiatric Publishing.

6. Which is TRUE about cognitive impairment in schizophrenia?

A. It affects processing speed and executive functioning, not memory.
B. It begins more than a decade after the first episode of psychosis.
C. It tends to be stable in severity.
D. It is not a central feature of schizophrenia.
E. It resolves with control of positive symptoms.

ANSWER: C

Cognitive impairment is a central feature of schizophrenia, usually present prior to the prodromal phase. Attention, processing speed, executive functioning, memory, language, and social cognition are impaired. The impairment is not reversed by antipsychotics or by resolution of positive symptoms. In some patients the deficit progresses over several years. but usually it stays relatively stable throughout disease course. Cognitive impairment exhibits limited fluctuation in association with positive symptoms.

REFERENCE

Nasrallah, H., & Smeltzer, D. (2011). *Contemporary diagnosis and management of schizophrenia* (2nd ed., pp. 79–80). Newtown, PA: Handbooks in Health Care.

7. Which option is TRUE regarding obsessive–compulsive symptoms in schizophrenia?

A. They are associated with poorer prognosis.
B. They are associated with a later schizophrenia onset.
C. They are associated with less neurocognitive impairment.
D. They resolve with treatment with antipsychotics.
E. Their occurrence in schizophrenia reduces suicide risk.

ANSWER: A

Obsessive–compulsive symptoms are associated with poorer prognosis in schizophrenia, worse neurocognitive impairment, greater depression severity, and more suicidal ideation. They also are associated with an earlier onset of disease. These symptoms are inconsistently relieved (or at times worsened) with neuroleptics.

REFERENCE

Nasrallah, H., & Smeltzer, D. (2011). *Contemporary diagnosis and management of schizophrenia* (2nd ed., p. 81). Newtown, PA: Handbooks in Health Care.

8. Which one is TRUE about late-onset schizophrenia?

A. It presents with more positive symptoms and lower burden of negative symptoms.
B. Thought disorganization is more common with late-onset schizophrenia.
C. Catatonia is more common when schizophrenia has a late onset.
D. There is a female predominance.

ANSWER: D

Late-onset schizophrenia often starts after age 45, and most patients are female. It tends to have fewer or equivalent positive symptoms as does schizophrenia that presents earlier but a greater burden of negative symptoms. Catatonia is less common in these patients.

REFERENCE

Nasrallah, H., & Smeltzer, D. (2011). *Contemporary diagnosis and management of schizophrenia* (2nd ed., p. 137). Newtown, PA: Handbooks in Health Care.

SECTION D: MOOD DISORDERS/ BIPOLAR DISORDERS/ DEPRESSIVE DISORDERS

1. Which of the following is a key symptom of depression with melancholic features?

A. Weight gain
B. Absence of mood reactivity
C. Depression that is worse in the evening
D. Interpersonal rejection sensitivity
E. Subjective heaviness of extremities

ANSWER: B

Depression with melancholic features presents with either loss of pleasure in nearly all activities or loss of mood reactivity, even in situations in which something highly desired occurs. Three or more of the following symptoms are also required for the diagnosis: distinct quality of depressed mood that is characterized by profound despondency or despair, depression that is worse in the morning, early morning awakening, psychomotor agitation or retardation, significant weight loss/anorexia, and excessive/inappropriate guilt. Weight gain, interpersonal rejection sensitivity, and subjective heaviness of extremities are features of atypical depression.

REFERENCE

American Psychiatric Association. (2013). *Diagnostic and statistical manual of mental disorders* (5th ed., p. 185). Arlington, VA: American Psychiatric Publishing.

2. The diagnosis of disruptive mood dysregulation disorder requires symptom onset prior to what age?

A. 6 years
B. 10 years
C. 13 years
D. 18 years
E. 21 years

ANSWER: B

Disruptive mood dysregulation disorder (DMDD) is a new diagnosis that was added to the depressive disorders chapter in *DSM-5*. This diagnosis was added to prevent overdiagnosis of bipolar disorder in children and was placed in the depressive disorders chapter with the thought that children labeled with DMDD will more likely go on to develop unipolar rather than bipolar depression. The key feature of DMDD is severe, recurrent temper outbursts out of proportion to the situation. The diagnosis should not be made in anyone younger than age 6 or older than 18, and the onset of symptoms in the patient must have occurred prior to the age of 10.

REFERENCE

American Psychiatric Association. (2013). *Diagnostic and statistical manual of mental disorders* (5th ed., pp. 156–160). Arlington, VA: American Psychiatric Publishing.

3. The rapid cycling specifier for bipolar disorder requires which of the following?

A. Four mood episodes in a year, at least one of which is mania
B. Four mood episodes of any kind in a year
C. Four mood episodes of any kind in 6 months
D. Four mood episodes of any kind in 6 months for at least 2 years
E. Four mood episodes of any kind in a year with at least one episode from each pole (i.e., depressed and elevated) being required

ANSWER: C

The rapid cycling specifier can be applied to either bipolar I or bipolar II disorder and is defined as four distinct mood episodes in a year. These episodes can be major depressive, hypomanic, or manic. Although the diagnosis of bipolar disorder requires both poles of symptoms to be present (i.e., depressive and hypomania/mania), it is not necessary for symptoms to be present from both poles to be characterized as rapid cycling.

REFERENCE

American Psychiatric Association. (2013). *Diagnostic and statistical manual of mental disorders* (5th ed., pp. 150–151). Arlington, VA: American Psychiatric Publishing.

4. Which of the following distinguishes bereavement from a major depressive episode?

A. Guilt
B. Insomnia
C. Feelings of sadness
D. Feelings of worthlessness
E. Longing to join the departed

ANSWER: E

Patients with bereavement generally do not feel worthless. Guilt may be present in bereavement; however, this often centers on the fact that one did not spend enough time with the deceased or failed to communicate to the deceased how much he or she was loved. Thoughts of wanting to die may be present both in bereavement and during a major depressive episode; however, the thought of wanting to die in bereavement usually involves a desire to be with or join the loved one rather than wanting to commit suicide secondary to feelings of worthlessness as seen in major depression.

REFERENCES

American Psychiatric Association. (2013). *Diagnostic and statistical manual of mental disorders* (5th ed., pp. 125–126). Arlington, VA: American Psychiatric Publishing.
Steffens, D. C., Blazer, D. G., & Thakur, M. E. (Eds.). (2015). *The American Psychiatric Publishing textbook of geriatric psychiatry* (5th ed., pp. 418–420). Arlington, VA, American Psychiatric Publishing.

5. Which of the following sleep changes is seen in patients with depression?

A. Reduced REM latency
B. Reduced REM density
C. Decreased sleep latency
D. Increased N3 (deep) sleep
E. Decreased number of awakenings

ANSWER: A

Patients with depression have reduced REM latency, meaning they have a shorter time from sleep onset to first REM than do nondepressed individuals. Depressed patients also have more awakenings during the night (i.e., greater sleep fragmentation); increased REM density or REM frequency during sleep, resulting in vivid dreams; and decreased N3 (deep or slow-wave) sleep. Decreased sleep latency (choice C) is seen in narcolepsy.

REFERENCE

Fleming, J. A. (1994). REM sleep abnormalities and psychiatry. *Journal of Psychiatry & Neuroscience, 19*, 335–344.

6. A 23-year-old woman is brought to your outpatient clinic by her friend, who states that the patient has been acting "different" for the past 4 days. The friend reports that the patient has had elevated mood with increased energy. On interview, the patient reports that she has not slept more than 3 hours per night during this time but says she feels great. Her speech is pressured, and her thoughts are racing. The patient denies any previous history of similar or depressive symptoms but does report a family history of major depressive disorder. What is the most likely diagnosis?

A. Bipolar I disorder
B. Bipolar II disorder
C. Cyclothymia
D. Bipolar II disorder, with rapid cycling
E. Other specified bipolar and related disorder

ANSWER: E

This patient's symptoms are consistent with a hypomanic episode. Bipolar II disorder requires the presence of at least one hypomanic episode and at least one major depressive episode; the patient's absence of the latter rules out this diagnosis. Cyclothymia is incorrect because the symptoms have been present for 4 days. The rapid cycling specifier cannot be applied at this time because the patient has not been diagnosed with bipolar I or II disorder. Furthermore, this is her first episode, and rapid cycling requires four or more distinct mood episodes over a 1-year period. The best answer in this case is other specified bipolar and related disorder.

REFERENCE

American Psychiatric Association. (2013). *Diagnostic and statistical manual of mental disorders* (5th ed., p. 148). Arlington, VA: American Psychiatric Publishing.

7. A 19-year-old man with no psychiatric history who has been experiencing 4 days of irritable mood and increased goal-directed activity is brought to the emergency department and subsequently hospitalized. The patient says that he feels so good that he "doesn't need sleep," and he has racing thoughts. He is grandiose and recently maxed out his credit card by purchasing several opulent watches. What is the most likely diagnosis?

A. Bipolar I disorder
B. Bipolar II disorder
C. Cyclothymia
D. Bipolar II disorder, with rapid cycling
E. Other specified bipolar and related disorder

ANSWER: A

Hypomanic and manic episodes are distinguished in a few key ways. Hypomania requires at least 4 days of symptoms, whereas mania requires a week *or less* if the symptoms are severe enough to warrant psychiatric hospitalization. Delusions exclude a diagnosis of hypomania and would favor a diagnosis of mania. Hypomania is not severe enough to cause significant impairment; in fact, many patients with hypomania are remarkably productive (but may drive their spouses, friends, and coworkers crazy in the process!). The presence of a manic episode warrants a diagnosis of bipolar I disorder.

REFERENCE

American Psychiatric Association. (2013). *Diagnostic and statistical manual of mental disorders* (5th ed., pp. 123–125). Arlington, VA: American Psychiatric Publishing.

8. Which of the following is the strongest predictor of developing depressive symptoms during pregnancy?

A. Minority ethnicity
B. Financial hardship
C. Unmarried status
D. Historical depression
E. Higher socioeconomic status

ANSWER: D

Lower socioeconomic status, financial hardship, and being unmarried may contribute to the development of depressive symptoms during pregnancy, but the strongest risk factor for the development of depression during pregnancy is the presence of a past history of depression. Minority status per se does not predict depression during pregnancy.

REFERENCES

Marcus, S. M., Flynn, H. A., Blow, F. C., & Barry, K. L. (2003). Depressive symptoms among pregnant women screened in obstetrics settings. *Journal of Women's Health, 12*, 373–380.

Rich-Edwards, J. W., Kleinman, K., Abrams, A., Harlow, B. L., McLaughlin, T. J., & Joffe, H. (2006). Socio-demographic predictors of antenatal and postpartum depressive symptoms among women in a medical group practice. *Journal of Epidemiology & Community Health, 60*, 221–227.

9. What is the lifetime prevalence of bipolar I disorder?

A. 1:10
B. 1:100
C. 5:100
D. 1:1,000
E. 1:10,000

ANSWER: B

Data from the National Comorbidity Survey Replication found a lifetime prevalence of bipolar I disorder of 1%. The lifetime prevalence of bipolar II was 1.1%, and the lifetime prevalence for any bipolar-related disorder was 4.4%.

REFERENCE

Merikangas, K. R., Akiskal, H. S., Angst, J., Greenberg, P. E., Hirschfeld, R. M., Petukhova, M., & Kessler, R. C. (2007). Lifetime and 12-month prevalence of bipolar spectrum disorder in the National Comorbidity Survey replication. *Archives of General Psychiatry, 64*, 543–552.

SECTION E: ANXIETY DISORDERS/OCD/TRAUMA-RELATED DISORDERS

1. Which of the following is the most common form of trauma that causes post-traumatic stress disorder in women?

A. Sexual assault
B. Car accident
C. Natural disaster
D. Diagnosis of terminal illness
E. Loss of loved one

ANSWER: A

Sexual assault is the most common form of trauma leading to post-traumatic stress disorder (PTSD) in women. Approximately one in three women will experience a lifetime sexual assault. Women are more than twice as likely to develop PTSD than are men (10% versus 4%).

REFERENCE

US Department of Veterans Affairs: National Center for PTSD. Retrieved from http://www.ptsd.va.gov/public/PTSD-overview/women/women-trauma-and-ptsd.asp

2. A 34-year-old man presents to your outpatient office with worsening anxiety for the past 6 months to the point that it has been affecting his work. His primary concern is that others are judging him intensely, so he has been avoiding situations where he has to be around his colleagues, including business meetings and conferences. Which of the following is the most likely diagnosis?

A. Avoidant personality disorder
B. Generalized anxiety disorder
C. Social anxiety disorder
D. Schizoid personality disorder
E. Panic disorder

ANSWER: C

The key feature of social anxiety disorder is marked or intense fear in social situations in which the individual is concerned about being scrutinized or judged by others (also known as social evaluatism). Avoidant and schizoid personality disorders are pervasive and have been present since the age of 18, which is not the case in this vignette. Generalized anxiety disorder may have social anxiety, but it is characterized by global worry involving a variety of stressors. Panic disorder is defined by recurrent panic attacks that come "out of the blue" and significant fear of having further panic attacks. Notably, "with panic" is a new *DSM-5* specifier that can be added to most other *DSM-5* diagnoses.

REFERENCE

American Psychiatric Association. (2013). *Diagnostic and statistical manual of mental disorders* (5th ed., pp. 202–208). Arlington, VA: American Psychiatric Publishing.

3. A 55-year-old Latin American woman is brought to your office by her daughter, who explains that her mother has episodes of shouting, anger, and "heat in the chest rising to the head." Which of the following

culture-bound syndromes is most consistent with her symptoms?

A. *Dhat* syndrome
B. *Ataque de nervios*
C. *Khyal cap*
D. *Susto*
E. *Kufungisia*

ANSWER: B

Ataque de nervios is a culture-bound syndrome described in Latino populations and is characterized by acute anxiety, anger, and uncontrollable screaming or shouting. Symptoms also include attacks of crying, trembling, and heat in the chest rising into the head. Another key features is feeling "out of control." It is unclear yet whether *ataque de nervios* may be more accurately understood as simply recurrent panic attacks. *Dhat* is a South Asian term that describes semen loss as a way of explaining any distressing symptoms. *Khyal cap* is a Cambodian syndrome whose symptoms are mainly those of panic attacks, such as dizziness, shortness of breath, and palpitations. *Susto* is a cultural explanation for distress seen in Mexico, Central America, and South America. *Kufungisia* describes distress in the Shona people of Zimbabwe.

REFERENCE

American Psychiatric Association. (2013). *Diagnostic and statistical manual of mental disorders* (5th ed., pp. 833–837). Arlington, VA: American Psychiatric Publishing.

4. Which of the following is an example of a compulsion?

A. Scruples
B. Checking
C. Contamination
D. Pathological doubt
E. Intrusive thoughts of violence

ANSWER: B

A compulsion is a repetitive behavior or mental act done in response to an obsession (intrusive, unwanted, distressing thought) because the individual feels compelled to perform the action. Compulsions typically reduce the distress caused by obsessions; however, some compulsions are performed as stereotyped behaviors based on idiosyncratic rules that a patient feels compelled to do *in the absence of an obsession*. In fact, a diagnosis of obsessive–compulsive disorder (OCD) requires the presence of *either* obsessions *or* compulsions because either can exist independent of the other. Obsessions and compulsions are nevertheless comorbid in the vast majority of patients with OCD. Checking is a compulsion, often in response to the obsession of doubt (i.e., Were the lights left on? Is the door locked?). The other choices are examples of obsessions.

REFERENCE

American Psychiatric Association. (2013). *Diagnostic and statistical manual of mental disorders* (5th ed., pp. 235–242). Arlington, VA: American Psychiatric Publishing.

5. Which of the following brain regions is the site of psychosurgery in patients with refractory obsessive–compulsive disorder?

A. Anterior cingulate
B. Prefrontal cortex
C. Arcuate fasciculus
D. Hippocampus
E. Mammillary bodies

ANSWER: A

Neurosurgery is a last resort treatment option for patients with OCD. Anterior cingulotomy is one such surgical option.

REFERENCE

Sheth, S. A., Neal, J., Tangherlini, F., Mian, M. K., Gentil, A., Cosgrove, G. R., Eskandar, E. N. & Dougherty, D. D. (2013). Limbic system surgery for treatment-refractory obsessive–compulsive disorder: A prospective long-term follow-up of 64 patients. *Journal of Neurosurgery, 118*, 491–497.

6. An attractive 31-year-old woman presents with excessive complaints about her appearance and a belief that her nose is "hideous." As a result, she no longer goes out with friends, which distresses her. Which of the following is her most likely diagnosis?

A. Body dysmorphic disorder
B. Social anxiety disorder
C. Generalized anxiety disorder

D. Illness anxiety disorder
E. Somatic symptom disorder

ANSWER: A

Patients with body dysmorphic disorder are preoccupied with their appearance and self-perceived flaws despite being told otherwise by friends and family. These flaws are generally mild or not noticeable to others. Social anxiety disorder is incorrect because the woman's avoidance of social interaction is directly related to her perceived appearance. In generalized anxiety disorder, worry is pervasive rather than specifically focused on appearance. Patients with illness anxiety are anxious specifically over having a medical diagnosis.

REFERENCE

American Psychiatric Association. (2013). *Diagnostic and statistical manual of mental disorders* (5th ed., pp. 242–247). Arlington, VA: American Psychiatric Publishing.

7. Which of the following distinguishes acute stress disorder (ASD) from PTSD?

A. ASD can have delayed expression.
B. Dissociative features may be diagnosed in PTSD but not ASD.
C. Significant distress is required for PTSD but not ASD.
D. The index trauma must be directly experienced in PTSD but not ASD.
E. PTSD requires 1 month of symptoms, but ASD requires resolution in 1 month.

ANSWER: E

Several features distinguish PTSD and ASD, although they both have the same criteria for index trauma (ruling out choice D). *DSM-5* describes this trauma as being experienced directly, witnessing it happen to others, learning that it has happened to a close family member or friend, *or* experiencing repeated exposure to aversive details of the event. Dissociative features may be seen in either disorder: In ASD these are among the core features, whereas in PTSD they may be identified with the specifier "with dissociative features." Both diagnoses require clinically significant distress. Duration and timing of onset are the key distinguishing factors between these conditions. ASD can be present from 3 to 30 days after the trauma; PTSD is diagnosed after 30 days of symptoms and may actually have a delayed onset (specifier "with delayed expression").

REFERENCE

American Psychiatric Association. (2013). *Diagnostic and statistical manual of mental disorders* (5th ed., pp. 271–280). Arlington, VA: American Psychiatric Publishing.

8. A 24-year-old man is afraid of flying and has been for years, and he presents at the request of his work supervisor. The patient describes how he has been driving to all his appointments even when he has to drive several states away. Which of the following is the most likely diagnosis?

A. Social phobia
B. Specific phobia
C. Generalized anxiety disorder
D. Delusional disorder
E. Panic disorder

ANSWER: B

Fear of flying (or aviophobia) is a specific phobia.

REFERENCE

American Psychiatric Association. (2013). *Diagnostic and statistical manual of mental disorders* (5th ed., pp. 197–202). Arlington, VA: American Psychiatric Publishing.

SECTION F: SOMATIC SYMPTOM AND RELATED DISORDERS

1. Which of the following best characterizes the shift from "somatoform disorders" in *DSM-IV-TR* to "somatic symptom and related disorders" in *DSM-5*?

A. Elimination of conversion disorder
B. A refined focus on psychological distress
C. An increased number of specific diagnoses
D. An emphasis on medically unexplainable symptoms
E. A renewed emphasis on ruling out medical conditions

ANSWER: B

The overarching shift in diagnosis from *DSM-IV-TR* to *DSM-5* for this class of conditions is a refined focus on psychological distress. The somatoform disorders of *DSM-IV-TR* required that diagnoses be given in the absence of a medical cause (i.e., medically unexplained); however, this is very difficult—if not next to impossible—to operationalize. The somatic symptom and related disorders of *DSM-5* rather focus on the presence of distress and may be diagnosed as a comorbidity. In fact, studies suggest that patients do best when treated with close medical care *combined with* mental health care. Conversion disorder remains in *DSM-5*.

REFERENCES

American Psychiatric Association. (2013). *Diagnostic and statistical manual of mental disorders* (5th ed., p. 309). Arlington, VA: American Psychiatric Publishing.

Dimsdale, J. E., Creed, F., Escobar, J., Sharpe, M., Wulsin, L., Barsky, A., et al. (2013). Somatic symptom disorder: An important change in DSM. *Journal of Psychosomatic Research*, *75*, 223–228.

2. What is the key difference between illness anxiety disorder and somatic symptom disorder?

A. The presence of an associated medical condition
B. Whether they are a diagnosis of exclusion
C. Predominance of somatic symptoms
D. Presence of neurological deficits
E. Number of symptoms

ANSWER: C

Somatic symptom disorder requires the presence of clinically significant somatic symptoms, whereas illness anxiety disorder requires the absence of (or at most only minimal) somatic symptoms. They both may be diagnosed with or independent of medical illness, and neither is a diagnosis of exclusion. The presence of neurological deficits is a diagnostic feature of conversion disorder provided neurological syndromes are adequately ruled out. Unlike somatization disorder in *DSM-IV-TR*, neither of these *DSM-5* diagnoses has a criterion related to number of symptoms.

REFERENCE

American Psychiatric Association. (2013). *Diagnostic and statistical manual of mental disorders* (5th ed., pp. 314, 317). Arlington, VA: American Psychiatric Publishing.

3. Which of the following best unifies the somatic symptom and related disorders category of disorders in *DSM-5*?

A. High state anxiety
B. Excessive illness behavior
C. Denial of psychogenic cause
D. Prominent physical symptoms
E. Symptoms lack a medical explanation

ANSWER: B

The unifying theme of somatic symptom and related disorders (SSRDs) in *DSM-5* is the presence of excessive illness behavior. Illness behavior encompasses the "intra- and interpersonal reactions of a patient to a disease or injury," which can be adaptive (e.g., guarding to prevent re-injury) or maladaptive (e.g., continued sedentarism long after a bout of illness, leading to obesity). Although most SSRDs have high anxiety, conversion disorder is classically characterized by *la belle indifference* (French for "beautiful indifference"). That is, patients are inappropriately unconcerned about their often glaring neurological impairment or episodes. Although denial is not uncommonly seen in many patients with SSRDs, it is not a diagnostic criterion. Illness anxiety disorder specifically requires limited to no physical symptoms related to distress. Overall, the *DSM-5* has shifted away from "psychogenic" conditions, although conversion disorder retains this feature.

REFERENCES

American Psychiatric Association. (2013). *Diagnostic and statistical manual of mental disorders* (5th ed., p. 309). Arlington, VA: American Psychiatric Publishing.

Hamilton, J. C., Hedge, K. A., & Feldman, M. D. (2015). Excessive illness behavior. In B. S. Fogel & D. B. Greenberg (Eds.), *Psychiatric care of the medical patient* (3rd ed., pp. 743–744). New York, NY: Oxford University Press.

Mechanic, D. (1966). Response factors in illness: The study of illness behavior. *Social Psychiatry*, *1*(1), 11–20.

4. A patient is suspected of functional paralysis. On examination, the physician gives instructions to the patient, who is lying supine on the hospital bed. Initially, the doctor places his hands under the patient's heels and asks the patient to raise each leg, one at a time. Then the doctor places his hands on the outside of the patient's ankles, applies adducting pressure, and asks the patient to abduct each leg. Which of the following would lend strongest support to a diagnosis of functional LEFT lower extremity weakness?

A. Request to raise the right leg involves no downward force of the left leg
B. Request to raise the left leg involves downward force of the right leg
C. Request to raise the left leg involves no downward force of the right leg
D. Request to abduct the right leg involves no outward force of the left leg
E. Request to abduct the left leg involves no adduction of the right leg

ANSWER: C

The correct answer is C, which is a positive Hoover sign, originally described more than a century ago. The possible answer choices, though, assess knowledge of the Hoover and abductor signs. The Hoover sign is predicated on the fact that in order to raise one leg, the other naturally pushes downward for support. A truly paretic left leg would not produce a downward force when the patient is asked to raise the right (sound) leg, and there should be downward force from the right (sound) leg when the patient is asked to raise the left (paretic) leg. The abductor sign involves requests to abduct both legs and then each leg independently. A positive abductor sign occurs when a request to abduct the paretic leg while the examiner applies adducting force to both legs yields adduction of the sound leg as though overcompensating. Choices D and E would be expected in true paralysis.

REFERENCES

Hoover, C. F. (1908). A new sign for the detection of malingering and functional paresis of the lower extremities. *JAMA, 51*, 746–747.

Sonoo, M. (2004). Abductor sign: A reliable new sign to detect unilateral non-organic paresis of the lower limb. *Journal of Neurology, Neurosurgery & Psychiatry, 75*, 121–125.

5. The most important aspect of medical care for patients with illness anxiety disorder should be:

A. Avoiding iatrogenic harm
B. Fewer medical appointments
C. Referral to medical specialists
D. Elimination of physical symptoms
E. Gaining insight into the absence of a medical condition

ANSWER: A

The foremost goal of a medical provider in the management of illness anxiety disorder is to prevent iatrogenic harm by way of preventing excessive testing and unnecessary procedures on the basis of anxiety. Management of illness anxiety disorder typically involves regular, scheduled appointments independent of anxiety burden, which often *increases* the frequency of medical visits among those of the care-avoidant type. Mental health care is recommended *in addition to* ongoing medical care rather than wholesale transfer of a patient from a primary care provider to a psychiatrist. Illness anxiety disorder is characterized by little to no somatic symptoms, so elimination of physical symptoms is moot. Patients may be referred to specialists for indicated workup, but this is not the foremost goal in managing this condition. Preventing excessive referrals is important. Illness anxiety disorder can be diagnosed in the presence of a medical condition (e.g., illness anxiety disorder in a person with chronic obstructive pulmonary disease and heart disease).

REFERENCE

Braun, I. M., Greenberg, D. B., Smith, F. A., & Cassem, N. H. (2010). Functional somatic symptoms, deception syndromes, and somatoform disorders. In T. A. Stern, G. L. Fricchione, N. H. Cassem, M. S. Jellinek, J. F. Rosenbaum. (Eds.), (2010). *Massachusetts General Hospital handbook of general hospital psychiatry* (6th ed., p. 182). Philadelphia, PA: Saunders Elsevier.

6. A 39-year-old woman is brought to a neurologist by her partner with complaints of episodic difficulty speaking. She says that during these episodes her voice has a "strangled" sound to it but then resolves spontaneously. She describes also seeing "sharp kitchen knives" in her vision when she develops this dysphonia. Further evaluation reveals a history of childhood abuse. Brain MRI during one of these episodes reveals no significant abnormalities. Which of the following diagnoses is most likely?

A. Somatic symptom disorder
B. Charles Bonnet syndrome
C. Illness anxiety disorder
D. Conversion disorder
E. Multiple sclerosis

ANSWER: D

The presence of vivid visual hallucinations in a young to middle-aged woman is rare and should raise the suspicion for either a neurocognitive disorder or dissociation. Conversion disorder (functional neurological disorder), which is phenomenologically dissociative in nature, is the most likely diagnosis here. The association of dysphonia with these symptoms cannot be explain with a single strategic central nervous system lesion, and as expected the MRI is unrevealing. Additional features that support conversion disorder are the stereotyped nature of her visual hallucinations and the predictability of their co-occurrence with dysphonia. A history of childhood abuse also significantly increases the likelihood of conversion disorder. One might imagine how this abuse involved both mechanical strangulation and enforcement with knives.

REFERENCE

American Psychiatric Association. (2013). *Diagnostic and statistical manual of mental disorders* (5th ed., pp. 318–319). Arlington, VA: American Psychiatric Publishing.

7. Which personality trait has been consistently linked with somatic symptom disorder?

A. Conscientiousness
B. Agreeableness
C. Neuroticism
D. Openness to experience
E. Extraversion

ANSWER: C

High trait neuroticism, or negative affectivity, has been associated with development of distress with somatic presentation. The other traits have not.

REFERENCE

American Psychiatric Association. (2013). *Diagnostic and statistical manual of mental Disorders* (5th ed., p. 313). Arlington, VA: American Psychiatric Publishing.

Hamilton, J. C., Hedge, K. A., & Feldman, M. D. (2015). Excessive illness behavior. In B. S. Fogel & D. B. Greenberg (Eds.), *Psychiatric care of the medical patient* (3rd ed., p. 746). New York, NY: Oxford University Press.

8. The Rome III disorders and criteria represent the international diagnostic system for which of the following class of functional disorders?

A. Pain syndromes (such as fibromyalgia)
B. Sexual disorders (such as dyspareunia)
C. Neurological disorders (such as conversion disorder)
D. Exertion-related syndromes (such as chronic fatigue syndrome)
E. Gastrointestinal dysfunction (such as irritable bowel syndrome)

ANSWER: E

The Rome Foundation is an international organization that defines functional gastrointestinal disorders (FGIDs). The Rome IV criteria were published in 2016 as a two-volume book and will be available online in 2017. They include separate diagnostic criteria for adults and children. The six FGID adult categories are esophageal, gastroduodenal, bowel, functional abdominal pain syndrome, biliary, and anorectal. This nosology notably includes diagnostic criteria for irritable bowel syndrome, functional dyspepsia, globus, and cyclical vomiting syndrome.

REFERENCES

Creed, F. (2006). Gastrointestinal disease. In M. Blumenfield & J. Strain (Eds.), *Psychosomatic medicine* (p. 146). Philadelphia, PA: Lippincott Williams and Wilkins.

D. A. Drossman, L. Chang, W. D. Chey, J. Kellow, J. Tack, W. E. Whitehead, Rome IV Committees. (Eds), (2016). *ROME IV: Functional Gastroinestinal Disorders, Disorders of Gut-Brain Interaction.*

SECTION G: DISSOCIATIVE DISORDERS

1. Which criterion best describes the difference between dissociative amnesia and transient global amnesia?

A. Transient global amnesia occurs in association with cerebrovascular disease.
B. Both resolve quickly over a few hours without residual cognitive symptoms.
C. Dissociative amnesia is characteristically anterograde.
D. Stressful life events can precede either of them.
E. Both can present with depersonalization.

ANSWER: A

Transient global amnesia is mostly seen in those 50 years old or older with a history of vascular disease, migraine, or epilepsy, and it is due to transient disruption of posterior cerebral blood flow. It tends to last for seconds to minutes and resolves without sequelae. During episodes, personal identity is preserved, and the patient typically perseverates over the same question(s), frequently accompanied by an awareness of memory loss. Dissociative amnesia is more commonly retrograde, though it may be anterograde. It commonly presents with depersonalization, idealization, regression, and somatic conversion symptoms, *including* loss of personal memory. Onset is common in adolescence or early adulthood. Most cases are associated with trauma, and a family history of dissociation may be seen.

REFERENCE

Sadock, B., & Sadock, V. (2015). Dissociative disorders. In *Synopsis of psychiatry* (11th ed., pp. 452–453). Wolters Kluwer.

2. Which of the following is a good prognostic factor for dissociative amnesia?

A. Prolonged, intermittent episodes with resolution
B. Comorbid conversion symptoms
C. Amnesia with depersonalization
D. Early onset of episodes
E. Comorbid depression

ANSWER: E

Few follow-up studies on this condition exist due to small patient numbers. These studies vary in follow-up rates and intervals, definitions of recovery or favorable outcome, and nature of neuropsychological assessment. Dissociative amnesia exhibits great heterogeneity in outcome and prognosis. Some amnesias remit spontaneously or after treatment, others decrease in symptoms and severity, and still others show a chronic or even deteriorating course. Variables that independently predict prognosis in dissociative amnesia have not been systematically studied, but brevity of symptoms and comorbid depression appear to be good prognostic factors.

REFERENCE

Markowitsch, H., & Staniloiu, A. (2013). 1687—Social cognition in patients with dissociative amnesia. *European Psychiatry*

3. Which of the following is true regarding dissociative fugue?

A. It is more common in women.
B. It starts in adolescence.
C. All affected patients develop depersonalization during fugue.
D. The fugue could be a purposeful journey away from home.
E. Most of the fugues remain refractory over time.

ANSWER: D

Dissociative fugues are mostly brief, lasting hours to days. They occur more commonly in men, particularly those with a military background. At the termination of the fugue, patients may experience depersonalization, derealization, confusion, perplexity, and trancelike behavior. Fugues may represent purposeful travel away from the place of daily activities. Most individuals recover, and refractory persistent cases are rare.

REFERENCE

Sadock, B., & Sadock, V. (2015). Dissociative disorders. In *Synopsis of psychiatry* (11th ed., pp. 457–458). Wolters Kluwer.

4. Which of the following treatment methods has been used to treat dissociative fugue with partial success?

A. Interpersonal therapy focusing on current relations and how to stop wandering
B. Cognitive behavioral therapy focusing on automatic thoughts of being injured
C. Group therapy with peers
D. Supportive therapy with development of ego strength
E. Psychodynamic therapy to integrate the identity that participated in fugue

ANSWER: E

Dissociative fugue has been successfully treated with psychodynamic psychotherapy with a focus on retrieval of memory during the fugue. Individuals may develop another identity to deal with trauma, stress, conflicts, and overwhelming emotions. In those cases, the most desirable outcome is fusion of identities by working through and integrating the experiences and memories that occurred during the fugue.

REFERENCE

Sadock, B., & Sadock, V. (2015). Dissociative disorders. In *Synopsis of psychiatry* (11th ed., p. 458). Wolters Kluwer.

5. Which personality disorder is commonly associated with dissociative identity disorder?

A. Borderline personality disorder
B. Antisocial personality disorder
C. Obsessive–compulsive personality disorder
D. Histrionic personality disorder
E. Paranoid personality disorder

ANSWER: C

Obsessive–compulsive personality trait is common in dissociative identity disorder. Concurrent OCD symptoms are often found in this disorder, with a subgroup of severe OCD symptoms related to trauma-associated compulsions such as checking doors.

REFERENCE

Sadock, B., & Sadock, V. (2015). Dissociative disorders. In *Synopsis of psychiatry* (11th ed., p. 460). Wolters Kluwer.

6. A 28-year-old prison inmate was brought to the emergency room after he had been confused and disoriented for a day and a half. He complained of seeing small animals on the floor, which were not real. On evaluation he was disoriented to person and place. His pupils are equal, round, and reactive to light and accommodation. His blood alcohol level and urine toxicology screen are negative. Routine blood tests are within normal limits. During mental status evaluation, he was asked, "What is the capital of the United States?" and responded, "New York." No focal neurological signs are found, and electroencephalogram reveals normal awake tracings. What is the most probable diagnosis?

A. Delirium
B. Complex partial seizure
C. Ganser syndrome
D. Transient ischemic attack
E. Depersonalization syndrome

ANSWER: D

Ganser syndrome is seen mostly in males. *Vorbeigehen* (literally "passing over"), as in passing over the correct answer, is the hallmark of the disorder. This symptom is also called "approximate answers." Disorientation, amnesia, and confusion are often seen. Some impairment of reality testing might occur. Visual and auditory hallucinations occur in half of patients. Neurological examination may show shifting hyperalgesia. The above case is inconsistent with a vascular event such as a transient ischemic attack because this resolves within hours. Normal EEG effectively rules out delirium. Depersonalization syndrome is not characteristically described in the above case.

REFERENCE

Sadock, B., & Sadock, V. (2015). Dissociative disorders. In *Synopsis of psychiatry* (11th ed., pp. 463–464). Wolters Kluwer.

7. Which one of the following statements is true about dissociative identity disorder?

A. There is a 5:1 male predominance.
B. Each identity may have a different cardiovascular response to external stimuli.
C. Each personality is aware of the autobiographical memories of the others.
D. Most of the symptoms improve with a 12-step program for incest survivors.

ANSWER: B

Dissociative identity disorder (DID) is more common in females, with a ratio of 5:1. Personalities typically have partial or no autobiographical memory of events that occurred while another personality was dominant. Clinical evaluation has suggested variation in heart rate, blood pressure, and cerebral blood flow (measured by PET scan) to the same trauma script across different personalities in DID. Psychoanalytic, psychodynamic, insight-oriented, cognitive behavioral, and family therapies may be helpful in treatment. Characteristically, 12-step groups for incest survivors worsen the symptoms due to their lack of clinical safeguards and lack of integrative approach between different personalities.

REFERENCES

Bryant, R. (1995). Autobiographical memory across personalities in dissociative identity disorder: A case report. *Journal of Abnormal Psychology, 104*, 625–631.
Reinders, A., Nijenhuis, E., Quak, J., Korf, J., Haaksma, J., Paans, A., ... Boer, J. (2006). Psychobiological characteristics of dissociative identity disorder: A symptom provocation study. *Biological Psychiatry, 60*, 730–740.
Sadock, B., & Sadock, V. (2015). Dissociative disorders. In *Synopsis of psychiatry* (11th ed., pp. 458–462). Wolters Kluwer.

SECTION H: SEXUAL DISORDERS/PARAPHILIA

1. Erections during which phase of sleep can help differentiate primary erectile disorder from erectile disorder due to vascular disease?

A. Rapid eye movement (REM)
B. Non-REM 1 (N1)
C. Non-REM 2 (N2)
D. Non-REM 3 (N3)

ANSWER: A

Nocturnal penile tumescence (NPT) reliably occurs during rapid eye movement (REM) sleep, and an overnight evaluation would differentiate a primary, psychogenic cause of erectile disorder (ED), in which NPT should occur in REM, from ED due to vascular disease, in which NPT will be limited to absent. ED in men 40 years and older predicts heart disease later in life.

REFERENCES

Hirshkowitz, M., & Schmidt, M. H. (2005). Sleep-related erections: Clinical perspectives and neural mechanisms. *Sleep Medicine Reviews*., *9*, 311–329.

Sadock, V. A. (2012). Normal human sexuality and sexual and gender identity disorders: Normal human sexuality. In B. J. Sadock, V. A. Sadock, & P. Ruiz (Eds.), *Kaplan and Sadock's comprehensive textbook of psychiatry* (9th ed., p. 2048). Wolters Kluwer.

2. You recommend high-dose sertraline for a man to prevent future episodes of indecent exposure. Therapeutic effect is most likely to occur due to activity at which serotonin receptor?

A. 1A
B. 1D
C. 2A
D. 3
E. 7

ANSWER: C

All antidepressants that inhibit serotonin reuptake can cause sexual side effects, including decreased libido (the therapeutic effect intended here) and delayed or absent orgasm, and these effects are thought to be mediated by 5-HT-2A. SSRIs have been used to treat paraphilias as well as hypersexuality in neurocognitive disorders. Conversely, mirtazapine, which acts in part as a 2A antagonist, generally does not inhibit sexual function, though it certainly may lead to severe weight gain. Other antidepressants not expected to have significant sexual side effects include bupropion, buspirone, lamotrigine, liothyronine, and psychostimulants.

REFERENCES

Guay, D. R. (2009). Drug treatment of paraphilic and nonparaphilic sexual disorders. *Clinical Therapeutics, 31*, 1–31.

Stahl, S. M. (2000). *Essential psychopharmacology of depression and bipolar disorder* (pp. 126–127). New York, NY: Cambridge University Press.

3. According to the National Health and Social Life Survey, one of the most authoritative surveys on sex in the United States, which of the following is TRUE of both men and women who were sexually abused as children relative to those without childhood sexual abuse?

A. More likely to have had more than 10 partners
B. Less likely to engage in group sexual activities
C. More likely to identify as heterosexual
D. Less likely to identify as bisexual
E. Comparable life satisfaction

ANSWER: A

The effect of childhood sexual abuse (CSA) is deep and often pervasive. CSA is frequently associated with several other factors that may account for a portion of the adverse outcomes seen in those with CSA, but growing evidence supports the pathogenic role of CSA, particularly on sexual identity and sexual activity throughout life.

REFERENCE

Sadock, V. A. (2012). Normal human sexuality and sexual and gender identity disorders. In B. J. Sadock, V. A. Sadock, & P. Ruiz (Eds.), *Kaplan and Sadock's comprehensive textbook of psychiatry* (9th ed., pp. 2035–2036). Wolters Kluwer.

4. Which of the following is the central principle of dual-sex therapy as developed by Masters and Johnson?

A. Individual psychotherapy is discouraged.

B. One of the partners is given the sick role.
C. Historical sexual dysfunction is de-emphasized.
D. Behavioral interventions are the principal treatment.
E. Sexual dysfunction represents relational disharmony.

ANSWER: E

Dual-sex therapy incorporates both partners in a form of couples-based therapy. This type of therapy posits that sexual dysfunction exists in the context of a relationship and is the result of relational disharmony. The difficulty is found in the couple, *not* in either one in isolation. (The "sick role" is a component of a different type of therapy: interpersonal psychotherapy.) Each individual, however, is encouraged to be in independent mental health care. The therapist collects a sex history from each partner independently, and these are then discussed jointly. Emphasis is placed on relational dynamics, not on behavioral interventions.

REFERENCE

Sadock, V. A. (2012). Normal human sexuality and sexual and gender identity disorders: Normal human sexuality. In B. J. Sadock, V. A. Sadock, & P. Ruiz (Eds.), *Kaplan and Sadock's comprehensive textbook of psychiatry* (9th ed., p. 2054). Wolters Kluwer.

5. Although paraphilias are much more common in men than in women, which of the following has the highest prevalence in women?

A. Sexual sadism disorder
B. Frotteuristic disorder
C. Fetishistic disorder
D. Pedophilic disorder
E. Voyeuristic disorder

ANSWER: A

Sadism and masochism are two paraphilias with the greatest prevalence in women. Certain paraphilic disorders—notably pedophilia—are found all but exclusively in men.

REFERENCE

Sorrentino, R. M. (2012). Normal human sexuality and sexual and gender identity disorders: Paraphilias. In B. J. Sadock, V. A. Sadock, & P. Ruiz (Eds.), *Kaplan and Sadock's comprehensive textbook of psychiatry* (9th ed., p. 2091). Wolters Kluwer.

6. A 22-year-old man presents to a psychiatrist for help with an intense desire that he has difficulty communicating. He describes a recent arrest for having rubbed up against several women on a city bus. He discloses having had sexual fantasies since his teens of doing this but only recently began acting on them. What is the correct diagnosis?

A. Voyeuristic disorder
B. Exhibitionistic disorder
C. Fetishistic disorder
D. Frotteuristic disorder
E. Unspecified paraphilic disorder

ANSWER: D

From the French word *frottage* for "rubbing" or "friction," frotteurism involves deriving sexual pleasure from rubbing against others, typically strangers. The activity occurs most commonly in public places where there are large crowds in order to evade notice, such as on crowded buses or subways or at concerts.

REFERENCE

Sorrentino, R. M. (2012). Normal human sexuality and sexual and gender identity disorders: Paraphilias. In B. J. Sadock, V. A. Sadock, & P. Ruiz (Eds.), *Kaplan and Sadock's comprehensive textbook of psychiatry* (9th ed., pp. 2093–2094). Wolters Kluwer.

7. A man with schizophrenia returns to the clinic after starting risperidone a month ago and complains, "My sex drive is gone." Further questioning reveals that the patient has noticed "wet nipples," but he had attributed this to sweating. Which laboratory value should be obtained at this appointment?

A. Testosterone level
B. Follicular stimulating hormone
C. Luteinizing hormone
D. Prolactin
E. Oxytocin

ANSWER: D

Antipsychotics—notably risperidone among atypicals—can cause hyperprolactinemia due to their effects on the tuberoinfundibular dopamine pathway. Dopamine acts as a prolactin-inhibiting hormone due to its effects on the pituitary gland, so D2 receptor blockade can cause disinhibition of prolactin release. High levels of serum prolactin are associated with decreased libido, impaired sexual arousal, impaired orgasm, galactorrhea (milk production), and over time gynecomastia (breast enlargement).

REFERENCE

Baggaley, M. (2008). Sexual dysfunction in schizophrenia: Focus on recent evidence. *Human Psychopharmacology: Clinical and Experimental, 23*, 201–209.

8. You evaluate an 11-year-old girl who is dressed in dirt-stained overalls and a plaid shirt. Her mother is concerned that she "only plays with boys" and likes rough-and-tumble sports and fishing. You learn that the girl's twin sister wears dresses, keeps her hair long and braided, and enjoys playing with dolls. Because of the sisters' divergent interests, the two rarely play together. The girl's mother says she is concerned that "there might be something wrong with my daughter." When you ask the girl, she says, "I just like getting dirty. So what?" She readily identifies as a girl. What is the most appropriate diagnosis?

A. Intersexuality
B. Gender dysphoria
C. Transvestic fetishism
D. Gender identity disorder
E. Normal child development

ANSWER: E

It is not uncommon for girls to be interested in conventionally male activities (or vice versa), particularly during early development. Aspects of this case that suggest a diagnosis is not warranted include the child's lack of distress and her clear identification as a girl. The *DSM-IV-TR* diagnosis of gender identity disorder was changed in *DSM-5* to gender dysphoria to emphasize gender incongruence rather than cross-gender identification per se. Two sets of diagnostic criteria are described for gender dysphoria: one for children and another for adolescents/adults. DSM-5 allows for gender dysphoria in adolescents or adults to be specified as "post-transition" if the person is living as the desired gender and has undergone or is preparing to undergo at least one cross-sex procedure or treatment. Intersexuality refers to ambiguous primary and secondary sexual characteristics such as ambiguous genitalia and may be the result of genetic abnormalities (e.g., XO or Turner syndrome) or aberrant hormone exposure in utero. Transvestic fetishism is a paraphilia.

REFERENCE

Green, R. (2012). Normal human sexuality and sexual and gender identity disorders: Gender identity disorders. In B. J. Sadock, V. A Sadock, & P. Ruiz (Eds.), *Kaplan and Sadock's comprehensive textbook of psychiatry* (9th ed., pp. 2093–2094). Wolters Kluwer.

9. Which of the following is the official position of the American Psychiatric Association regarding therapeutic techniques aimed at changing a homosexual orientation?

A. They are indicated for select patients.
B. They deserve greater attention in ongoing research.
C. They are indicated as long as the therapist has appropriate training.
D. They should be offered to patients undergoing gender reassignment surgery.
E. They should be opposed for assuming that homosexual orientation should be changed.

ANSWER: E

Since *DSM-II*, the American Psychiatric Association (APA) has eliminated the diagnosis of homosexuality as a mental disorder, and since that time gender identity and sexual orientation have been areas of increasing attention by the APA. The current position states, "The American Psychiatric Association opposes any psychiatric treatment, such as 'reparative' or 'conversion' therapy, which is based upon the assumption that homosexuality per se is a mental disorder, or based upon a prior assumption that the patient should change his/her homosexual orientation."

REFERENCE

See https://web.archive.org/web/20110407082738/http://www.psych.org/Departments/EDU/Library/APAOfficialDocumentsandRelated/PositionStatements/200001.aspx.

SECTION I: EATING DISORDERS

1. Which of the following diagnostic criteria for anorexia nervosa has been eliminated in *DSM-5*?

A. Intense fear of gaining weight or of becoming fat, or persistent behavior that interferes with weight gain, even though at a significantly low weight

B. Restriction of energy intake relative to requirement, leading to a significantly low body weight in the context of age, sex, developmental trajectory, and physical health
C. Disturbance in the way in which one's body weight or shape is experienced, undue influence of body weight or shape on self-evaluation, or persistent lack of recognition of the seriousness of the current low body weight
D. Amenorrhea (i.e., the absence of at least three consecutive menstrual cycles) in postmenarcheal females

ANSWER: D

Whereas the main diagnostic criteria have not been changed during the transition from the *DSM-IV-TR* to *DSM-5*, the requirement of amenorrhea has been eliminated.

REFERENCE

American Psychiatric Association. (2013). Feeding and eating disorders. In *Diagnostic and statistical manual of mental disorders* (5th ed., pp. 338–339). Arlington, VA: American Psychiatric Publishing.

2. A 36-year-old white female presented to the outpatient clinic with depressed mood, lack of interest in fun activities, and poor sleep. She reports discrete periods of time when she eats uncontrollably with a lack of control for the past 6 months. She often feels embarrassed and guilty after these episodes. She adds that she is somewhat concerned about her body weight, but her body mass index (BMI) is within normal limits for her height. She likes taking long walks in the evening, but she does not change the intensity of her exercise based on these episodes of excessive eating. What is the most likely disorder?

A. Other specified eating disorder
B. Bulimia nervosa
C. Anorexia nervosa
D. Binge eating disorder
E. Orthorexia

ANSWER: D

The patient meets the criteria for binge eating disorder: she has recurrent binges characterized by lack of self-control and guilt following these episodes. Her presentation meets the duration requirement of at least 3 months of symptoms. Although the patient expresses some concern about her weight, she maintains a normal BMI, ruling out anorexia nervosa. Patients with bulimia nervosa have recurrent binges with compensatory behaviors, which are not described in this vignette.

REFERENCE

American Psychiatric Association. (2013). Feeding and eating disorders. In *Diagnostic and statistical manual of mental disorders* (5th ed., pp. 350–351). Arlington, VA: American Psychiatric Publishing.

3. Which of the following medications is approved by the FDA for the treatment of bulimia nervosa?

A. Lisdexamfetamine
B. Fluoxetine
C. Sertraline
D. Bupropion
E. Lorcaserin

ANSWER: B

The only FDA-approved drug for the treatment of bulimia nervosa is fluoxetine. In addition to reducing binging and purging episodes, fluoxetine might also be useful for the treatment of co-occurring depression and anxiety disorders. Lisdexamfetamine was approved for moderate to severe binge eating disorder in 2015. The other medications are not indicated for the management of eating disorders.

REFERENCE

National Institutes of Health. (2016). Eating disorders. Retrieved October 23, 2015, from http://www.nimh.nih.gov/health/topics/eating-disorders/index.shtml
US Food and Drug Administration. (2015). FDA expands uses of Vyvanse to treat binge-eating disorder. Retrieved October 23, 2015, from http://www.fda.gov/NewsEvents/Newsroom/PressAnnouncements/ucm432543.htm

4. A 4-month-old boy was brought to a pediatrician for not ingesting "enough" milk and being underweight for his age. He was placed on nutrition in addition to breastfeeding to address the low milk intake. The child is distressed and vomits when feeding on these supplements. What is the next step in evaluating this child?

A. Educate the parents about the temperamental traits of a child

B. Propose a transactional model of intervention
C. Recommend evaluation for functional or structural GI disorder
D. Consider hospital admission for nutritional supplementation

ANSWER: C

The case describes an example of avoidant/restrictive food intake disorder (*DSM-5*) that is an extension of feeding disorder of infancy or early childhood (*DSM-IV*). The main diagnostic feature of this disorder is avoiding or restricting food intake, leading to clinically significant failure to meet nutritional requirements. Additional features present in this case are inability to gain age-appropriate weight and need for additional nutritional supplementation. Educating the parents using a transactional model (choices A and B) has proved effective in treating children who exhibit difficult temperamental traits, but it is not the appropriate next step. Given the history of vomiting, it will be valuable to recommend medical evaluation to rule out swallowing pathology before venturing into psychotherapeutic techniques.

REFERENCES

American Psychiatric Association. (2013). Feeding and eating disorders. In *Diagnostic and statistical manual of mental disorders* (5th ed., p. 334). Arlington, VA: American Psychiatric Publishing.

Sadock, B., & Ruiz, P. (2015). Feeding and eating disorders of infancy and early childhood. In *Kaplan and Sadock's synopsis of psychiatry: Behavioral sciences, clinical psychiatry* (11th ed., internet. ed., p. 1210). Philadelphia, PA: Wolters Kluwer.

5. A 30-year-old woman comes to your clinic with recurrent binge eating episodes for the past month, with a sense of lack of control during these episodes. On the days following her binge eating she runs 6 to 7 miles to compensate for the calorie intake. These episodes happen at least two or three times a week. Although she is able to maintain her weight, she still feels fat. What is your diagnosis for this patient?

A. Bulimia nervosa
B. Anorexia nervosa
C. Other specified feeding or eating disorder
D. Unspecified feeding or eating disorder

ANSWER: C

The patient meets all the criteria required for the diagnosis of bulimia nervosa (choice A) except that she has been experiencing these symptoms for only a month. Per *DSM-5*, a diagnosis of bulimia nervosa requires 3 months of symptoms. In instances like these, the diagnosis of other specified feeding or eating disorder (choice C) could be given by mentioning the reason for not giving a diagnosis of bulimia nervosa ("1 month of symptoms"). When there are insufficient data to diagnose a specific eating disorder, a diagnosis of unspecified feeding or eating disorder can be given.

REFERENCE

American Psychiatric Association. (2013). Feeding and eating disorders. In *Diagnostic and statistical manual of mental disorders* (5th ed., pp. 350, 353, 354). Arlington, VA: American Psychiatric Publishing.

6. The *DSM-5* recommends patients below what age should not generally be given the diagnosis of pica?

A. 6 months
B. 1 year
C. 2 years
D. 3 years
E. 5 years

ANSWER: C

Pica is characterized by persistent eating of nonnutritive substances and can lead to medical problems such as intestinal infection, intestinal obstructions, or lead poisoning. Pica can be diagnosed in children, adolescents, and adults; however, to rule out developmentally appropriate mouthing of objects, a minimum age of 2 years is required for the diagnosis.

REFERENCE

Sadock, B., & Ruiz, P. (2015). Feeding and eating disorders of infancy and early childhood. In *Kaplan and Sadock's synopsis of psychiatry: Behavioral sciences, clinical psychiatry* (11th ed., internet. ed., p. 1206). Philadelphia, PA: Wolters Kluwer.

7. Which of the following laboratory or clinical abnormalities can be found in patients with anorexia nervosa?

A. ST segment and T-wave changes in ECG
B. High serum cholesterol
C. Mild hypothyroidism
D. All of the above

ANSWER: D

Patients with anorexia nervosa (especially those with purging type) commonly have electrolyte imbalances that can lead to ST segment and T-wave changes in ECG. They may also have high serum cholesterol and mild hypothyroidism.

REFERENCE

Sadock, B., & Ruiz, P. (2015). Feeding and eating disorder. In *Kaplan and Sadock's synopsis of psychiatry: Behavioral sciences, clinical psychiatry* (11th ed., internet. ed., p. 513). Philadelphia, PA: Wolters Kluwer.

8. Which eating disorder may be complicated by bezoar, toxoplasmosis, intestinal perforation, or lead intoxication?

A. Trichotillomania
B. Binge eating disorder
C. Pica
D. Rumination disorder
E. Diabulimia

ANSWER: C

Pica involves the eating of nonnutritive, nonfood substances, and it may be complicated by bezoar (a concretion forming in the stomach, as opposed to trichobezoars [informally "hairballs"] seen with hair ingestion often in association with trichotillomania), toxoplasmosis due to ingesting feces or dirt, perforation due to ingestion of sharp or hard objects, or lead intoxication from eating lead-paint chips. Binge eating disorder may rarely present with intestinal perforation. Rumination disorder often presents with malnutrition, and *diabulimia* is an informal term describing patients with insulin-dependent diabetes and bulimia nervosa. These patients underadminister insulin to prevent weight gain but may suffer many complications due to acute and chronic hyperglycemia.

SECTION J: PERSONALITY DISORDERS

1. Which of the following statement is/are TRUE about personality disorders?

A. About 10% to 20% of the general population has a personality disorder.
B. Half of those with psychiatric disorders have a personality disorder.
C. Symptoms of personality disorders are alloplastic.
D. Symptoms of personality disorder are ego-syntonic.
E. All of the above are true.

ANSWER: E

Personality disorders are chronic disorders that tend to be ego-syntonic (i.e., the patient perceives the personality to be acceptable). Given the ego-syntonic nature of the symptoms, patients with personality disorders typically do not seek help except when they realize their personality creates recurrent conflict with others. More commonly, they seek to alter the environment in which they live to adapt it to themselves (alloplastic adaptation). About 10% to 20% of the general population is considered to have a personality disorder. The prevalence of personality disorders is about 50% among patients with psychiatric disorders.

REFERENCE

Sadock, B., & Ruiz, P. (2015). Personality disorders. In *Kaplan and Sadock's synopsis of psychiatry: Behavioral sciences, clinical psychiatry* (11th ed., internet ed., p. 742). Philadelphia, PA: Wolters Kluwer.

2. Which of the following personality disorders is most prevalent among relatives of patients diagnosed with schizophrenia?

A. Schizoid personality disorder
B. Schizotypal personality disorder
C. Paranoid personality disorder
D. Narcissistic personality disorder

ANSWER: B

Schizotypal personality disorder, which is characterized by odd and peculiar thinking and behavior, is more common among first-degree relatives of patients with schizophrenia. Alternatively, there is an increase in prevalence of schizophrenia and other psychotic disorders among relatives of patients with schizotypal personality disorder. Several endophenotypes such as impairment in smooth pursuit eye movement or prepulse inhibition provide further evidence of the biological link between schizophrenia and schizotypal personality.

REFERENCE

American Psychiatric Association. (2013). Personality disorders. In *Diagnostic and statistical manual of mental disorders* (5th ed., pp. 656–657). Arlington, VA: American Psychiatric Publishing.

3. Which of the following associations between a personality disorder and a comorbid psychiatric disorder is NOT correct?

A. Antisocial personality disorder: alcohol use disorder
B. Histrionic personality disorder: somatic symptom disorder
C. Avoidant personality disorder: generalized anxiety disorder
D. Narcissistic personality disorder: bipolar II disorder

ANSWER: D

Antisocial personality disorder is highly comorbid with substance use disorders. In fact, antisocial personality disorder is present in 70% of patients with alcohol use disorder; compare that with the 75% prevalence among prison populations. Somatic symptom disorder is sometimes comorbid in patients with histrionic personality disorder. Patients with avoidant personality disorder are prone to having generalized anxiety, which should be treated in these patients. There is no known association between narcissistic personality disorder and bipolar II disorder.

REFERENCE

Sadock, B., & Ruiz, P. (2015). Personality disorders. In *Kaplan and Sadock's synopsis of psychiatry: Behavioral sciences, clinical psychiatry* (11th ed., internat. ed., pp. 748,752, 754). Philadelphia, PA: Wolters Kluwer.

4. A 23-year-old man with paranoid personality disorder sees you in a clinic for long-term psychodynamic psychotherapy. You are late for one of the appointments by 5 minutes. The patient becomes visibly angry and accuses you of being unprofessional. What will be a reasonable response to this patient?

A. Have I ever been late before?
B. I couldn't help it; I was stuck in traffic.
C. You've been late for several of your sessions. This is my first time being late.
D. I apologize for being late. I had an unexpected emergency I had to attend to.

ANSWER: D

While working with patients with paranoid personality disorder, being honest and straightforward when met with inconsistencies or faults is essential. Being defensive (as in choices A, B, and C) can be interpreted as hostility and can lead to a rupture in the therapeutic relationship.

REFERENCE

Sadock, B., & Ruiz, P. (2015). Personality disorders. In *Kaplan and Sadock's synopsis of psychiatry: Behavioral sciences, clinical psychiatry* (11th ed., internet ed., p. 745). Philadelphia, PA: Wolters Kluwer.

5. Mr. D is a 45-year-old single male who works as a nighttime museum guard and enjoys fishing at the lake near his house. Other than attending family gatherings every summer, he socializes little and has few friends. On the night that he does not work, he goes stargazing and maintains a blog related to finding the best places to spot the aurora borealis. What personality disorder is most likely in this patient?

A. Avoidant personality disorder
B. Antisocial personality disorder
C. Schizoid personality disorder
D. Schizotypal personality disorder
E. Paranoid personality disorder

ANSWER: C

Patients with schizoid personality disorder prefer solitary work over work involving interaction with other people. They do not feel the need to have emotional ties, a key difference with those who have avoidant personality disorder, who long to have close relationships and to be involved in group activities. A key difference between patients with schizoid and schizotypal personality disorder is the lack of odd behavior, perceptions, and thought disorders in schizoid personality. Patients with schizotypal personality resemble more closely patients with schizophrenia than do patients with schizoid personality disorder.

REFERENCE

Sadock, B., & Ruiz, P. (2015). Personality disorders. In *Kaplan and Sadock's synopsis of psychiatry: Behavioral sciences, clinical psychiatry* (11th ed., internat. ed., pp. 746–747) Philadelphia, PA: Wolters Kluwer.

6. Which of the following therapies is effective for impulsive behaviors in borderline personality disorder?

A. Short-term psychodynamic therapy
B. Dialectical behavior therapy
C. Cognitive behavior therapy
D. Transference-based therapy
E. Exposure therapy

ANSWER: B

Dialectical behavior therapy is effective for impulsive behaviors in borderline personality disorder, including self-injurious behaviors and so-called parasuicidal gestures.

REFERENCE

Sadock, B., & Ruiz, P. (2015). Personality disorders. In *Kaplan and Sadock's synopsis of psychiatry: Behavioral sciences, clinical psychiatry* (11th ed., internat. ed., p. 751). Philadelphia, PA: Wolters Kluwer.

7. Which of the following personality disorders has a higher prevalence in males?

A. Histrionic personality disorder
B. Borderline personality disorder
C. Antisocial personality disorder
D. Schizoid personality disorder
E. Both C and D

ANSWER: E

Both antisocial and schizoid personality disorders are more prevalent in males, whereas the other choices are more prevalent in females.

REFERENCE

Sadock, B., & Ruiz, P. (2015). Personality disorders. In *Kaplan and Sadock's synopsis of psychiatry: Behavioral sciences, clinical psychiatry* (11th ed., internet ed., pp. 746–750). Philadelphia, PA: Wolters Kluwer.

8. A 45-year-old female presents to the clinic with symptoms of anxiety. She reports that she has always liked to be by herself and was not active in activities involving social gathering. Despite wanting to be close with people, she fears that she will be rejected if she tries to form friendships. What is her most likely personality disorder?

A. Dependent personality disorder
B. Avoidant personality disorder
C. Obsessive–compulsive personality disorder
D. Counterdependent personality disorder
E. Antisocial personality disorder

ANSWER: B

Patients with avoidant personality disorder desire to be in relationships and have social interaction but avoid these interactions for fear of being rejected. This is in contrast to persons with schizoid personality disorder, who prefer to be by themselves and do not express any interest in forming relationships.

REFERENCE

Sadock, B., & Ruiz, P. (2015). Personality disorders. In *Kaplan and Sadock's synopsis of psychiatry: Behavioral sciences, clinical psychiatry* (11th ed., internat. ed., pp. 746–753). Philadelphia, PA: Wolters Kluwer.

SECTION K: OTHER CONDITIONS THAT MAY BE A FOCUS OF CLINICAL ATTENTION

1. A 65-year-old woman with no prior psychiatric history was brought to the emergency room by her children over a concern that she was "not taking care of herself." She had been in bed virtually the entire time over the past 3 weeks since her husband's death the month prior. On evaluation, she is dehydrated, anergic, gloomy, and preoccupied with thoughts of her own death. She is convinced her "life is over" and is unable to entertain any reasonable hope for herself in the future. What is the appropriate diagnosis?

A. Major depressive disorder, single episode, severe with psychotic features
B. Adjustment disorder, with depressed mood
C. Dysthymic disorder
D. Uncomplicated bereavement
E. Persistent complex bereavement disorder

ANSWER: A

The appropriate diagnosis is severe major depression with psychosis (here, nihilistic delusions). This question differentiates between bereavement and major depression. This woman has depression accompanied by prominent neurovegetative features. Her conviction that her life is over combined with dense hopelessness bespeak of nihilism—a common delusional feature often overlooked in the diagnosis of major depression. Persistent complex bereavement disorder is a proposed diagnosis in *DSM-5* that requires that symptoms of bereavement persist for at least a year in adults (6 months in children). One of the more publicized and contested changes in *DSM-5* was elimination of the "bereavement exclusion." A series of reviews and studies challenged the validity of this exclusion, ultimately laying the groundwork for eliminating this exclusion in *DSM-5*. *DSM-5* offers a detailed footnote describing the distinction between major depression and bereavement.

REFERENCES

American Psychiatric Association. (2013). *Diagnostic and statistical manual of mental disorders* (5th ed., p. 161). Arlington, VA: American Psychiatric Publishing.

Iglewicz, A., Seay, K., Zetumer, S. D., & Zisook, S. (2013). The removal of the bereavement exclusion in the *DSM-5*: Exploring the evidence. *Current Psychiatry Reports, 15*, 413.

Zisook, S., & Kendler, K. S. (2007). Is bereavement-related depression different than non-bereavement-related depression? *Psychological Medicine, 37*, 779–794.

2. A woman is brought from her surprise 75th birthday party to the hospital by ambulance with a presentation that includes new ST segment elevation concerning for acute coronary syndrome. An urgent coronary angiogram reveals no significant coronary atherosclerosis, but anterior wall hypokinesis with apical involvement is appreciated. She is diagnosed with apical ballooning syndrome. What psychiatric diagnosis is most likely appropriate?

A. Panic disorder
B. Acute stress disorder
C. Somatic symptom disorder
D. Adjustment disorder with anxiety
E. Psychological factor affecting other medical condition

ANSWER: E

The vignette presents a prototypical presentation for what may be more commonly called *tako-tsubo* (Japanese for "octopus pot," which the ballooning cardiac apex in this condition resembles) cardiomyopathy or, colloquially, "broken heart syndrome." The condition occurs after a psychological stressor and may even occur after a positive event such as a surprise party. The diagnosis of psychological factors affecting other medical conditions, which was moved into the somatic symptom and related disorders section in *DSM-5*, would be most appropriate because there is a medical condition present, and the psychological stress of the party served as the direct psychophysiological precipitant of this condition.

REFERENCES

American Psychiatric Association. (2013). *Diagnostic and statistical manual of mental disorders* (5th ed., p. 322). Arlington, VA: American Psychiatric Publishing.

Prasad, A., Lerman, A., & Rihal, C. S. (2008). Apical ballooning syndrome (Tako-Tsubo or stress cardiomyopathy): A mimic of acute myocardial infarction. *American Heart Journal, 155*, 408–417.

SECTION L: MENTAL DISORDERS DUE TO A GENERAL MEDICAL CONDITION

1. You are performing an outpatient intake a 26-year-old male military veteran with a chief complaint of "angry outbursts" for the past year. He describes how he had been a "laid-back person" before his service in the armed forces, but since he has returned home from the Middle East, he has had a hot temper and is often very irritable. He denies anhedonia, significant change in sleep, or suicidal thoughts. He denies intrusion symptoms or avoidance. He returned stateside after his convoy was hit by a roadside bomb. He has no recollection of the event and no memory for the month after the incident. On review of systems he says that "food doesn't taste the same" since this event. What is the most likely diagnosis?

A. Bipolar II disorder
B. Acute stress disorder
C. Post-traumatic stress disorder, chronic
D. Adjustment disorder with disturbance of conduct
E. Personality change due to traumatic brain injury, aggressive type

2. What brain region is most likely damaged?

A. Ventromedial prefrontal cortex

B. Dorsolateral prefrontal cortex
C. Orbitofrontal cortex
D. Raphe nuclei
E. Hippocampus

QUESTION 1 ANSWER: E.

This veteran describes personality change after experiencing a blast injury, which is a type of traumatic brain injury. In this case, the most prominent feature is affective dysregulation. Olfactory loss is commonly seen in patients with diffuse axonal injury, likely due to the shear force on olfactory bulbs and tracts during the concussive force (Schofield, Moore, & Gardner, 2014). This often presents as food tasting blander because olfaction plays a large role in taste. There is no evidence from the vignette that the patient has behavioral indiscretion. In the absence of re-experiencing symptoms, a diagnosis of post-traumatic stress disorder (PTSD) is inappropriate. In fact, individuals who have lost consciousness may have a reduced likelihood of developing PTSD after a trauma because they have limited if any encoding of traumatic material. The temporal association of the injury with a month of post-traumatic amnesia, duration of symptoms, and presence of taste change all favor a diagnosis of personality change over bipolar II disorder.

REFERENCES

American Psychiatric Association. (2013). *Diagnostic and statistical manual of mental disorders* (5th ed., p. 682). Arlington, VA: American Psychiatric Publishing.

Schofield, P. W., Moore, T. M., & Gardner, A. (2014). Traumatic brain injury and olfaction: A systematic review. *Frontiers in Neurology.*, 5(5), 1–22.

QUESTION 2 ANSWER: C.

Traumatic brain injury (TBI) that involves rapid acceleration/deceleration traditionally causes significant torque around the brainstem, leading to rotation of the neuraxis and ultimately direct trauma of the orbitofrontal cortices due to mechanical trauma against bony prominences beneath them. This patient presents with emotional disinhibition, characteristic of orbitofrontal injury, as when Phineas Gage endured a traumatic incident with a tamping iron. TBI traditionally involves frontal and anterior temporal pole damage. Ventromedial damage typically presents as anergia, abulia, and poor self-awareness. Injury to the dorsolateral prefrontal cortex causes dysexecutive syndrome, consisting of impaired sequencing, organizing, abstraction, and planning. Raphe nuclei are not traditionally implicated in TBI, and hippocampal damage is associated with poor registration.

REFERENCE

Silver, J. M., Yudofsky, S. C., & Anderson, K. E. (2011). Aggressive disorders. In J. M. Silver, T. W. McAllister, & S. C. Yudofsky (Eds.), *Textbook of traumatic brain injury* (2nd ed., p. 22). Arlington, VA: American Psychiatric Association Publishing.

3. While evaluating a patient for elevated mood over the week leading up to your current evaluation, you discover that the patient was started on high-dose prednisone 2 weeks prior. The patient speaks in humorous voices and borders on being silly. Family members confirm that the patient has had increased self-confidence and self-importance, but they have no safety concerns. In addition to considering a medication for acute mood stabilization and close psychiatric follow-up, which of the following is also indicated?

A. Recommend the lowest prednisone dose feasible.
B. Recommend discontinuation of prednisone.
C. Admit the patient to a psychiatric hospital.
D. Provide a diagnosis of bipolar II disorder.
E. Refer the patient to cognitive behavioral therapy.

ANSWER: A

The propensity of corticosteroids to cause psychiatric symptoms, often mood elevation and psychosis, is dose dependent. Early work by the Boston Collaborative Drug Surveillance Program found that psychiatric features occurred in 1.3% of those on 40 mg/day or less of prednisone, in 4.6% of those receiving 41 to 80 mg/day, and in 18.4% of those on more than 80 mg/day. Investigating whether a lower dose is feasible for the patient's medical condition, then, is appropriate. Abrupt discontinuation should not be recommended without collaboration with the treating medical provider. No indication for psychiatric admission is presented in the vignette. Bipolar II disorder should not be given because (A) one cannot be confident of a primary mood episode in this patient with recent start of prednisone, and (B) a diagnosis of bipolar II requires a history of major depressive episode. Cognitive behavioral therapy would not be first-line treatment for short-term prednisone-induced mood elevation.

REFERENCES

Boston Collaborative Drug Surveillance Program. (1972). Acute adverse reactions to prednisone in relation to dosage. *Clinical Pharmacology & Therapeutics, 13*, 694–698.

Warrington, T. P., & Bostwick, J. M. (2006). Psychiatric adverse effects of corticosteroids. *Mayo Clinic Proceedings, 81*, 1361–1367.

QUESTIONS AND ANSWERS

This chapter has accompanying questions and answers which are available to subscribers as part of the Oxford eLearning platform. To access the questions, follow the link below, or go to http://oxford-elearning.oup.com/books.

http://oxford-elearning.oup.com/books/test/67/10.1093/med/9780190265557.003.0005

6.

TREATMENT OF PSYCHIATRIC DISORDERS

Neha Gupta

1. Abrupt withdrawal of which of the following medications can cause headaches, dizziness, myalgia, rhinorrhea, diarrhea, chills, agitation, irritability, and crying spells?

A. Haloperidol
B. Atomoxetine
C. Olanzapine
D. Citalopram
E. Lithium

ANSWER: D

Abrupt withdrawal of SSRIs like citalopram can lead to withdrawal symptoms. Signs and symptoms of sudden withdrawal of SSRI include feelings of disequilibrium such as dizziness and vertigo; flu-like symptoms; gastrointestinal disturbances; sensory disturbances such as paresthesias and electrical shock sensation; and sleep disturbances such as insomnia, fragmented sleep, and vivid and frightening dreams. Psychological symptoms can also occur, including agitation, irritability, anxiety, and crying episodes. An acronym for SSRI discontinuation symptoms is FINISH, for flu-like symptoms, insomnia, nausea, imbalance, sensory disturbances, and hyperarousal.

REFERENCE

Fava, M., Rosenbaum, J., Stern, T., & Wilens, T. (Eds.). (2016). *Massachusetts General Hospital comprehensive clinical psychiatry* (2nd ed., p. 569). New York, NY: Elsevier.

2. A 24-year-old woman with an eating disorder that involves purging was recently diagnosed with major depressive disorder. The patient would like to be started on a psychotropic medication for depression. Which medication is contraindicated in this patient?

A. Fluoxetine
B. Venlafaxine
C. Fluvoxamine
D. Escitalopram
E. Bupropion

ANSWER: E

Bupropion has an increased risk for seizures and should not be used in those with a seizure disorder or those with an increased risk for seizures such as eating disorders, head trauma, or alcohol abuse. The risk of seizure with the immediate-release preparation is 0.1% at doses of less than 300 mg/day and 0.4% at doses from 300 to 400 mg/day. The risk for seizures may be lower with longer acting formulations, but in general the guidelines recommend keeping the total daily dose at or below 450 mg/day.

REFERENCE

Fava, M., Rosenbaum, J., Stern, T., & Wilens, T. (Eds.). (2016). *Massachusetts General Hospital comprehensive clinical psychiatry* (2nd ed., pp. 571). New York, NY: Elsevier.

3. Which of the following is the only SSRI without an indication in the United States for depression?

A. Fluvoxamine
B. Paroxetine
C. Fluoxetine
D. Sertraline
E. Citalopram

ANSWER: A

Fluvoxamine in the only SSRI not approved by the FDA for the treatment of depression in United States; it is approved only for obsessive–compulsive disorder. However, several clinical trials have demonstrated efficacy of fluvoxamine in major depressive disorder. Notably, it has the shortest half-life among the SSRIs approved in the United States and is the worst tolerated among them.

REFERENCE

Fava, M., Rosenbaum, J., Stern, T., & Wilens, T. (Eds.). (2016). *Massachusetts General Hospital comprehensive clinical psychiatry* (2nd ed., pp. 494–496). New York, NY: Elsevier.

4. Which of the following diagnostic tests should be performed before starting a Tricyclic Antidepressant (TCA) in a healthy adult?

A. EEG
B. EKG
C. Chest X-ray
D. Echocardiogram
E. Lung function test

ANSWER: B

TCAs inhibit the fast sodium channels, resulting in electrocardiographic changes in those at risk such as post–myocardial infarction patients or those with bifascicular heart block, left bundle branch block, or a prolonged QT interval. TCA overdose can cause third-degree heart block due to its class IA antiarrhythmic properties. The EKG changes can be seen at therapeutic dosages, and therefore TCAs should generally be avoided in such patients. Furthermore, due to the inhibition of sodium channels and cholinergic receptors, TCAs also increase the risk for seizures.

REFERENCE

Fava, M., Rosenbaum, J., Stern, T., & Wilens, T. (Eds.). (2016). *Massachusetts General Hospital comprehensive clinical psychiatry* (2nd ed., pp. 500–502). New York, NY: Elsevier.

5. How often should kidney and thyroid tests be checked in a patient who is started on lithium for Bipolar Disorder?

A. Only once before starting lithium
B. One week after starting lithium
C. Before starting lithium and then 1 year after starting lithium
D. Before starting, then 3 months, 6 months, and then every 6 to 12 months after starting lithium
E. Before starting lithium and then every 3 months until discontinuation

ANSWER: D

These tests should be done before starting lithium, then 3 months, 6 months, and then every 6 to 12 months after starting lithium. Laboratory assessments for lithium therapy include a baseline pregnancy test, electrocardiogram (in patients over the age of 40), renal function tests (blood urea nitrogen, serum creatinine, and electrolytes), and thyroid function tests (TSH), with re-evaluation of renal and thyroid indices at 3 and 6 months and then every 6 to 12 months and as clinically indicated. Lithium serum levels are usually assessed when the medication is at steady state, which is approximately 5 days after a dose change and then as clinically indicated. More frequent monitoring is needed in those with medical issues and those with abnormal lithium levels.

REFERENCE

Hales, R. E., Yudofsky, S. C., & Roberts, L. W. (Eds.). (2014). *The American Psychiatric Publishing textbook of psychiatry* (6th ed., p. 335). Washington, DC: American Psychiatric Publishing.

6. Which of the following medications is FDA approved for bipolar depression?

A. Olanzapine/fluoxetine combination
B. Aripiprazole
C. Lamotrigine
D. Divalproex
E. Lithium

ANSWER: A

The three medications approved by the FDA for bipolar depression are olanzapine/fluoxetine combination (2003), quetiapine (2006), and lurasidone (2013). Aripiprazole has been approved for bipolar acute mania and maintenance, lamotrigine has been approved for bipolar maintenance, divalproex has been approved for bipolar acute mania, and lithium has been approved for bipolar acute mania and maintenance.

REFERENCE

Hales, R. E., Yudofsky, S. C., & Roberts, L. W. (Eds.). (2014). *The American Psychiatric Publishing textbook of psychiatry* (6th ed., p. 334). Washington, DC: American Psychiatric Publishing.

7. Which of the following medications is FDA approved for panic disorder?

A. Bupropion
B. Fluoxetine
C. Duloxetine
D. Venlafaxine
E. Escitalopram

ANSWER: D

In 2005, venlafaxine received FDA approval for the treatment of panic disorder. Venlafaxine Extended Release has been shown to be effective for panic attacks at doses from 75 to 225 mg/day. Venlafaxine is the only SNRI that is FDA approved for panic disorder. Bupropion has not been shown to be an effective agent for the treatment of panic episodes and may be anxiogenic in some individuals. Of the SSRIs, paroxetine and sertraline are the only ones approved by the FDA for panic disorder.

REFERENCE

Schatzberg, A. F., & DeBattista, C. (2015). *Manual of clinical psychopharmacology* (8th ed., pp. 431–432). Washington, DC: American Psychiatric Publishing.

8. A 22-year-old man has been prescribed diazepam 15 mg four times a day for the past year for generalized anxiety disorder. The patient runs out of his current prescription and decides not to refill it because he no longer wishes to continue with the medication. The patient is in danger of developing seizures how long after discontinuation?

A. 1 to 2 hours
B. 8 to 12 hours
C. 1 to 2 days
D. 2 to 4 days
E. More than 5 days

ANSWER: E

Discontinuation of a benzodiazepine can result in debilitating withdrawal symptoms. Common symptoms of benzodiazepine withdrawal include anxiety, sweating, nausea, altered mental status, and increased sensitivity to light and sound. Seizures are the most dangerous of the withdrawal symptoms, though they are rare. Seizures after discontinuation of diazepam are rare given the long half-life of its metabolite nordiazepam (also known as desmethyldiazepam; half-life of 75 to 200 hours), but if present they would be very unlikely to occur within 5 days of discontinuation. With shorter acting benzodiazepines such as lorazepam and alprazolam, seizures can be seen within 2 to 3 days. Any sign of withdrawal should be taken seriously, and special precautions should be taken when considering either restarting or tapering benzodiazepines.

REFERENCE

Schatzberg, A. F., & DeBattista, C. (2015). *Manual of clinical psychopharmacology* (8th ed., p. 428). Washington, DC: American Psychiatric Publishing.

9. What was the first second-generation antipsychotic approved for the treatment of acute mania?

A. Ziprasidone
B. Risperidone
C. Olanzapine
D. Aripiprazole
E. Quetiapine

ANSWER: C

Olanzapine was the first second-generation antipsychotic approved for the treatment of acute mania. After lithium and lamotrigine, it was the third drug to show benefit in the prevention of mania and depression in patients with bipolar I disorder. Also, olanzapine in combination with fluoxetine became the first drug approved for the treatment of bipolar depression. The intramuscular form of olanzapine has been approved for the acute treatment of agitation in patients with schizophrenia and bipolar disorder.

REFERENCE

Schatzberg, A. F., & DeBattista, C. (2015). *Manual of clinical psychopharmacology* (8th ed., p. 241). Washington, DC: American Psychiatric Publishing.

10. Which of the following antipsychotics has been FDA approved to treat recurrent suicidal behavior in patients with schizophrenia or schizoaffective disorder?

A. Olanzapine
B. Quetiapine
C. Aripiprazole
D. Clozapine
E. Haloperidol

ANSWER: D

Clozapine has been FDA approved for the treatment of recurrent suicidal behavior in patients with schizophrenia or schizoaffective disorder. Although other second-generation antipsychotics, such as olanzapine, have also been shown to decrease suicidal behavior, clozapine appears to be the most effective. Clozapine is more efficacious overall than any of the other second-generation antipsychotics in reducing impulsive aggression, which in turn reduces symptoms of self-aggression, self-mutilation, and suicide attempts. Because of its side effect profile, clozapine is typically not used as a first- or second-line medication. However, there have been multiple cases where clozapine was effectively used to reduce self-destructive behavior in schizophrenia, bipolar disorder, and borderline personality disorder. By way of parallel, lithium can decrease suicidality in bipolar disorder.

REFERENCE

Schatzberg, A. F., & DeBattista, C. (2015). *Manual of clinical psychopharmacology* (8th ed., p. 226). Washington, DC: American Psychiatric Publishing.

11. Which of the following psychotropic medications is the only medication to be approved for binge eating disorder?

A. Fluoxetine
B. Risperidone
C. Lithium
D. Methylphenidate
E. Lisdexamfetamine

ANSWER: E

Binge eating disorder (BED) is a new diagnosis added to *DSM-5* to differentiate repeated binging without purging from bulimia nervosa. Lisdexamfetamine was reported to be more effective than placebo in BED in Phase III multicenter trials. In January 2015, it received FDA approval for treating BED in adults and is the first drug approved for BED. Lisdexamfetamine for BED is started at 30 mg/day, with increased dosing to 50 to 70 mg/day.

REFERENCE

Schatzberg, A. F., & DeBattista, C. (2015). *Manual of clinical psychopharmacology* (8th ed., p. 511). Washington, : American Psychiatric Publishing.

12. In addition to antihistaminic effects, what pharmacodynamic property of trazodone, mirtazapine, olanzapine, and quetiapine also causes sedation?

A. Agonist at 5-HT1 receptor
B. Antagonist at 5-HT1 receptor
C. Agonist at 5-HT2 receptor
D. Antagonist at 5-HT2 receptor
E. Agonist at D2 receptor

ANSWER: D

Trazodone, mirtazapine, and second-generation antipsychotics such as olanzapine and quetiapine are potent antagonists at the 5-HT2 receptor. Trazodone at dosages of 50 to 200 mg at nighttime is more often used for insomnia rather than for its original FDA-approved indication of depression. Quetiapine at low doses of 25 to 100 mg/day causes significant sedation as well, but off-label use of quetiapine for insomnia *alone* is generally discouraged because of its potential for weight gain, treatment-emergent diabetes, and neuroleptic malignant syndrome (NMS).

REFERENCE

Schatzberg, A. F., & DeBattista, C. (2015). *Manual of clinical psychopharmacology* (8th ed., p. 471). Washington, DC: American Psychiatric Publishing.

13. Which of the following is an opioid receptor antagonist that is used in the treatment of opioid dependence?

A. Methadone
B. Levo-alpha-acetylmethadol (LAAM)
C. Buprenorphine
D. Naltrexone
E. Clonidine

ANSWER: D

Naltrexone is a full opioid receptor antagonist, binding to the opioid receptor, preventing the euphoric effects seen with opioids such as heroin and oxycodone. Therefore, patients taking naltrexone will not feel the euphoric effects when using an opioid, resulting in decreased use of the opioid. Naltrexone should be administered 7 to 10 days after last opioid use to prevent precipitated withdrawal symptoms. In 2010, an injectable form of naltrexone (Vivitrol) was approved by the FDA; it has proved to be a safe, effective alternative and has resulted in increased patient adherence and reduced relapse rates. Methadone, LAAM, and buprenorphine are all opioid substitutes. Clonidine is an alpha-2 adrenergic agonist.

REFERENCE

Fava, M., Rosenbaum, J., Stern, T., & Wilens, T. (Eds.). (2016). *Massachusetts General Hospital comprehensive clinical psychiatry* (2nd ed., pp. 298–299). New York, NY: Elsevier.

14. A 47-year-old man with a long history of alcohol use disorder, cirrhosis, and hypertension now seeks pharmacological intervention for treatment of alcohol use. Which of the following medications is the best choice for this patient?

A. Acamprosate
B. Clonazepam
C. Naltrexone
D. Naloxone
E. Disulfiram

ANSWER: A

Acamprosate is FDA approved for relapse prevention among those suffering from alcohol use disorder. It serves as a partial glycine antagonist at glycine-dependent NMDA receptors, thereby reducing glutamatergic activity and moderating symptoms related to prolonged alcohol withdrawal. It may be most effective for those who have recently completed alcohol detoxification. It is preferred over naltrexone and disulfiram for patients with liver damage because acamprosate is cleared through the kidneys, unlike naltrexone and disulfiram, which are hepatically metabolized. Naloxone and clonazepam are not indicated for the treatment of alcohol addiction. Off-label topiramate would be another consideration because it has minimal hepatic metabolism, and randomized clinical trials support its efficacy for alcohol use disorder. Gabapentin, which is exclusively renally cleared, may have a role for alcohol use disorder as well.

REFERENCE

Fava, M., Rosenbaum, J., Stern, T., & Wilens, T. (Eds.). (2016). *Massachusetts General Hospital comprehensive clinical psychiatry* (2nd ed., pp. 286–287). New York, NY: Elsevier.

15. When choosing medication for acute agitation, which of the following is most likely to produce symptoms of restlessness such as the need to be in constant motion, rocking from foot to foot, and pacing?

A. Lorazepam IM
B. Chlorpromazine PO
C. Ziprasidone IM
D. Haloperidol IM
E. Olanzapine PO

ANSWER: D

Haloperidol is a high-potency typical antipsychotic that has the advantage of not causing significant adrenergic blockade in the acute setting. However, among the side effects of high-potency typical antipsychotics are symptoms of akathisia such as the need to be in constant motion, rocking from foot to foot, and pacing. An effective strategy to avoid akathisia in the acute setting is to alternate the antipsychotic with a benzodiazepine. Haloperidol is often combined with lorazepam (PO, IM, or IV) for synergistic sedation, and lorazepam may also reduce the likelihood of developing extrapyramidal symptoms (EPS) with haloperidol. For young men who are demographically at the greatest risk for EPS, benztropine or diphenhydramine (PO, IM, or IV) can be added to haloperidol and lorazepam to prevent EPS, including acute dystonia in particular. Benzodiazepines and atypical second-generation antipsychotics (with the exception of aripiprazole) are unlikely to cause akathisia.

REFERENCE

Schatzberg, A. F., & DeBattista, C. (2015). *Manual of clinical psychopharmacology* (8th ed., p. 584). Washington, DC: American Psychiatric Publishing.

16. Offspring exposed to valproate during pregnancy are at known increased risk of which of the following teratogenic effects?

A. Lower IQ
B. Renal failure

C. Increased birth weight
D. Development of psychosis
E. Postnatal pulmonary hypertension

ANSWER: A

Besides the increased risk of neural tube defects, valproate use in pregnancy is associated with lower IQs in children exposed to the medication in utero. Studies have revealed an inverse correlation between higher doses of maternal valproate and lower IQ in exposed offspring. The growing evidence showing correlations between maternal valproate use and higher rates of intellectual disability in exposed offspring indicates that valproate should not be used in pregnancy as a first-line agent in bipolar patients.

REFERENCE

Schatzberg, A. F., & DeBattista, C. (2015). *Manual of clinical psychopharmacology* (8th ed., p. 637–639). Washington, DC: American Psychiatric Publishing.

17. By which of the following time periods should cognition have returned to baseline following electroconvulsive therapy?

A. 1 hour
B. 24 hours
C. 2 days
D. 1 week
E. 2 weeks

ANSWER: E

Although there has been no evidence showing structural brain damage as a result of electroconvulsive therapy (ECT), there are known effects on cognition. Anterograde amnesia is a common effect of ECT and is more commonly associated with bilateral electrode placement, high stimulus intensity, continuous versus brief pulse treatement, inadequate oxygenation, prolonged seizure activity, older age, alcohol abuse, and lower premorbid cognitive function. Brief anterograde amnesia after each session is common, but permanent retrograde amnesia is much less common. Studies have shown significant cognitive decline 0 to 3 days after completion of ECT. However, after 2 weeks, improvements compared with baseline were seen in processing speed, working memory, anterograde memory, and executive function.

REFERENCE

Fava, M., Rosenbaum, J., Stern, T., & Wilens, T. (Eds.). (2016). *Massachusetts General Hospital comprehensive clinical psychiatry* (2nd ed., p. 514). New York, NY: Elsevier.

18. Which form of psychotherapy encourages the patient to speak "whatever comes to mind"?

A. Cognitive behavioral therapy
B. Supportive psychotherapy
C. Interpersonal psychotherapy
D. Psychodynamic psychotherapy
E. Dialectical behavior therapy

ANSWER: D

Psychodynamic psychotherapy is also known as insight-oriented or expressive psychotherapy, and its more structured form is known as psychoanalysis. It can be brief or time-limited, but it is usually open-ended and done in a long-term setting. Sessions usually take place one or two times per week, with the patient being encouraged to speak about "whatever comes to mind." The goal of psychodynamic psychotherapy is to recognize, interpret, and work through unconscious thoughts and urges that are maladaptive to develop more mature defense mechanisms.

REFERENCE

Fava, M., Rosenbaum, J., Stern, T., & Wilens, T. (Eds.). (2016). *Massachusetts General Hospital comprehensive clinical psychiatry* (2nd ed., p. 102). New York, NY: Elsevier.

19. What is the average number of sessions in cognitive behavioral therapy?

A. 5 to 7
B. 8 to 10
C. 12 to 20
D. 25 to 30
E. 40 to 50

ANSWER: C

Cognitive behavioral therapy (CBT) is usually a short-term approach, typically with 12 to 20 sessions. CBT is a collaborative, structured, and goal-oriented intervention that targets core components of a given disorder. The "cognitive" element involves cognitive restructuring and problem-solving that addresses automatic thoughts. The "behavioral" component involves versions of monitoring, exposure, scheduling, and skills training.

REFERENCE

Fava, M., Rosenbaum, J., Stern, T., & Wilens, T. (Eds.). (2016). *Massachusetts General Hospital comprehensive clinical psychiatry* (2nd ed., pp. 154–155). New York, NY: Elsevier.

20. Which of the following treatments encourages participation in organized groups that help achieve and maintain recovery from alcohol use disorder?

A. Al-Anon
B. Cognitive behavioral therapy
C. Narcotics Anonymous
D. Twelve-step facilitation
E. Interpersonal psychotherapy

ANSWER: D

Twelve-step facilitation (TSF) is an empirically supported therapy that, as its name suggests, facilitates attendance at recovery groups, including Alcoholics Anonymous, Narcotics Anonymous, Gamblers Anonymous, and so forth. TSF involves educating the patient about the content, format, and structure of mutual help groups early during treatment and then continuing to monitor the patient's reactions and responses to meeting attendance. Interventions that incorporate TSF have been shown to enhance patients' outcomes by approximately 10% to 20% over, outcomes achieved with standard CBT. Al-Anon is a support group for close family and friends of those with alcohol use disorder.

REFERENCE

Fava, M., Rosenbaum, J., Stern, T., & Wilens, T. (Eds.). (2016). *Massachusetts General Hospital comprehensive clinical psychiatry* (2nd ed., p. 288). New York, NY: Elsevier.

QUESTIONS AND ANSWERS

This chapter has accompanying questions and answers which are available to subscribers as part of the Oxford eLearning platform. To access the questions, follow the link below, or go to http://oxford-elearning.oup.com/books.

http://oxford-elearning.oup.com/books/test/67/10.1093/med/9780190265557.003.0006

PART II

NEUROLOGY AND NEUROSCIENCES

Edited by Shirshendu Sinha

7.

NEURAL DEVELOPMENT THROUGH THE LIFE CYCLE

Rajesh R. Tampi, Juan Young, Mohsina Ahmed, Raman Marwaha

1. At what time does the nervous system first appear in the human embryo?

A. 1st week of gestation
B. 2.5 to 4 weeks of gestation
C. 4.5 to 6 weeks of gestation
D. 6.5 to 8 weeks of gestation
E. 8.5 to 10 weeks of gestation

ANSWER: B

The nervous system first appears in the human embryo between 2.5 and 4 weeks of gestation.

REFERENCE

DiCicco-Bloom, M., & Falluel-Morel, A. (2009). Neural development and neurogenesis. In B. J. Sadock, V. A. Sadock, & P. Ruiz (Eds.), *Kaplan and Sadock's comprehensive textbook of psychiatry* (9th ed., p. 43). Philadelphia, PA: Lippincott Williams and Wilkins.

2. Which of the following does not develop from the differentiation of the neural tube in the human brain?

A. Prosencephalon
B. Midbrain
C. Cerebellum
D. Pachymeninx
E. Spinal cord

ANSWER: D

The neural tube, which derives from ectoderm, differentiates into prosencephalon, mesencephalon (midbrain), rhombencephalon (medulla, pons, and cerebellum), and the spinal cord. The pachymeninx (another term for dura mater) is derived from mesoderm.

REFERENCE

DiCicco-Bloom, M., & Falluel-Morel, A. (2009). Neural development and neurogenesis. In B. J. Sadock, V. A. Sadock, & P. Ruiz (Eds.), *Kaplan and Sadock's comprehensive textbook of psychiatry* (9th ed., p. 45). Philadelphia, PA: Lippincott Williams and Wilkins.

3. In children, which of the following is the most serious neurological complication of lead poisoning?

A. Apathy
B. Ataxia
C. Delirium
D. Headache
E. Irritability

ANSWER: C

The most serious neurological complication of lead poising in children is delirium and its associated potential for lasting neurocognitive deficits.

REFERENCE

Dapul, H., & Laraque, D. (2014). Lead poisoning in children. *Advances in Pediatrics., 61*, 313–333.

4. Which of the following terms describes the disruption of normal neuronal migration during gestation?

A. Macrocephaly
B. Lissencephaly
C. Anencephaly
D. Microcephaly
E. Hydrocephaly

ANSWER: A

The term *lissencephaly* describes the disruption of normal neuronal migration during gestation, which leads to four cortical layers instead of the normal six and a smooth cortical surface without the normal pattern of sulci and gyri.

REFERENCE

DiCicco-Bloom, M., & Falluel-Morel, A. (2009). Neural development and neurogenesis. In B. J. Sadock, V. A. Sadock, & P. Ruiz (Eds.), *Kaplan and Sadock's comprehensive textbook of psychiatry* (9th ed., pp. 57–58). Philadelphia, PA: Lippincott Williams and Wilkins.

5. Approximately at what age does the human brain reach its maximum weight?

A. 5 years
B. 8 years
C. 12 years
D. 15 years
E. 20 years

ANSWER: E

The human brain reaches its maximum weight at around 20 years of age.

REFERENCE

Galasko, D. R. (2009). The aging brain. In B. J. Sadock, V. A. Sadock, & P. Ruiz (Eds.), *Kaplan and Sadock's comprehensive textbook of psychiatry* (9th ed., p. 3975). Philadelphia: Lippincott Williams and Wilkins.

6. Which of the following are markers for Alzheimer's disease in the human brain?

A. Neurofibrillary tangles
B. Lipofuscin
C. Corpora amylacea
D. Neuromelanin
E. All of the above

ANSWER: A

In the human brain, neurofibrillary tangles and amyloid deposits are markers of Alzheimer's disease. Lipofuscin, corpora amylacea, and neuromelanin represent cellular responses to aging, but their clinical consequence is unclear.

REFERENCE

Galasko, D. R. (2009). The aging brain. In B. J. Sadock, V. A. Sadock, & P. Ruiz (Eds.), *Kaplan and Sadock's comprehensive textbook of psychiatry* (9th ed., p. 3976–3977). Philadelphia: Lippincott Williams and Wilkins.

7. Which of the following is not considered an important predictor for successful aging?

A. High education level
B. Absence of alcohol abuse
C. Social class
D. Regular exercise
E. Social support

ANSWER: C

Predictors for successful aging include higher education level, absence of alcohol abuse and cigarette smoking, absence of depression, maintenance of appropriate weight, regular exercise, and social supports. However, social class does not appear to be an important predictor for successful aging.

REFERENCE

Galasko, D. R. (2009). The aging brain. In B. J. Sadock, V. A. Sadock, & P. Ruiz (Eds.), *Kaplan and Sadock's comprehensive textbook of psychiatry* (9th ed., p. 3987). Philadelphia: Lippincott Williams and Wilkins.

8. Which of the following tasks would a normally developing 3-year-old child be unable to complete on testing?

A. Builds towers of four or more blocks
B. Walks alone

C. Dresses and undresses self
D. Copies a triangle and other geometric shapes
E. Carries on a conversation using two or three sentences

ANSWER: D

A normally developing child is able to copy a triangle and other geometric shapes by the age of 5 years. By 3 years of age, a child is able to build towers of four or more blocks, walk alone, dress and undress him- or herself, and carry on a conversation using two- or three-word sentences.

REFERENCE

Developmental Milestones. http://www.cdc.gov/ncbddd/actearly/milestones/index.html. Accessed January 28, 2016.

9. Which of the following is NOT true of individuals who develop alcohol-related dementia (ARD)?

A. Female predominance
B. Psychiatric comorbidity
C. Medical comorbidity
D. Social isolation
E. Identified during hospital admissions

ANSWER: A

Individuals who develop ARD are predominantly male, have comorbid psychiatric and medical conditions (including liver and digestive diseases), are socially isolated, and are often identified through hospital admissions.

REFERENCE

Ridley, N J., Draper, B., & Withall, A. (2013). Alcohol-related dementia: An update of the evidence. *Alzheimer's Research & Therapy*., *25*, 3.

10. Which of the following is NOT correct regarding fetal alcohol syndrome (FAS)?

A. The prevalence is 0.5 to 2 per 1,000 births in the United States.
B. Affected children present with minor facial abnormalities.
C. Affected children have prenatal and postnatal growth retardation.
D. The frontal cortex is the most commonly affected brain region.
E. The majority of children with FAS meet the criteria for attention deficit hyperactivity disorder.

ANSWER: D

In children with FAS, neuroimaging studies indicate that the brain regions most clearly affected are the corpus callosum, cerebellum, and basal ganglia. The rest of the choices are correct regarding FAS.

REFERENCE

Teicher, M. H. (2009). Psychiatric aspects of child neurology. In B. J. Sadock, V. A. Sadock, & P. Ruiz (Eds.), *Kaplan and Sadock's comprehensive textbook of psychiatry* (9th ed., p. 581). Philadelphia, PA: Lippincott Williams and Wilkins.

11. A 34-year-old woman gives birth to a child who has short palpebral fissures, a smooth philtrum, and microcephaly. Based on the child's physical appearance, which one of the following substances is this woman most likely to have abused during pregnancy?

A. Crack cocaine
B. Marijuana
C. Alcohol
D. Nicotine
E. Heroin

ANSWER: C

Fetal alcohol syndrome affects about one third of all infants born to alcoholic women. It is characterized by growth retardation, microphthalmia, short palpebral fissures, midface hypoplasia (smooth or short philtrum and a thin upper lip), microcephaly, intellectual deficits, and seizures. The incidence of infants born with fetal alcohol syndrome is about 0.5 per 1,000 live births. Marijuana use in pregnancy is associated with low birth weight, prematurity, and withdrawal symptoms, including excessive crying, tremors, and hyperemesis. Crack cocaine use by the mother causes increased irritability and crying spells in infants. Heroin leads to withdrawal syndrome in infants. Nicotine causes low birth weight and premature births.

REFERENCE

Sadock, B. J., & Sadock, V. A. (2007). *Kaplan and Sadock's synopsis of psychiatry* (10th ed., p. 20). Philadelphia, PA: Lippincott Williams and Wilkins.

12. A child can go up and down the stairs alone, builds a tower of six or seven cubes, and refers to him- or herself by name. What is the age of this child presuming that he or she is exhibiting age-appropriate development?

A. 2 years
B. 3 years
C. 4 years
D. 5 years
E. 6 years

ANSWER: A

A 2-year-old child runs well, can go up and down stairs alone, can build a tower of 6 to 7 cubes, can draw a line, refers to him- or herself by name, and can engage in parallel play. A 3-year-old child can ride a tricycle, can build a tower of 9 or 10 cubes, can copy a circle, and is able to feed him- or herself. A 4-year-old child is able to stand on one foot for 5 to 8 seconds, copy a cross, and play cooperatively with other children. At 5 years of age, a child can skip using feet alternately, copy a square, and dress and undress him- or herself. At 6 years of age, a child can ride a bicycle, copy a triangle, and print his or her name.

REFERENCE

Sadock, B. J., & Sadock, V. A. (2007). *Kaplan and Sadock's synopsis of psychiatry* (10th ed., p. 23). Philadelphia, PA: Lippincott Williams and Wilkins.

13. Which of the following has been incorrectly paired?

A. Mesencephalon → cerebral peduncles, colliculi, and tegmentum
B. Diencephalon → thalamus and hypothalamus
C. Metencephalon → pons and cerebellum
D. Telencephalon → cerebral cortex
E. Myelencephalon → basal ganglia and hippocampus

ANSWER: E

Telencephalon gives rise to cortex, basal ganglia, and hippocampus, whereas the medulla is derived from the myelencephalon.

REFERENCE

DiCicco-Bloom, M., & Falluel-Morel, A. (2009). Neural development and neurogenesis. In B. J. Sadock, V. A. Sadock, & P. Ruiz (Eds.), *Kaplan and Sadock's comprehensive textbook of psychiatry* (9th ed., p. 45). Philadelphia, PA: Lippincott Williams and Wilkins.

14. Which of the following is FALSE regarding neural patterning?

A. It involves transcription of genes responsible for cellular proliferation, migration, or differentiation.
B. It is insensitive to environmental factors.
C. Patterning genes exhibit distinct temporal sequences of expression and function, acting in hierarchical fashion.
D. Patterning gene expression is regulated by growth factors released from regional signaling centers.
E. The numerous transcription factors and proteins involved in patterning the embryonic nervous system have been highly conserved through evolution.

ANSWER: B

Neural patterning is the process by which cells of the nervous system differentiate based on specific spatial positions. Patterning gene expression in the nervous system is sensitive to environmental factors.

REFERENCE

DiCicco-Bloom, M., & Falluel-Morel, A. (2009). Neural development and neurogenesis. In B. J. Sadock, V. A. Sadock, & P. Ruiz (Eds.), *Kaplan and Sadock's comprehensive textbook of psychiatry* (9th ed., p. 50). Philadelphia, PA: Lippincott Williams and Wilkins.

15. Heterotopias have been found in which areas of the brain in dyslexia?

A. Thalamus
B. Amygdala
C. Hippocampus
D. Planum temporale
E. Angular gyrus

ANSWER: D

Heterotopias are ectopic masses (incorrectly placed neurons). During neuronal migration, certain errors may lead to failure of neurons to reach cerebral cortex, resulting in heterotopias. In a study of four patients with dyslexia, heterotopias were a common finding in the planum temporale, which is located just posterior to the auditory cortex and represents a key portion of Wernicke's area.

REFERENCE

Sadock, B. J., & Sadock, V. A. (2007). The brain and behavior. In *Kaplan and Sadock's synopsis of psychiatry* (10th ed., pp. 70–132). Philadelphia, PA : Lippincott Williams and Wilkins.

16. Which of the following occurs during synaptic pruning?

A. Decrease in cholinergic neurons
B. Decrease in glutamatergic neurons
C. Decrease in GABAergic neurons
D. Increase in cholinergic neurons
E. Increase in glutamatergic neurons

ANSWER: B

Synaptic pruning is the process of synapse elimination that starts in early childhood. During pruning, there is loss of excitatory glutamatergic neurons in prefrontal cortex.

REFERENCE

R. A. (2007). Normal development. In A. Martin & F. R. Volkmar (Eds.), *Lewis's Child and adolescent psychiatry* (4th ed., pp. 252–290). Philadelphia, PA: Lippincott Williams and Wilkins.

17. Which of the following could a normally developing 3-year-old child do?

A. Build a tower of nine cubes
B. Copy a cross
C. Copy a triangle
D. Skip
E. Stand on one foot

ANSWER: A

A normally developing 3-year-old child is able to ride a tricycle, alternate feet going up stairs, build a tower of nine cubes, copy a circle, unbutton clothing, and feed him- or herself.

REFERENCE

Sadock, B. J., & Sadock, V. A. (2007). Human development throughout the life cycle. In *Kaplan and Sadock's synopsis of psychiatry* (10th ed., pp. 12–69). Philadelphia, PA: Lippincott Williams and Wilkins.

18. At what age does the need for independence for a child alternate with the need for closeness?

A. 10 months
B. 14 months
C. 18 months
D. 24 months
E. 30 months

ANSWER: C

Rapprochement, which occurs around 18 months of age, is a phase of separation-individuation proposed by Margaret Mahler in which children move away from their mothers and then come back for reassurance.

REFERENCE

Sadock, B. J., & Sadock, V. A. (2007). Human development throughout the life cycle. In *Kaplan and Sadock's synopsis of psychiatry* (10th ed., pp. 12–69). Philadelphia, PA: Lippincott Williams and Wilkins.

19. Which of the following may improve neurogenesis and neuronal stem cell proliferation?

A. Calcium
B. Iron
C. Zinc
D. Folic acid
E. Vitamin B12

ANSWER: C

Animal studies have demonstrated that zinc supplementation increases adult neuronal stem cell proliferation and increases the stem cell marker nestin in newborns. Additionally, zinc deficiency has been found to decrease the proliferation of stem cells during brain development in mice.

REFERENCE

Levenson, C. W., & Morris, D. (2011). Zinc and neurogenesis: Making new neurons from development to adulthood. *Advances in Nutrition: An International Review Journal.*, *2*, 96–100.

20. Which of the following is a consistent abnormal finding in the brains of individuals with autism spectrum disorder?

A. Lewy bodies
B. Elevated mercury levels
C. Decreased cerebral gray matter
D. Increased head circumference at birth
E. Significant decrease in Purkinje cells

ANSWER: E

A robust literature details abnormal cerebellar development in patients with autism spectrum disorder, which may manifest as dysfunction in both fine and gross motor skills. However, one of the more consistent findings related to cerebellar abnormalities is a decrease in the number of Purkinje cells, specifically in the posterolateral neocerebellar cortex and adjacent archicerebellar cortex of the cerebellar hemispheres.

REFERENCE

Fatemi, S. H., Aldinger, K. A., Ashwood, P., Bauman, M. L., Blaha, C. D., Blatt, G. J., & Welsh, J. P. (2012). Consensus paper: Pathological role of the cerebellum in autism. *Cerebellum*, *11*, 777–807.

QUESTIONS AND ANSWERS

This chapter has accompanying questions and answers which are available to subscribers as part of the Oxford eLearning platform. To access the questions, follow the link below, or go to http://oxford-elearning.oup.com/books.

http://oxford-elearning.oup.com/books/test/67/10.1093/med/9780190265557.003.0007

8.

BASIC NEUROSCIENCES

Rajesh Tampi

1. Which of the following findings is inherently pathological in an aging brain?

A. Lewy bodies
B. Reduction in the weight of the brain
C. Reduced blood flow to the brain
D. Sulcal widening
E. Ventricular enlargement

ANSWER: A

Reduction of weight and blood flow are features of the normal aging brain. Additionally, there is widening of sulci and associated ventricular enlargement. Lewy bodies are inclusions found in neurons of individuals with Parkinson's disease, Parkinson-plus syndromes, and dementia with Lewy bodies.

REFERENCE

Ropper, A. H., Samuels, M. A., & Klein, J. P. (2014). The neurology of aging. In *Adams and Victor's principles of neurology* (10th ed.). New York: McGraw-Hill Education. Retrieved from http://accessmedicine.mhmedical.com/content.aspx?bookid=690&sectionid=50910879

2. Hydroxylation of tryptophan is the rate-limiting step of which neurotransmitter?

A. Acetylcholine
B. Histamine
C. Dopamine
D. Serotonin
E. Epinephrine

ANSWER: D

Serotonin is synthesized by the hydroxylation of tryptophan via the enzyme tryptophan hydroxylase. Acetylcholine is synthesized from acetyl coenzyme A by the transfer of an acetyl group. Histamine is synthesized from histidine. Epinephrine and dopamine are synthesized from tyrosine.

REFERENCE

Berger, M., Honig, G., Wade, J. M., & Tecott, L. (2009). Monoamine neurotransmitters. In B. J. Sadock, V. A. Sadock, & P. Ruiz (Eds.), *Kaplan and Sadock's comprehensive textbook of psychiatry* (9th ed., pp. 65–76). Philadelphia, PA: Lippincott Williams and Wilkins.

3. Which one of the following is not a monoamine neurotransmitter?

A. Glutamate
B. Serotonin
C. Dopamine
D. Acetylcholine
E. Histamine

ANSWER: A

There are six monoamine neurotransmitters: serotonin, epinephrine, norepinephrine, dopamine, acetylcholine, and histamine. Glutamate and gamma-aminobutyric acid (GABA) are neurotransmitters derived from amino acids.

REFERENCE

Berger, M., Honig, G., Wade, J. M., & Tecott, L. (2009). Monoamine neurotransmitters. In B. J. Sadock, V. A. Sadock, & P. Ruiz (Eds.), *Kaplan and Sadock's comprehensive textbook of psychiatry* (9th ed., pp. 65–76). Philadelphia, PA: Lippincott Williams and Wilkins.

4. Which of the following cells constitute myelin in the central nervous system (CNS)?

A. Schwann cells
B. Oligodendrocytes
C. Microglia
D. Astrocytes
E. All of the above

ANSWER: B

Myelin is formed in the CNS by oligodendrocytes. Schwann cells form myelin in the peripheral nervous system (PNS). Microglia are derived from macrophages and act as scavengers that eliminate debris from neuronal injury and death. Astrocytes are cells that form the blood–brain barrier, remove certain neurotransmitters from the synaptic cleft, buffer extracellular potassium concentration, and serve a nutritive function.

REFERENCE

Melchitzky, D., & Lewis, D. A. (2009). Functional neuroanatomy. In B. J. Sadock, V. A. Sadock, & P. Ruiz (Eds.), *Kaplan and Sadock's comprehensive textbook of psychiatry* (9th ed., p. 9). Philadelphia, PA: Lippincott Williams and Wilkins.

5. Which of the following chromosomes is mapped to the apolipoprotein E (apoE) lipoprotein gene in late-onset Alzheimer's disease?

A. Chromosome 1
B. Chromosome 14
C. Chromosome 19
D. Chromosome 21
E. None of the above

ANSWER: D

The apolipoprotein E (ApoE) gene is mapped to the long arm of chromosome 19 in individuals with late-onset Alzheimer's disease (AD). Chromosome 1 is linked with the presenilin-2 (PS-2) gene in early-onset familial AD. The presenilin-1 (PS-1) gene on chromosome 14 has been recognized as a major locus for early-onset familial AD. Chromosome 21 is considered to be an excellent candidate region for genetic studies of individuals with AD because individuals with Down syndrome (trisomy 21) develop an early-onset dementia that is clinically and histopathologically indistinguishable from Alzheimer's disease.

REFERENCE

Karch, C. M., Cruchaga, C., & Goate, A. M. (2014). Alzheimer's disease genetics: From the bench to the clinic. *Neuron, 83*, 11–26.

6. Which of the following is TRUE regarding the hypothalamus?

A. A lesion to the supraoptic nucleus can result in diabetes mellitus.
B. A lesion to the ventromedial nucleus can result in anorexia.
C. A lesion to the suprachiasmatic nucleus can lead to a loss of the circadian rhythm.
D. A lesion to the arcuate nucleus can impair the secretion of vasopressin.
E. All of the above.

ANSWER: C

The hypothalamus regulates the release of major hormones and is involved in temperature regulation, control of food and fluid intake, sexual behavior, reproduction, circadian rhythm, and the mediation of emotional responses. The supraoptic region of the hypothalamus contains the supraoptic and paraventricular nuclei, which secrete vasopressin or the antidiuretic hormone (ADH), oxytocin, and corticotropin-releasing hormone (CRH). Damage to the supraoptic nucleus blocks the production of ADH, resulting in diabetes insipidus. The ventromedial nucleus of the hypothalamus regulates satiety, and bilateral lesions result in hyperphagia and aggressive behavior (termed *hypothalamic rage*), whereas bilateral lesions of the lateral hypothalamic area result in anorexia. The suprachiasmatic nucleus is responsible for maintaining the circadian rhythm. The arcuate nucleus of the hypothalamus contains many of the neurons that regulate the release of hormones. These neurons produce the "releasing factors," which influence the release of the growth hormone, ACTH, thyrotropin, the gonadotropins (FSH and LH), and prolactin.

REFERENCE

Jacobson, S., & Marcus, E. M. (2008). Hypothalamus, neuroendocrine system, and autonomic nervous system. In *Neuroanatomy for the neuroscientist*. Springer Science and Business Media. Retrieved from http://download.springer.com/static/pdf/550/chp%253A10.1007%252F978-0-387-70971-0_7.pdf?auth66=1425855429_5638c88f1d79024f7267d0ff10df23e3&ext=.pdf

7. Which one of the following are ion-channel linked receptors?

A. Dopamine receptors
B. Nicotinic receptors
C. Noradrenaline receptors
D. Muscarinic receptors
E. All of the above

ANSWER: B

Nicotinic receptors are ion-channel linked receptors. Dopamine, noradrenaline, and muscarinic receptors are all G-protein receptors. Most serotonin receptors except 5 HT3 receptors are G-protein receptors. 5 HT3 receptors are directly coupled to ion channels.

REFERENCE

Südhof, T. C., & Starke, K. (2007). Neurotransmitter release. In *Pharmacology of neurotransmitter release*. Berlin: Springer Science and Business Media. Retrieved from http://download.springer.com/static/pdf/90/bok%253A978-3-540-74805-2.pdf?auth66=1425864457_7876bb8e61b0e0ad0ee57a8043210f98&ext=.pdf

8. Which of the following neurotransmitters is associated with impulsive aggression?

A. Dopamine
B. Norepinephrine
C. Acetylcholine
D. Serotonin
E. Histamine

ANSWER: D

Disruption of serotonin neurotransmission is thought to be associated with impulsive aggression. Low cerebrospinal fluid (CSF) levels of 5-hydroxyindoleacetic acid (5-HIAA), the main metabolite of serotonin (representing low brain serotonin activity), has been found in individuals with impulsive aggression.

REFERENCE

Lee, R. J., Gill, A., Chen, B., McCloskey, M., & Coccaro, E. F. (2012). Modulation of central serotonin affects emotional information processing in impulsive aggressive personality disorder. *Journal of Clinical Psychopharmacology*, *32*, 329–335.

9. Brain biopsy in an individual with Parkinson's disease would show which of the following characteristic histopathological finding?

A. Lewy bodies
B. Beta amyloid plaques
C. Neurofibrillary tangles
D. Hirano bodies
E. Spongiform degeneration

ANSWER: A

Lewy bodies are the characteristic histopathological finding seen on the brain autopsy of an individual with Parkinson's disease.

REFERENCE

Alafuzoff, I., & Parkkinen, L. (2014). Staged pathology in Parkinson's disease. *Parkinsonism & Related Disorders*, *20*(suppl. 1), S57–S61.

10. Which of the following is NOT correct regarding the ventricular system in the human brain?

A. There are two lateral ventricles.
B. There is singular third ventricle.
C. There is singular fourth ventricle.
D. The cerebral aqueduct connects the third ventricle to the fourth ventricle.
E. Cerebrospinal fluid is produced by the arachnoid villi.

ANSWER: E

Cerebrospinal fluid is produced by the choroid plexus within each ventricle and reabsorbed by the arachnoid villi.

REFERENCE

Melchitzky, D., & Lewis, D. A. (2009). Functional neuroanatomy. In B. J. Sadock, V. A. Sadock, & P. Ruiz (Eds.), *Kaplan and Sadock's comprehensive textbook of psychiatry* (9th ed., pp. 5–42). Philadelphia, PA: Lippincott Williams and Wilkins.

11. Which of the following arteries supplies Wernicke's area of the brain?

A. Anterior cerebral artery
B. Middle cerebral artery
C. Posterior cerebral artery
D. Posterior communicating artery
E. Vertebral artery

ANSWER: B

The middle cerebral artery is the main continuation of the internal carotid artery and supplies two thirds of the lateral surface of the brain, including the Broca's and Wernicke's areas.

REFERENCE

Netter, F. H. (2004). *Atlas of human anatomy* (3rd ed., plate 135). Teterboro, NJ: ICON Learning Systems.

12. Which of the following is part of the limbic system?

A. Cingulate gyrus
B. Caudate nucleus
C. Corpus striatum
D. Subthalamic nucleus
E. Substantia nigra

ANSWER: A

The basal ganglia comprise the caudate nucleus, putamen, globus pallidus, subthalamic nucleus, and substantia nigra. The limbic system consists of cingulate gyrus, hippocampus, parahippocampal gyri, amygdala, mammillary body, anterior thalamus, septal area, and hypothalamus.

REFERENCE

Melchitzky, D., & Lewis, D. A. (2009). Functional neuroanatomy. In B. J. Sadock, V. A. Sadock, & P. Ruiz (Eds.), *Kaplan and Sadock's comprehensive textbook of psychiatry* (9th ed., pp. 5–42). Philadelphia, PA: Lippincott Williams and Wilkins.

13. Which of the following combinations is NOT paired correctly?

A. Acetylcholine; nucleus basalis of Meynert
B. Norepinephrine; locus ceruleus
C. Serotonin; midline raphe nucleus
D. Dopamine; substantia nigra
E. Histamine; ventral tegmental area

ANSWER: E

The cell bodies of histaminergic neurons are located within the tuberomammillary nucleus of the hypothalamus. Dopaminergic neurons are most widely distributed in substantia nigra and ventral tegmental area but are also located in the tuberoinfundibular pathway.

REFERENCE

Melchitzky, D., & Lewis, D. A. (2009). Functional neuroanatomy. In B. J. Sadock, V. A. Sadock, & P. Ruiz (Eds.), *Kaplan and Sadock's comprehensive textbook of psychiatry* (9th ed., pp. 5–42). Philadelphia, PA: Lippincott Williams and Wilkins.

14. Which of the following is NOT correct regarding glial cells in the human nervous system?

A. Glial cells are more numerous than neurons.
B. Oligodendrocytes form the myelin sheath in the central nervous system.
C. Astrocytes form the myelin sheath in the peripheral nervous system.
D. Astrocytes are the most numerous of glial cells.
E. Microglia serve as scavenger cells.

ANSWER: C

The myelin sheath is formed by Schwann cells in the peripheral nervous system, not by the astrocytes. Astrocytes help in the formation of the blood–brain barrier, neurotransmitter removal from the synaptic cleft, buffering extracellular potassium, and providing nutrition to the neurons.

REFERENCE

Melchitzky, D., & Lewis, D. A. (2009). Functional neuroanatomy. In B. J. Sadock, V. A. Sadock, & P. Ruiz (Eds.), *Kaplan and Sadock's comprehensive textbook of psychiatry* (9th ed., pp. 5–42). Philadelphia, PA: Lippincott Williams and Wilkins.

15. Which of the following is TRUE of oxytocin?

A. It is synthesized in the pituitary gland.
B. It acts only as a peripheral hormone.
C. It is an amino acid.
D. It has been shown to be involved in processing of social information.
E. All of the above.

ANSWER: D

Oxytocin is synthesized in the paraventricular and supraoptic nuclei of the hypothalamus. It is a neuropeptide that acts as a central neurotransmitter and as a peripheral hormone. In addition to its peripheral effects of uterine contraction during childbirth and lactation, oxytocin has been shown to have anxiolytic effects and to be involved in social attachment and processing of social information.

REFERENCE

Hofmann, S. G., Fang, A., & Brager, D. N. (2015). Effect of intranasal oxytocin administration on psychiatric symptoms: A meta-analysis of placebo-controlled studies. *Psychiatry Research*, *228*, 708–714.

16. Which of the following is TRUE of circadian rhythms?

A. They persist in the absence of time cues.
B. The primary circadian oscillator in humans is the suprachiasmatic nucleus.
C. Circadian light variation serves as the primary zeitgeber.
D. Melatonin is a circadian-regulating hormone.
E. All of the above.

ANSWER: E

All of the above statements are true of circadian rhythms. Notably, melatonin is a chronobiotic, not a hypnotic, agent. It may be instrumental in resetting or entraining circadian rhythms but rarely works as a "sleeping pill."

REFERENCE

Videnovic, A., Lazar, A. S., Barker, R. A., & Overeem S. (2014). 'The clocks that time us': Circadian rhythms in neurodegenerative disorders. *Nature Reviews Neurology.*, *10*, 683–693.

17. Which of the following disorders involves excessive trinucleotide repeats?

A. Fragile X syndrome
B. Huntington's disease
C. Myotonic dystrophy
D. Spinocerebellar ataxia
E. All of the above

ANSWER: E

All of these disorders occur due to the presence of excessive trinucleotide repeats. They are inherited through autosomal dominant mode of transmission.

REFERENCE

Adkinson, L. (2011). Mechanisms of inheritance. In L. Adkinson (Ed.), *Elsevier's Integrated Review Genetics* (2nd ed., pp. 28–50). Philadelphia, PA: Saunders.

18. Which of the following is the main excitatory neurotransmitter in the human central nervous system?

A. Glutamate
B. Glycine
C. Histamine
D. GABA
E. Norepinephrine

ANSWER: A

Glutamate is the main excitatory transmitter in the human central nervous system.

REFERENCE

Zhou, Y., & Danbolt, N. C. (2013). Glutamate as a neurotransmitter in the healthy brain. *Journal of Neural Transmission.*, *121*, 799–817.

19. Which one of the following describes the procedure by which pedigree data are examined to determine whether a disease phenotype is co-segregating with a genetic marker of known chromosomal location?

A. Path analysis
B. Segregation analysis
C. Linkage analysis

D. Genome-wide association studies
E. Twin studies

ANSWER: C

Linkage analysis is a statistical procedure by which pedigree data are examined to determine whether a disease phenotype is co-segregating with a genetic marker of known chromosomal location.

REFERENCE

Ott, J., Wang, J., & Leal, S. M. (2015). Genetic linkage analysis in the age of whole-genome sequencing. *Nature Reviews Genetics.*, *16*, 275–284.

20. Which of the following immunologic changes differentiates chronic from acute stress?

A. Increase in white blood cell (WBC) count
B. No change in lymphocyte count
C. No change in monocyte count
D. Decrease in T lymphocyte count
E. All of the above

ANSWER: D

A decrease in T lymphocyte count is seen in chronic stress but not in acute stress. All the other changes mentioned in the choices above are seen in both acute and chronic stress.

REFERENCE

Raison, C. L., Cowles, M. K., & Miller, A. H. (2009). Immune systems and central nervous system interactions. In B. J. Sadock, V. A. Sadock, & P. Ruiz (Eds.), *Kaplan and Sadock's comprehensive textbook of psychiatry* (9th ed., p. 187). Philadelphia, PA: Lippincott Williams and Wilkins.

QUESTIONS AND ANSWERS

This chapter has accompanying questions and answers which are available to subscribers as part of the Oxford eLearning platform. To access the questions, follow the link below, or go to http://oxford-elearning.oup.com/books.

http://oxford-elearning.oup.com/books/test/67/10.1093/med/9780190265557.003.0008

9.

DIAGNOSTIC PROCEDURES

Kristina Zdanys

1. Which of the following is a strength of the Mini Mental State Examination (MMSE) when used to assess cognitive decline in a clinical setting?

A. It is a detailed test of executive function.
B. The time to complete the assessment is brief.
C. Results are independent of mood.
D. It can be self-administered by the patient.
E. There is no bias from educational level.

ANSWER: B

The MMSE is a cognitive assessment tool in which patients are scored on a 30-point scale, with 30 points indicating the best cognitive performance and 0 points indicating the worst cognitive deficit. The time required for administering this exam is brief (5 to 10 minutes), making it easy to incorporate into an assessment. Limitations of this assessment include that it is a poor measure of executive function; it does not account for the impact of mood symptoms on cognitive performance; and patients with a higher education level tend to have higher scores in a narrower range. It is a clinician-administered examination.

REFERENCES

Buckingham, D. N., Mackor, K. M., Miller, R. M., Pullam, N.N., Molloy, K.N., Grigsby, C.C....& Winningham, R.G. (2013). Comparing the cognitive screening tools: MMSE and SLUMS. *PURE Insights*, *2*, article 3.

Folstein, M. F., Holstein, S. E., & McHugh, P. R. (1975). Mini-Mental State: A practical guide for grading the cognitive state of patients for the clinician. *Journal of Psychiatric Research*, *12*, 189–198.

Ridha, B., & Rossor, M. (2005). The Mini-Mental State Examination. *Practical Neurology*, *5*, 298–303.

2. Which of the following would not be a reason to refer a patient for neuropsychological assessment?

A. To inform the differential diagnosis of neurocognitive impairment
B. To follow decline longitudinally
C. To measure treatment response following traumatic brain injury
D. To confirm diagnosis of a specific neurocognitive disorder
E. To estimate a patient's functional potential

ANSWER: D

Neuropsychological testing is meant to aid in the differential diagnosis by providing diagnostic information but not to confirm diagnosis of a specific neurocognitive disorder. Diagnostically, it is used in conjunction with other aspects of workup (clinical criteria, history, physical examination, brain imaging, and ultimately brain autopsy). It is also valuable to measure the course of cognitive decline, measure treatment response, and assess functional potential.

REFERENCE

Harvey, P. D. (2012). Clinical applications of neuropsychological assessment. *Dialogues Clinical Neuroscience*, *14*, 91–99.

3. A 54-year-old woman with alcohol use disorder and cirrhosis presents to the emergency room for altered mental status. On exam she moves slowly, is disoriented to time and place, and demonstrates asterixis. Ammonia level is elevated. Which of the following findings may be seen on electroencephalogram (EEG)?

A. Triphasic waves
B. Periodic sharp-wave complexes
C. 3 Hz spike-and-wave complexes
D. Increased occipital alpha activity
E. Phase reversal

ANSWER: A

This woman's presentation is suggestive of hepatic encephalopathy. Triphasic waves are a characteristic finding on EEG in this disorder.

REFERENCE

Ellul, M. A., Gholkar, S. A., & Cross T. J. (2015). Hepatic encephalopathy due to liver cirrhosis. *British Medical Journal, 351*, h4187.

4. A 7-year-old boy is referred to a psychiatrist for evaluation of inattention. Several times during the interview, the boy stares blankly with eyes rolled upward. He blinks at regular intervals during these episodes and stops speaking. The psychiatrist believes that the patient may be having seizures. What finding would be expected on electroencephalogram (EEG)?

A. Triphasic waves
B. Periodic sharp-wave complexes
C. 3 Hz spike-and-wave complexes
D. Increased occipital alpha activity
E. Phase reversal

ANSWER: C

This boy's presentation is suspicious for absence (historically "petit mal") seizures, which begin in childhood and may be accompanied by automatisms such as blinking. EEG during absence seizures demonstrates bilateral 3 Hz spike-and-wave complexes.

REFERENCE

Hughes, J. R. (2009). Absence seizures: A review of recent reports with new concepts. *Epilepsy & Behavior, 15*, 404–412.

5. A 20-year-old man sustains a knife wound to his back and is medically stabilized. Neurological exam reveals paralysis of his right leg and loss of temperature and pain sensation on his left leg. There is a positive Babinski sign on the right. What is the likely lesion?

A. Left-sided spinal cord hemitransection
B. Right-sided spinal cord hemitransection
C. Left-sided spinothalamic tract lesion
D. Left-sided corticospinal tract lesion
E. Bilateral dorsal column lesion

ANSWER: B

The neurological examination is consistent with Brown–Séquard syndrome, which occurs in individuals who suffer hemitransection of the spinal cord. These patients present with paralysis ipsilateral to the lesion and contralateral sensory loss. The hemitransection involves both the spinothalamic tract and the corticospinal tract. In this case, the injury must be on the right side given right leg paralysis.

REFERENCE

Ranga, U., & Aiyappan, S. K. (2014). Brown–Séquard syndrome. *Indian Journal of Medical Research, 140*, 572–573.

6. An 8-year-old girl with a history of Chiari I malformation presents to her neurologist for follow-up. On exam, the patient has pain and temperature sensory loss in her bilateral shoulders and arms (what the neurologist notes to be a "cape-like" distribution). Her symptoms can be attributed to involvement of what part of the spinal cord?

A. Fasciculus cuneatus
B. Fasciculus gracilis
C. Central canal
D. Bilateral corticospinal tracts
E. Bilateral spinocerebellar tracts

ANSWER: C

Syringomyelia is observed in patients with Chiari I malformation, among other conditions. This is characterized by the cavitation of the central canal of the spinal cord, which then compresses the anterolateral spinothalamic tracts, causing bilateral pain and temperature sensory loss in a cape-like distribution of arms and shoulders.

REFERENCE

Pindrik, J., & Johnston, J. M. (2015). Clinical presentation of Chiari I malformation and syringomyelia in children. *Neurosurgery Clinics of North America, 26*, 509–514.

7. Which of the following is a "lower motor neuron" sign?

A. Hyperactive deep tendon reflexes
B. Muscle spasticity
C. Positive Babinski sign
D. Muscle flaccidity
E. Hemisensory loss

ANSWER: D

Lower motor neuron signs include weakness or paralysis with muscle flaccidity, hyporeflexia, and muscle atrophy. Upper motor neuron signs include spastic paralysis, hypertonia, spasticity, positive Babinski sign, and hyperreflexia.

REFERENCE

Doherty, J. G., Burns, A. S., O'Ferrall, D. M., & Ditunno, J.F. (2002). Prevalence of upper motor neuron vs. lower motor neuron lesions in complete lower thoracic and lumbar spinal cord injuries. *Journal of Spinal Cord Medicine*, *25*, 289–292.

8. A 32-year-old woman presents to the emergency room for eye pain and vision loss. Neurological examination is notable for tremor and dysarthria. She undergoes a lumbar puncture, which reveals oligoclonal bands in the cerebrospinal fluid (CSF). What would be expected on magnetic resonance imaging (MRI)?

A. Multiple ring-enhancing lesions of the basal ganglia
B. Acute posterior cerebral artery (PCA) infarct
C. Acute anterior cerebral artery (ACA) infarct
D. Bilateral ventricular dilation
E. Demyelinating lesions in the brain and/or spinal cord

ANSWER: E

This patient likely has multiple sclerosis (MS), the diagnosis of which is supported by presence of oligoclonal bands in the CSF. In most cases, lesions of MS are visible in the spinal cord and the periventricular, juxtacortical, and/or infratentorial areas.

REFERENCE

Polman, C. H., Reingold, S. C., Banwell, B., Clanet, M., Cohen, J.A., Filippi, M.... & Wolinsky, J.S. (2011). Diagnostic criteria for multiple sclerosis: 2010 revisions to the McDonald criteria. *Annals of Neurology*, *69*, 292–302.

9. Compared with computerized tomography (CT), magnetic resonance imaging (MRI) has which of the following?

A. Lower spatial resolution
B. More radiation exposure
C. Faster time to complete scan
D. Greater soft tissue detail
E. Less expensive

ANSWER: D

A benefit of MRI over CT is that images have more detail for soft tissue structures. MRI images also have higher spatial resolution. There is no radiation involved in MRI. MRI typically takes a longer time to perform and usually costs more than CT scan.

REFERENCE

Wang S., Thakur M. E., & Doraiswamy P. M. (2015). Use of the laboratory in the diagnostic workup of older adults. In D. C. Steffens, D. G. Blazer, & M. E. Thakur (Eds.), *The American Psychiatric Publishing textbook of geriatric psychiatry* (5th ed., pp. 107–126). Arlington, VA: American Psychiatric Publishing.

10. A 31-year-old woman presents to the emergency room believing she is having a stroke. She reports "double vision" and is concerned that her eyelids are drooping. Physical exam reveals proximal muscle weakness. The emergency room physician applies an ice cube to her eyes, and the ptosis improves. Edrophonium test is positive. Which of the following laboratory findings would be consistent with her likely diagnosis?

A. Oligoclonal bands in cerebrospinal fluid (CSF)
B. Increased tau protein in CSF
C. Decreased amyloid protein in CSF
D. Serum anti-Hu antibodies
E. Serum acetylcholine receptor antibodies

ANSWER: E

The patient's likely diagnosis is myasthenia gravis. Immunoassay in most cases reveals the presence of serum acetylcholine receptor antibodies. Oligoclonal bands in CSF are consistent with multiple sclerosis (MS). Increased tau protein and decreased amyloid protein in CSF are biomarkers for Alzheimer's disease. Anti-Hu antibodies are seen in paraneoplastic syndromes.

REFERENCE

Oger, J., & Frykman, H. (2015). An update on laboratory diagnosis in myasthenia gravis. *Clinica Chimica Acta*, *449*, 43–48.

QUESTIONS AND ANSWERS

This chapter has accompanying questions and answers which are available to subscribers as part of the Oxford eLearning platform. To access the questions, follow the link below, or go to http://oxford-elearning.oup.com/books.

http://oxford-elearning.oup.com/books/test/67/10.1093/med/9780190265557.003.0009

10.

CLINICAL ASPECTS OF NEUROPSYCHIATRIC DISORDERS

Shirshendu Sinha, Kristina Zdanys

1. Which of the following conditions is commonly associated with rapid eye movement (REM) sleep behavior disorder?

A. Central sleep apnea
B. Attention deficit hyperactivity disorder
C. Alcohol use disorder
D. Synucleinopathies
E. Bipolar disorder

ANSWER: D

Idiopathic REM sleep behavior disorder is commonly associated with later appearance of neurodegenerative disorders such as synucleinopathies (Parkinson's disease or so-called Parkinson-plus syndromes, including multiple system atrophy or major or mild neurocognitive disorder with Lewy bodies). Consequently, the neurological status of patients with REM sleep behavior disorder should be closely monitored and managed accordingly. Melatonin is considered among the first-line interventions for REM sleep behavior disorder.

REFERENCE

American Psychiatric Association. (2013). *Diagnostic and statistical manual of mental disorders* (5th ed., p. 408). Arlington, VA: American Psychiatric Publishing

2. The essential feature of insomnia disorder is characterized by:

A. Daytime fatigue
B. Sleep inertia
C. Dissatisfaction with sleep quantity or quality
D. Cognitive impairment
E. Anxiety

ANSWER: C

The essential feature of insomnia disorder is characterized by dissatisfaction with sleep quantity or quality with complaints of difficulty of initiating or maintaining sleep. The sleep complaints must cause clinically significant distress or impairment in social, occupational, or other important areas of functioning. The sleep disturbance may occur during the course of another mental or medical disorder, or it may occur independently.

REFERENCE

American Psychiatric Association. (2013). *Diagnostic and statistical manual of mental disorders* (5th ed., p. 363). Arlington, VA: American Psychiatric Publishing.

3. Which of the following class of medications is most commonly associated with rebound insomnia?

A. Sedative, hypnotic, or anxiolytic substances
B. Second-generation antipsychotics
C. Stimulants
D. Selective serotonin reuptake inhibitors
E. Tricyclic antidepressants

ANSWER: A

Rebound insomnia, a condition of an exacerbation of insomnia, often occurs in the context of abrupt discontinuation of chronic sedative, hypnotic, or anxiolytic medication. Sedative, hypnotic, or anxiolytic drugs with short durations of action are most commonly associated with the complaints of rebound insomnia.

REFERENCE

American Psychiatric Association. (2013). *Diagnostic and statistical manual of mental disorders* (5th ed., p. 417). Arlington, VA: American Psychiatric Publishing.

4. What is the most common cause of excessive daytime sleepiness (EDS)?

A. Sleep restriction from social and vocational pressure
B. Narcolepsy
C. Obstructive sleep apnea
D. Caffeine withdrawal
E. Idiopathic hypersomnolence

ANSWER: A

Although various sleep disorders listed above and conditions like caffeine withdrawal can result in EDS, sleep deprivation from social and vocational pressure (i.e., "everyday life stressors") is the most common cause of EDS. EDS can be measured by the Epworth Sleepiness Scale.

REFERENCE

Kaufman, D. M. (2013). *Clinical neurology for psychiatrists* (7th ed., pp. 368–369). Philadelphia, PA: Elsevier Health Sciences.

5. You are evaluating a 25-year-old woman at a sleep clinic for insomnia. She reports a peculiar creeping feeling in her legs, particularly in the late evening or at night. This uncomfortable feeling is worse when her legs are still and improves with movement. The symptoms interfere with getting to sleep. Which of the following laboratory tests should be ordered?

A. Potassium
B. Ferritin
C. Magnesium
D. Sodium
E. TSH

ANSWER: B

Patients with restless legs syndrome (RLS) often have iron deficiency with a low level of serum ferritin. Iron is a cofactor for tyrosine hydroxylase, which is essential for dopamine synthesis. Alpha-2 delta agonists (such as gabapentin) and dopamine receptor agonists (such as levodopa, pramiprexole, or ropirinole) are commonly used to treat RLS. Patients on dopamine receptor agonists should be monitored for pathological gambling and augmentation (i.e., worsening) of RLS symptoms.

REFERENCE

Sinha, S., Jhaveri, R., & Banga, A. (2015). Sleep disturbances and behavioral disturbances in children and adolescents. *Psychiatric Clinics of North America*, *38*, 705–721.

6. An adult patient with narcolepsy complains of excessive disruption of sleep at night, which is interfering with daytime functioning. What is the most appropriate pharmacological intervention?

A. Dextroamphetamine
B. Modafinil
C. Armodafinil
D. Sodium oxybate
E. Fluoxetine

ANSWER: D

In the treatment of narcolepsy, pharmacological treatment interventions have traditionally involved the administration of stimulant compounds, such as dextroamphetamine, to target reduction of daytime sleepiness and to suppress sleep attacks. In recent years, the nonstimulant compounds modafinil and armodafinil have become widely accepted as "wake-promoting" compounds, although they have limited efficacy to alleviate episodes of cataplexy. To obtain control of cataplexy with narcolepsy, an antidepressant drug with potent REM suppressant effects may be added. Fluoxetine has been studied most extensively among the antidepressant drugs. A recent pharmacological option that has been approved for use in adults with narcolepsy who experience prominent disruption of sleep at night is sodium oxybate, which is marketed for the treatment of sleep disturbance in narcolepsy patients as Xyrem. Patients prescribed Xyrem must be registered in an online database because, notably, Xyrem not only has a narrow therapeutic index but actually is gamma-hydroxybutyrate (GHB, the infamous date-rape drug).

REFERENCE

Sinha, S., Jhaveri, R., & Banga, A. (2015). Sleep disturbances and behavioral disturbances in children and adolescents. *Psychiatric Clinics of North America, 38*, 705–721.

7. Which of the following is the most accepted method of diagnosing narcolepsy?

A. Cerebrospinal fluid orexin level
B. Multiple sleep latency test
C. Nocturnal pulse oximetry
D. Actigraphy
E. None of the above

ANSWER: B

The clinical suspicion of narcolepsy should be confirmed by laboratory testing. The most accepted method of diagnosing narcolepsy is by means of the multiple sleep latency test (MSLT) to document quantitatively the extent of excessive daytime sleepiness (EDS) and to determine the presence of sleep-onset rapid eye movement (SOREM) during the four to five 20-minute nap opportunities that are evaluated as part of the MSLT procedure. Conventionally, the MSLT is conducted on the day after an overnight polysomnography (PSG) evaluation to document a night of adequate sleep before the MSLT, as well as to rule out the presence of another primary sleep disorder that might account for the presence of EDS. A low level of orexin A in the cerebrospinal fluid has become an additional diagnostic criterion for narcolepsy according to the second edition of the International Classification of Sleep Disorders and has been included in *DSM-5* as an alternative supportive feature to cataplexy.

REFERENCE

Sinha, S., Jhaveri, R., & Banga, A. (2015). Sleep disturbances and behavioral disturbances in children and adolescents. *Psychiatric Clinics of North America, 38*, 705–721.

8. Suvorexant is a dual orexin receptor antagonist recently approved by the US Food and Drug Administration for the treatment of sleep onset and sleep maintenance insomnia. Which one of the following conditions is an absolute contraindication for use of suvorexant?

A. Sleep apnea
B. Narcolepsy
C. Post-traumatic stress disorder
D. Substance-induced sleep disorder
E. Circadian rhythm sleep–wake disorders

ANSWER: B

Suvorexant blocks the orexin system, thereby reducing arousals and improving sleep consolidation. The orexin system is located in the lateral hypothalamus and plays a crucial role in arousal. In normal animal models, there is a diurnal variation of orexin activity, with increased activity during wakefulness and reduced activity during sleep. A well-established connection between orexin mutations and narcolepsy has been demonstrated in humans and animals. Patients with narcolepsy have a low level of orexin in the cerebrospinal fluid. Thus, suvorexant is contraindicated in patients with narcolepsy or suspected narcolepsy, with a potential to accentuate daytime sleepiness in these already sleepy individuals. In fact, side effects of suvorexant may resemble features of narcolepsy, including sleep paralysis, hypnogogic hallucinations, cataplexy, and excessive daytime sleepiness.

REFERENCE

Lee-Iannotti, J. K., & Parish, J. M. (2016). Suvorexant: A promising, novel treatment for insomnia. *Neuropsychiatric Disease and Treatment, 12*, 491.

9. Which of the following is suggestive of non-REM sleep?

A. Decreased recall of thought content
B. Vivid dreaming
C. Decreased movement
D. Increased cerebral perfusion
E. Increased sympathetic activity

ANSWER: A

Individuals have very little or no recall of thought content that might be present during their non-REM sleep.

Individuals can recall their dreams that occur during REM sleep. REM sleep is also associated with decreased body movements, increased cerebral blood flow, and increased sympathetic activity.

REFERENCE

Kaufman, D. M. (2013). *Clinical neurology for psychiatrists* (7th ed., p. 366). Philadelphia, PA: Elsevier Health Sciences.

10. A 55-year-old man presents to a sleep clinic for evaluation of sleep apnea. He complains of daytime sleepiness, fatigue, and impaired concentration. His wife reports that he snores and gasps during sleep at night. His medical history is significant for obesity and hypertension. Which polysomnographic (PSG) finding confirms the diagnosis of obstructive sleep apnea/hypopnea syndrome (OSAHS)?

A. PSG evidence of at least 5 apnea or hypopnea episodes per hour of sleep
B. PSG evidence of at least 10 apnea or hypopnea episodes per hour of sleep
C. PSG evidence of at least 15 apnea or hypopnea episodes per hour of sleep
D. PSG evidence of at least 20 apnea or hypopnea episodes per hour of sleep
E. None of the above

ANSWER: A

OSAHS is the most common breathing-related sleep disorder. OSAHS in adults is diagnosed on the basis of clinical symptoms and polysomnographic findings. The diagnosis is based on (A) nocturnal breathing disturbances (i.e., snoring, snorting/gasping, breathing pauses during sleep), or (B) daytime sleepiness, fatigue, or unrefreshing sleep despite sufficient opportunities to sleep that are not better explained by another mental disorder and not attributable to another medical condition, along with (C) evidence by polysomnography of 5 or more obstructive apneas or hypopneas per hour of sleep (Criterion A1). Diagnosis can be made in the absence of these symptoms if there is evidence by polysomnography of 15 or more obstructive apneas and/or hypopneas per hour of sleep (Criterion A2). Obesity and male sex are major risk factors for OSAHS. Hypertension is one of the most common comorbidities (present in up to 60% of cases). A common clinical screen for OSAHS is known by its acronymic name: STOP-BANG.

REFERENCE

American Psychiatric Association. (2013). *Diagnostic and statistical manual of mental disorders* (5th ed., pp. 378–380). Arlington, VA: American Psychiatric Publishing.

11. A 25-year-old woman presents with anxiety and sleep disturbances. On clinical interview she meets diagnostic criteria for generalized anxiety disorder. In terms of sleep, she gets to bed around midnight; it takes her at least a couple of hours to fall asleep at night, and upon awakening around 11:00 a.m. she feels "drunk" for an hour or so. Her sleep phase has caused her to lose at least two jobs over the past 6 months. She practices good sleep hygiene, avoids daytime naps, does not drink caffeinated beverages past noon, and denies any feelings of restless legs. She is not overweight and does not snore. Which of the following is the likely diagnostic impression?

A. Unspecified anxiety disorder with sleep issues
B. Generalized anxiety disorder
C. Insomnia disorder
D. Generalized anxiety disorder and circadian rhythm sleep disorder, delayed sleep phase type
E. Circadian rhythm sleep disorder, delayed sleep phase type

ANSWER: D

In the above case, per *DSM-5*, both diagnoses should be coded, even though insomnia can be considered a symptom of generalized anxiety disorder. The circadian rhythm sleep disorder, delayed sleep phase type is suggested by a history of a delay in the timing of the major sleep period (usually more than 2 hours) in relation to the desired sleep and wake-up time, resulting in symptoms of insomnia and excessive sleepiness. When allowed to set their own schedule, individuals with delayed sleep phase type exhibit normal sleep quality and duration for age. Patients commonly experience sleep-onset insomnia, difficulty waking in the morning, and excessive early day sleepiness.

REFERENCE

American Psychiatric Association. (2013). *Diagnostic and statistical manual of mental disorders* (5th ed., pp. 390–391). Arlington, VA: American Psychiatric Publishing.

12. Which of the following medications is associated with parasomnias?

A. Zolpidem
B. Doxepin
C. Quetiapine
D. Fluoxetine
E. Dextroamphetamine

ANSWER: A

Parasomnias are associated with use of benzodiazepine receptor agonists such as zolpidem. This could happen when these medications are taken at higher doses (intoxication) and when they are combined with other sedative drugs (polypharmacy).

REFERENCE

American Psychiatric Association. (2013). *Diagnostic and statistical manual of mental disorders* (5th ed., p. 417). Arlington, VA: American Psychiatric Publishing.

13. Which of the following is not a key diagnostic feature of delirium?

A. Chronic onset
B. Fluctuating course
C. Impaired attention
D. Cognitive disturbance
E. Reduced awareness

ANSWER: A

According to Criterion B of Delirium, the disturbance develops over a short period of time, usually hours to a few days. It also tends to fluctuate through the day, often worsening in the evening and at night. Mild and major neurocognitive disorders that increase the risk of delirium usually have a chronic course.

REFERENCE

American Psychiatric Association. (2013). *Diagnostic and statistical manual of mental disorders* (5th ed., pp. 596–598). Arlington, VA: American Psychiatric Publishing.

14. Which of the following is usually NOT a risk factor for the development of delirium?

A. Febrile illness
B. Mild and major neurocognitive disorder
C. Young adult
D. Hospitalized older individuals
E. Infancy and childhood

ANSWER: C

The prevalence of delirium is highest among hospitalized older individuals. Mild and major neurocognitive disorders increase the risk of delirium. Susceptibility to delirium in infancy and childhood may be greater than in the early (young) and middle adult population. Childhood delirium may happen in the context of febrile illness.

REFERENCE

American Psychiatric Association. (2013). *Diagnostic and statistical manual of mental disorders* (5th ed., pp. 600–601). Arlington, VA: American Psychiatric Publishing.

15. A 45-year-old woman with major depressive disorder and borderline personality disorder is admitted to the intensive care unit after an attempted overdose of a tricyclic antidepressant (TCA). Which of the following is not a manifestation of possible clinical condition?

A. Dilated pupils
B. Hypertension
C. Dry skin
D. Hypothermia
E. Delirium

ANSWER: D

The patient most likely suffers from anticholinergic toxicity from TCA overdose. With anticholinergic toxicity, the patient develops anticholinergic syndrome, which is characterized by dilated pupils, elevated pulse rate and blood pressure, dry skin, hyperthermia (not hypothermia), and delirium. The dry skin of the anticholinergic toxidrome differentiates it from that of stimulants or other sympathomimetic ingestants, which present with diaphoresis.

REFERENCE

Kaufman, D. M. (2013). *Clinical neurology for psychiatrists* (7th ed., p. 507). Philadelphia, PA: Elsevier Health Sciences.

16. The clinical presentation of Wernicke encephalopathy (WE) may be overlooked due to low index of

suspicion. Which of the following conditions is associated with WE?

A. Hyperemesis gravidarum
B. Prolonged total parenteral nutrition
C. HIV infection
D. Alcohol use disorder
E. All of the above

ANSWER: E

Wernicke encephalopathy, caused by vitamin B1 deficiency, is not diagnosed in about 80% of cases. This may in part be because clinicians are looking for the full triad, which *rarely* occurs in the same patient. Alcohol use disorder is the most common cause of WE, but this can be present in other conditions associated with vitamin B1 deficiency such as hyperemesis gravidarum, prolonged total parenteral nutrition, and infection with HIV.

REFERENCE

Donnino, M. W., Vega, J., Miller, J., & Walsh, M. (2007). Myths and misconceptions of Wernicke's encephalopathy: What every emergency physician should know. *Annals of Emergency Medicine, 50*, 715–721.

17. The classic clinical triad of Wernicke encephalopathy (WE) consists of mental status changes, ophthalmoplegia, and gait ataxia. This triad is present in what percentage of cases?

A. In almost all cases
B. In 80% of cases
C. In 50% of cases
D. In 25% of cases
E. In 10% of cases

ANSWER: E

The classic triad of WE is present in only 10% of cases. Conversely, other signs of disease such as hypothermia, vestibular dysfunction, and other ocular abnormalities can be present. Thus, reliance on the presence of the clinical triad as the sole criterion for disease is often inadequate and may lead to underdiagnosis.

REFERENCE

Donnino, M. W., Vega, J., Miller, J., & Walsh, M. (2007). Myths and misconceptions of Wernicke's encephalopathy: What every emergency physician should know. *Annals of Emergency Medicine, 50*, 715–721.

18. Which of the following is the most common ocular finding present in Wernicke encephalopathy (WE)?

A. Nystagmus
B. Bilateral sixth nerve palsy
C. Conjugate gaze palsy
D. Pupillary abnormality
E. Retinal hemorrhage

ANSWER: A

Ophthalmoplegia is part of the classic WE triad. However, ophthalmoplegia remains only one of a variety of ocular findings that include nystagmus, sixth nerve palsy, ptosis, retinal hemorrhage, papilledema, and (less commonly) anisocoria or miosis. Complete ophthalmoplegia rarely occurs and likely represents progressive disease, and nystagmus (usually horizontal) is the most common ocular abnormality.

REFERENCE

Donnino, M. W., Vega, J., Miller, J., & Walsh, M. (2007). Myths and misconceptions of Wernicke's encephalopathy: What every emergency physician should know. *Annals of Emergency Medicine, 50*, 715–721.

19. A 35-year-old male investment banker suffers traumatic brain injury from a motor vehicle accident. The patient is quite apathetic and has not been able to perform at work. He is currently on short-term disability. He does not engage in much conversation with his family and friends. At times his appears very irritable and aggressive, and he makes inappropriate comments and exhibits out-of-character sexual urges. Where is the likely site of the injury?

A. Hippocampus
B. Parietal lobe
C. Frontal lobe
D. Temporal lobe
E. Amygdalae

ANSWER: C

Frontal lobes contain the primary centers of personality, emotions, and executive decision. Damage to the orbitofrontal prefrontal cortex (PFC) leads to disinhibition of instinctive behaviors, aggression, and sexual urges. Damage to the ventromedial PFC leads to inanition and apathy. Damage to the dorsolateral PFC causes executive dysfunction (difficulty at work, including impaired sequencing, organizing, abstraction, and planning).

REFERENCE

Kaufman, D. M. (2013). *Clinical neurology for psychiatrists* (7th ed., p. 123). Philadelphia, PA: Elsevier Health Sciences.

20. Where is the likely site of lesion in a middle-aged male patient who displays memory impairments, hyperphagia, hyperorality, and sexual promiscuity?

A. Temporal lobe
B. Frontal lobe
C. Parietal lobe
D. Mammillary bodies
E. Midbrain

ANSWER: A

The patient described here most likely suffers from Klüver–Bucy syndrome, which results from bilateral temporal lobe injury—more specifically the amygdalae. The usual causes include conditions that have a predilection for striking the temporal lobes such as herpes simplex encephalitis, frontotemporal dementia, or bilateral posterior cerebral artery infarction. The Klüver–Bucy syndrome is commonly manifested by memory impairments, a variety of oral exploration (compulsive eating, drinking, or smoking), and increase in sexual activity (in at least 50% of cases).

REFERENCE

Kaufman, D. M. (2013). *Clinical neurology for psychiatrists* (7th ed., pp. 357–358). Philadelphia, PA: Elsevier Health Sciences.

21. A 60-year-old man with no medical history suffers from sudden memory loss. His physical examination is normal, with no focal neurological findings. The laboratory studies are unremarkable. He has no history of substance use and does not take any medications besides multivitamins. His MRI study indicates moderate changes in white matter. He appears anxious. Which of the following is the most likely diagnosis?

A. Alzheimer dementia
B. Wernicke encephalopathy
C. Transient global amnesia
D. Carbon monoxide toxicity
E. Anterior cerebral artery transient ischemic attack

ANSWER: C

The patient in the above case likely suffers from transient global amnesia (TGA). TGA results from transient ischemic attack (TIA) involving the posterior cerebral arteries, which supply the temporal lobes. The temporal lobes contain part of the limbic system, particularly hippocampi. Hence TIA in posterior circulation may cause temporary amnesia and personality change (anxiety). TGA is characterized by sudden development of amnesia. Affected individuals suffer from both anterograde amnesia (cannot memorize or learn new things) and retrograde amnesia (cannot recall recently acquired information). The anterograde amnesia is more profound and causes more impairments and distress. Some patients may become agitated, distraught, or panicked. By definition the total duration of the amnestic period must not exceed 24 hours.

REFERENCE

Kaufman, D. M. (2013). *Clinical neurology for psychiatrists* (7th ed., pp. 241–243). Philadelphia, PA: Elsevier Health Sciences.

22. A patient who is recovering from a stroke displays paucity of speech with excessive pauses or interruptions. He cannot repeat phrases. He can follow written commands. He appears quite frustrated with his situation. What is the most likely diagnosis?

A. Wernicke aphasia
B. Broca aphasia
C. Global aphasia
D. Transcortical motor aphasia
E. Alexia without agraphia

ANSWER: B

The clinical presentation here is consistent with Broca (by location) aphasia, which is also known as nonfluent or motor or expressive (by function) aphasia. The etiology is usually a middle cerebral artery stroke or another discrete structural lesion. The patient displays decreased production of words with pauses and cannot repeat phrases but has intact comprehension so that he or she can follow written commands. The patient is also aware of his or her problem, which causes frustration.

REFERENCE

Kaufman, D. M. (2013). *Clinical neurology for psychiatrists* (7th ed., pp. 157–158). Philadelphia, PA: Elsevier Health Sciences.

23. A 70-year-old man with a history of recent stroke speaks nonsensical words. His rate of speech is normal. He cannot follow spoken or written commands. He does not seem to be bothered by his impairment. What is the most likely diagnosis?

A. Wernicke aphasia
B. Broca aphasia
C. Global aphasia
D. Conductive aphasia
E. Transcortical expressive aphasia

ANSWER: A

The clinical presentation is consistent with Wernicke aphasia (by location), also known as fluent, comprehension, or sensory (by function) aphasia. The hallmark feature is paraphasias, which are incorrect, meaningless, or nonsensical words. Patients speak at a normal rate. They cannot repeat phrases and follow through verbal or written commands. They have no awareness of the problem and so do not appear to be bothered by it.

REFERENCE

Kaufman, D. M. (2013). *Clinical neurology for psychiatrists* (7th ed., p. 160). Philadelphia, PA: Elsevier Health Sciences.

24. A patient who remains fluent in speech and retains comprehension but is unable to repeat short sentences most likely has a lesion in which of the following structures?

A. Arcuate fasciculus
B. Broca's area
C. Wernicke's area
D. Planum temporale
E. Anterior cingulate gyrus

ANSWER: A

Lesions in the tract, the arcuate fasciculus that connects Broca's and Wernicke's areas, result in conduction aphasia. Patients with conduction aphasia remain fluent and retain comprehension but cannot repeat short sentences or even short phrases. The most frequent cause is embolic stroke in the parietal or posterior temporal lobe, but the condition may also be seen with a strategically located tumor.

REFERENCE

Kaufman, D. M. (2013). *Clinical neurology for psychiatrists* (7th ed., p. 161). Philadelphia, PA: Elsevier Health Sciences.

25. Global aphasia is characterized by

A. Intact comprehension but loss of repetition
B. Intact comprehension and repetition
C. Intact comprehension but loss of naming
D. Loss of comprehension and intact repetition
E. Loss of comprehension and repetition

ANSWER: E

Global aphasia, which results from extensive dominant-hemispheric damage, causes an extreme form of nonfluent aphasia in which patients have impaired comprehension, expression, repetition, and naming. Patients often become mute and present with right hemiplegia, right homonymous hemianopsia, and conjugate deviation of eyes to the left.

REFERENCE

Kaufman, D. M. (2013). *Clinical neurology for psychiatrists* (7th ed., pp. 158–159). Philadelphia, PA: Elsevier Health Sciences.

26. Which of the following is NOT consistent with the clinical presentation of anomia?

A. Inability to name objects
B. Use of paraphasias
C. Ignorance of object function
D. Intact comprehension is intact
E. Intact repetition is intact

ANSWER: C

Anomia or anomic aphasia is a variety of fluent aphasia characterized by inability to name objects. Agnosia is not present so that the patient knows the function of the object but is not able to name it. The patient also often uses paraphasias as a way to offer substitutes. Comprehension and repetition remain intact.

REFERENCE

Kaufman, D. M. (2013). *Clinical neurology for psychiatrists* (7th ed., p. 160). Philadelphia, PA: Elsevier Health Sciences.

27. Which of the following is the first to improve with treatment in patients with normal pressure hydrocephalus?

A. Dementia
B. Gait apraxia
C. Urinary urgency
D. Urinary frequency
E. Visual acuity

ANSWER: B

Normal pressure hydrocephalus (NPH) is characterized by dementia, urinary incontinence (urgency and frequency), and gait apraxia. Vision is not typically impaired in NPH. Gait apraxia is the initial, most consistent, and most prominent feature of NPH. Gait apraxia is also the first to improve with treatment.

REFERENCE

Kaufman, D. M. (2013). *Clinical neurology for psychiatrists* (7th ed., p. 127). Philadelphia, PA: Elsevier Health Sciences.

28. Which of the following clinical syndromes is characterized by cortical blindness, anosognosia, and confabulation?

A. Anton syndrome
B. Gerstmann syndrome
C. Wernicke–Korsakoff syndrome
D. Split-brain syndrome
E. Marchiafava–Bignami syndrome

ANSWER: A

Anton syndrome presents with cortical blindness, anosognosia, and confabulation. Patients deny having lost vision, but this is thought to be related to anosognosia of deficit. They at times blame external factors such as a dark room for their problem. They also confabulate by describing their room, clothing, and various other objects.

REFERENCE

Kaufman, D. M. (2013). *Clinical neurology for psychiatrists* (7th ed., p. 266). Philadelphia, PA: Elsevier Health Sciences.

29. A patient presents with an impaired ability to calculate, write, and identify fingers and right/left confusion. What is most likely site of injury?

A. Frontal lobe
B. Nondominant parietal lobe
C. Dominant parietal lobe
D. Temporal lobe
E. Mammillary bodies

ANSWER: D

The above case is consistent with clinical presentation of Gerstmann syndrome, which is characterized by the presence of four neuropsychological deficits: acalculia (impaired arithmetic skills), finger agnosia (inability to identify fingers), left/right confusion, and agraphia (inability to write). A lesion in the arcuate gyrus of the dominant parietal lobe is usually the cause.

REFERENCE

Kaufman, D. M. (2013). *Clinical neurology for psychiatrists* (7th ed., p. 163). Philadelphia, PA: Elsevier Health Sciences.

30. Which of the following is not an indication of polysomnogram (PSG)?

A. Sleep apnea
B. Narcolepsy
C. REM sleep behavior disorder
D. Periodic limb movement disorder
E. Restless legs syndrome (RLS)

ANSWER: E

RLS is a sensorimotor disorder in which the patient complains of a peculiar creepy or crawling feeling in the extremities. The undesirable sensation is worse or only occurs in the evening or at night, is exacerbated by keeping the limbs still, and is relieved or partially relieved by movement. The symptoms interfere with initiation and maintenance of sleep. The diagnosis of RLS is clinical, based solely on reported symptoms or symptoms observed in the patient.

REFERENCES

Kaufman, D. M. (2013). *Clinical neurology for psychiatrists* (7th ed., p. 384). Philadelphia, PA: Elsevier Health Sciences.

Sinha, S., Jhaveri, R., & Banga, A. (2015). Sleep disturbances and behavioral disturbances in children and adolescents. *Psychiatric Clinics of North America, 38*, 705–721.

31. A 72-year-old man who requires assistance in most instrumental activities of daily living presents to a geriatric psychiatrist with reports of vivid visual hallucinations. He describes seeing children and dogs in his living room. The Mini Mental State Examination score was 19 out of 30. His wife reports he has been "acting out his dreams." When prescribed a low-dose antipsychotic, the patient became heavily sedated with muscle rigidity. The most likely diagnosis is:

A. Major neurocognitive disorder with Lewy bodies
B. Major neurocognitive disorder due to Alzheimer's disease
C. Mild neurocognitive disorder
D. Major neurocognitive disorder due to Huntington's disease
E. Major frontotemporal neurocognitive disorder

ANSWER: A

Lewy body dementia (in *DSM-5*, major neurocognitive disorder with Lewy bodies) is characterized by progressive cognitive decline, well-formed and detailed visual hallucinations, fluctuating cognition, spontaneous parkinsonism, REM sleep behavior disorder (i.e., acting out dreams), neuroleptic sensitivity, and low dopamine transporter uptake on imaging. Cognitive symptoms precede motor symptoms.

REFERENCES

Folstein, M. F., Folstein, S. E., & McHugh, P. R. (1975): "Mini-Mental State": A practical method for grading the cognitive state of patients for the clinician. *Journal of Psychiatric Research, 12*, 189–198.

McKeith, I. G., Dickson, D. W., Lowe, J., Emre, M., O'Brien, J.T., Feldman, H...Consortium on DLB. (2005). Diagnosis and management of dementia with Lewy bodies: Third report of the DLB consortium. *Neurology, 65*, 1863–1872.

32. A 78-year-old woman with major neurocognitive disorder due to Alzheimer disease of moderate severity accuses her husband of marital infidelity. Her husband leaves the house for several hours each day while the patient is cared for by an adult son. The husband insists he is not unfaithful to his wife and explains that he uses those hours to run errands and exercise at the gym. The adult son corroborates the husband's report. The patient has no other delusional thoughts. The first step in treatment would be:

A. Initiate risperidone 0.25 mg twice daily.
B. Initiate sertraline 25 mg daily and titrate as tolerated.
C. Provide caregiver education and reassurance to the patient.
D. Refer the patient and her husband for marital therapy.
E. Explore options for long-term placement of the patient in a skilled nursing facility.

ANSWER: C

Nonpharmacological strategies are first-line treatment for behavioral disturbances and misinterpretations in major neurocognitive disorder due to Alzheimer disease and other neurocognitive disorders. Marital therapy would not be helpful given there is no evidence of true infidelity and this perception is in the context of moderate cognitive decline. There is no indication of behavioral disturbances that would necessitate placement in a skilled nursing facility at this time.

REFERENCE

Tampi, R., Williamson, D., Mittal, V., McEnerney, N., Thomas, J., & Cash, M. (2011). Behavioral and psychological symptoms of dementia: Part 2—Treatment. *Clinical Geriatrics, 19*, 31–40.

33. An 82-year-old woman returns to her home following hospitalization for an MRI-confirmed stroke and subsequent rehabilitation. Family members notice she is forgetful and has new-onset difficulty managing her finances and medications. Her primary care doctor performs a Mini Mental State Examination, and the

patient earns 18 out of 30 points. She was previously living independently with no history of cognitive impairment. Her most likely diagnosis is:

A. Major neurocognitive disorder with Lewy bodies
B. Major neurocognitive disorder due to Alzheimer disease
C. Major vascular neurocognitive disorder
D. Major neurocognitive disorder due to Huntington disease
E. Major frontotemporal neurocognitive disorder

ANSWER: C

The onset of major vascular neurocognitive disorder is temporally related to a vascular event and can be caused by a strategic infarct or small vessel disease, leading to the classic "stepwise decline" seen in the condition. There is evidence of the presence of cerebrovascular disease based on history, physical examination, and/or neuroimaging.

REFERENCES

Folstein, M. F., Folstein, S. E., & McHugh, P. R. (1975). "Mini-Mental State": A practical method for grading the cognitive state of patients for the clinician. *Journal of Psychiatric Research*, *12*, 189–198.

Gorelick, P. B., Scuteri, A., Black, S. E., Black, S.E., Decarli, C., Greenberg, S.M...American Heart Association Stroke Council, Council on Epidemiology and Prevention, Council on Cardiovascular Nursing, Council on Cardiovascular Radiology and Intervention, and Council on Cardiovascular Surgery and Anesthesia. (2011). Vascular contributions to cognitive impairment and dementia: A statement for healthcare professionals from the American Heart Association/American Stroke Association. *Stroke*, *42*, 2672–2713.

34. A 58-year-old man is diagnosed with major frontotemporal neurocognitive disorder. What are the two common clinical phenotypes of this disease?

A. Behavioral variant and language variant
B. Behavioral variant and processing speed variant
C. Behavioral variant and attentional variant
D. Attentional variant and language variant
E. Language variant and processing speed variant

ANSWER: A

Major frontotemporal neurocognitive disorder is grouped into two main clinical phenotypes. The behavioral variant is the most common presentation, with changes in social conduct, including disinhibited, impulsive, or inappropriate behavior. The language variant, known as primary progressive aphasia (PPA), presents with difficulty with naming, with word-finding, and eventually with reading and writing. Three variants of PPA have been described: disorders of grammatical processing, semantic processing, and a logopenic variant. Some patients preserve understanding of word meaning, whereas in other cases understanding of meaning is lost.

REFERENCE

McKhann, G. M., Albert, M. S., Grossman, M., Miller, B., Dickson, D., Trojanowski, J.Q... Work Group on Frontotemporal Dementia and Pick's Disease. (2001). Clinical and pathological diagnosis of frontotemporal dementia: Report of the Work Group on Frontotemporal Dementia and Pick's Disease. *Archives of Neurology*, *58*, 1803–1809.

35. A 62-year-old man is arrested for exposing his genitals to several riders on a public subway. He is brought to the emergency room for psychiatric clearance before arraignment. The psychiatrist contacts the man's partner, who reports he has a 1-year history of behavioral changes, including inappropriate sexual advances toward strangers, shoplifting, and swearing loudly during religious services and in other public venues. She reports the patient does not appear to have any remorse for these actions. She feels these behaviors are gradually worsening. There is no history of medical illness, substance abuse, or mood disorder. His presentation is suggestive of which neurocognitive disorder?

A. Major neurocognitive disorder with Lewy bodies
B. Major neurocognitive disorder due to Alzheimer disease
C. Major neurocognitive disorder co-morbid with antisocial personality disorder
D. Major neurocognitive disorder due to antisocial personality
E. Major frontotemporal neurocognitive disorder

ANSWER: E

Behavioral variant major frontotemporal neurocognitive disorder (colloquially "frontotemporal dementia") is characterized by behavioral changes that are inappropriate and impulsive. Symptoms are not better accounted for by medical illness, substance abuse, or other primary psychiatric disorder.

REFERENCE

McKhann, G. M., Albert, M. S., Grossman, M., Miller, B., Dickson, D., Trojanowski, J.Q... Work Group on Frontotemporal Dementia and Pick's Disease. (2001). Clinical and pathological diagnosis of frontotemporal dementia: Report of the Work Group on Frontotemporal Dementia and Pick's Disease. *Archives of Neurology, 58*, 1803–1809.

36. A 58-year-old woman presents to a neurologist with rapidly progressing dementia for 2 months and irregular, shock-like muscle contractions. The neurologist performs an electroencephalogram (EEG), which shows periodic sharp-wave complexes. What marker would be expected in cerebrospinal fluid (CSF)?

A. NMDA receptor antibodies
B. Increased amyloid protein
C. Positive venereal disease research laboratory (VDRL)
D. 14-3-3 protein
E. Increased measles antibody titer

ANSWER: D

Dementia and myoclonus in a middle-aged adult is characteristic of mild and major neurocognitive disorder due to prion disease, in this case Creutzfeldt–Jakob disease. Classically in this disorder, EEG demonstrates periodic sharp-wave complexes, and CSF is positive for 14-3-3 protein. CSF amyloid protein is decreased and tau protein increased in major neurocognitive disorder due to Alzheimer disease. Positive VDRL would be seen in neurosyphilis. Increased measles antibody titer would be seen in subacute sclerosing panencephalitis. NMDA receptor antibody encephalitis may show a range of EEG changes, including diffuse background slowing or generalized cortical excitability, but the most specific EEG signature is extreme delta brush (alpha waves superimposed on delta waves).

REFERENCE

Henry, C., & Knight, R. (2002). Clinical features of variant Creutzfeldt–Jakob disease. *Reviews in Medical Virology, 12*, 143–150.

37. Which of the following is NOT a risk factor for major and mild neurocognitive disorder due to HIV infection?

A. Long-term use of combined antiretroviral therapy
B. Co-morbid cytomegalovirus or toxoplasmosis
C. Duration of acquired immunodeficiency syndrome
D. Low CD4 nadir
E. High vial load

ANSWER: A

Combined antiretroviral therapy (cART; historically "highly active antiretroviral therapy," or HAART) improves cognitive function in patients experiencing neurocognitive disorder due to HIV infection. Co-morbid cytomegalovirus or toxoplasmosis may worsen cognition, as do comorbid hepatitis C infection and general vascular risk factors.

REFERENCE

Kaufman, D. M. (2001). Dementia. In *Clinical neurology for psychiatrists* (6th ed., p. 135). Philadelphia: Saunders.

38. A 37-year-old man presents to his neurologist with a 1-year history of motor symptoms, including involuntary jerky movements of the pelvis, limbs, and trunk with unsteady gait. For several months he has also experienced worsening cognitive function and depression. His father had similar symptoms in his early 40s. The most likely genetic basis of this disease is:

A. Apolipoprotein E, epsilon 4 allele
B. Apolipoprotein E, epsilon 2 allele
C. Prion protein PrP^{Sc}
D. Huntingtin gene with excessive CAG repeats
E. None of the above

ANSWER: D

This patient most likely has major neurocognitive disorder due to Huntington disease. This gene, which encodes the protein huntingtin (with an *i*), is found on the short arm of chromosome 4. Apolipoprotein E, epsilon 4 allele increases risk of late-onset Alzheimer's disease and is found on chromosome 19. Prion protein PrP^{Sc} is the mutation seen in sporadic major and minor neurocognitive disorder due to prion disease and is found on chromosome 20. Interestingly, the superscript "sc" stands for scrapie, an analogous fatal spongiform encephalopathy seen in sheep and goats so named because affected animals incorrigibly scrape themselves against posts and other objects to the point of rubbing themselves bare.

REFERENCE

Roos, R A. (2010). Huntington's disease: A clinical review. *Crphanet Joural of Rare Diseases*, 5, 40.

39. An 85-year-old woman presented to her neurologist for 6 months of worsening memory. For the past 8 years the neurologist has been treating the woman for motor symptoms, including tremor, rigidity, and slow movements. The neurologist notes that her Mini Mental State Examination score is 6 points lower than it was at her baseline evaluation 5 years ago. More intensive neuropsychological evaluation reveals deficits in the areas of visuospatial and executive function. The most likely diagnosis of her cognitive impairment is:

A. Major neurocognitive disorder with Lewy bodies
B. Major neurocognitive disorder due to Alzheimer disease
C. Major neurocognitive disorder due to Huntington disease
D. Major neurocognitive disorder due to Parkinson disease
E. Major frontotemporal neurocognitive disorder

ANSWER: D

This patient most likely has Parkinson disease based on the triad of tremor, rigidity, and bradykinesia. Major neurocognitive disorder due to Parkinson disease is a common, gradually developing complication of the condition, particularly as the patient ages and the disease progresses. Although this form of dementia is on the synucleinopathy spectrum of major neurocognitive disorder with Lewy bodies, a key distinguishing feature is that motor symptoms appear first in major neurocognitive disorder due to Parkinson disease.

REFERENCE

Cosgrove, J., Alty, J. E., & Jamieson, S. (2015). Cognitive impairment in Parkinson's disease. *Postgraduate Medical Journal, 91*, 212–220.

40. A 42-year-old woman sustains a traumatic brain injury in a motor vehicle accident. Six weeks later she returns to her job as a sales clerk. Two weeks later she is fired for making inappropriate comments to clients, inappropriate laughter, and a tendency to become distracted. When asked how she feels about losing her employment, she exhibits indifference and has no plans to seek other work. Based on these symptoms, which area of the brain was likely injured during the accident?

A. Frontal lobe
B. Parietal lobe
C. Temporal lobe
D. Occipital lobe
E. Hippocampus

ANSWER: A

This patient's presenting symptoms of disinhibition and apathy are characteristic of frontal lobe injury.

REFERENCE

Kaufman, D. M. (2001). Dementia. In *Clinical neurology for psychiatrists* (6th ed., p. 126). Philadelphia: Saunders.

41. A 78-year-old man with alcohol use disorder presents to the emergency room with acute confusion, ataxia, and nystagmus. Aside from monitoring and treating symptoms of alcohol withdrawal, what should be administered immediately in the emergency room to reduce risk of chronic sequelae?

A. Glucose
B. Thiamine
C. Cyanocobalamin
D. Niacin
E. Pyridoxine

ANSWER: B

The patient is presenting in the acute stages of Wernicke–Korsakoff syndrome, Wernicke encephalopathy. Thiamine administration may reduce the risk of chronic Korsakoff syndrome, although brain damage is often irreversible.

REFERENCE

Latt, N., & Dore, G. (2014). Thiamine in the treatment of Wernicke encephalopathy in patients with alcohol use disorders. *Internal Medicine Journal, 44*, 911–915.

42. Which of the following genes is associated with late-onset Alzheimer disease?

A. Presenilin 1
B. Presenilin 2
C. Amyloid precursor protein
D. Brain-derived neurotrophic factor
E. Apolipoprotein E, epsilon 4 allele

ANSWER: E

Presenilin 1 (on chromosome 14), presenilin 2 (on chromosome 1), and amyloid precursor protein (on chromosome 21) are all associated with early-onset Alzheimer disease. Brain-derived neurotrophic factor has not been associated with Alzheimer disease risk. Apolipoprotein E, epsilon 4 allele, is a susceptibility gene for late-onset Alzheimer disease, located on chromosome 19.

REFERENCE

Alonso Vilatela, M. E., Lopez-Lopez, M., & Yescas-Gomez, P. (2012). Genetics of Alzheimer's disease. *Archives of Medical Research, 43*, 622–631.

43. An 83-year-old man presents to the emergency room for confusion and falls. Assessment of gait is suggestive of apraxia. His partner notes that he has been increasingly incontinent of urine for several weeks. Computerized tomography (CT) scan of the head demonstrates enlarged ventricles. What surgical procedure may be helpful for this patient?

A. Deep brain stimulation to subthalamic nucleus
B. Shunt placement into the lateral ventricle
C. Vagal nerve stimulation
D. Focal resection of the right globus pallidus
E. Aneurysm coiling

ANSWER: B

This patient presents with the clinical triad of gait apraxia, urinary incontinence, and dementia, classically associated with normal pressure hydrocephalus (NPH). Typically patients undergo serial lumbar puncture to decrease the degree of hydrocephalus and may show some improvement with this intervention alone. For long-term treatment, neurosurgery involving shunt placement into the lateral ventricle is considered.

REFERENCE

Torsnes, L., Blafjelldal, V., & Poulsen, F. R. (2014). Treatment and clinical outcome in patients with idiopathic normal pressure hydrocephalus—a systematic review. *Danish Medical Journal, 61*, A4911.

44. A 75-year-old woman presents to her primary care physician with a 2-year history of gradually worsening forgetfulness affecting her ability to manage household chores efficiently and take her medications correctly. Her partner reports that the patient has not been driving for 6 months because she was getting lost in familiar surroundings. There is no history of vascular risk factors or behavioral symptoms. The patient is a high school graduate. She scores 22 out of 30 on the Mini Mental State Examination, missing all three words on delayed recall. What would be first-line treatment for this patient at this time?

A. N-methyl-D-aspartate (NMDA) receptor antagonist
B. Gamma-secretase inhibitor
C. Cholinesterase inhibitor
D. Amyloid-directed monoclonal antibody
E. Beta-secretase inhibitor

ANSWER: C

The patient's presentation is consistent with major neurocognitive disorder due to Alzheimer disease, likely mild severity based on her Mini Mental State Examination score, gradual decline, and current deficits. Alzheimer disease pathology typically begins in the hippocampus, leading to impaired recall. Cholinesterase inhibitors (donepezil, rivastigmine, and galantamine) are approved by the FDA for treatment of major neurocognitive disorder due to Alzheimer disease, mild to moderate severity. Donepezil and rivastigmine are also approved for severe stage of Alzheimer disease. Memantine, an NMDA receptor antagonist, is approved for moderate to severe stages of Alzheimer disease. The other options are currently in experimental stages.

REFERENCE

Schwarz, S., Froelich, L., & Burns, A. (2012). Pharmacological treatment of dementia. *Current Opinion in Psychiatry, 25*, 542–550.

45. An autopsy is performed on a 74-year-old patient who had a 3-year history of progressive cognitive decline. Based on the neuropathological findings, the pathologist concludes the patient likely suffered from major neurocognitive disorder with Lewy bodies. What is the neuropathological finding?

A. Amyloid plaques
B. Neurofibrillary tangles
C. Alpha-synuclein introcytoplasmic inclusions
D. Intranuclear eosinophilic inclusions
E. Spongiform encephalopathy

ANSWER: C

Lewy bodies are composed of alpha-synuclein intracytoplasmic inclusions. These also may be observed in major neurocognitive disorder due to Parkinson disease. Amyloid plaques and neurofibrillary tangles are characteristic neuropathology in Alzheimer disease. Intranuclear eosinophilic inclusions, or Cowdry bodies, are seen in subacute sclerosing panencephalitis. Spongiform encephalopathy is seen in major neurocognitive disorder due to prion disease, such as Creutzfeldt–Jakob disease.

REFERENCE

McKeith, I. G., Dickson, D. W., Lowe, J., Emre, M., O'Brien, J.T., Feldman, H.... Consortium on DLB. (2005). Diagnosis and management of dementia with Lewy bodies: Third report of the DLB consortium. *Neurology, 65*, 1863–1872.

46. In the fifth edition of the *Diagnostic and Statistic Manual of Mental Disorders* (*DSM*-5), neurocognitive impairment is now classified as mild or major neurocognitive disorder. What is an important distinction between these two categories?

A. Major neurocognitive disorder cannot be accounted for by delirium.
B. Deficits of mild neurocognitive disorder do not interfere with daily activities.
C. Major neurocognitive disorder requires subjective and objective concerns.
D. Major neurocognitive disorder represents a decline from a previous level of functioning.
E. Behavioral disturbances are observed only in major neurocognitive disorder.

ANSWER: B

One of the key distinctions between mild and major neurocognitive disorders in *DSM-5* is that patients with mild neurocognitive disorder do not have deficits that interfere with daily activities. Another distinction is that although patients with both conditions have some decline from their previous level of functioning, this decline is modest in mild neurocognitive disorder and significant in major neurocognitive disorder. Both groups show deficits on cognitive assessments, but mild neurocognitive disorder is classified by modest impairment, and major neurocognitive disorder is classified by substantial impairment. In both cases, symptoms cannot be accounted for by delirium, require subjective and objective concerns, and may or may not present with behavioral symptoms.

REFERENCE

American Psychiatric Association. (2013). *Diagnostic and statistical manual of mental disorders* (5th ed.). Arlington, VA: American Psychiatric Publishing.

47. A 65-year-old man presents to the emergency room for recurrent falls. On interview, his partner reports that he tends to fall backward. The partner also noted that the patient has had increasing difficulty solving puzzles in the past several months. Physical exam is notable for symmetric parkinsonism, axial rigidity, and vertical gaze palsy. The patient's gait is somewhat broad-based, and his facial expression appears surprised. What is the likely diagnosis?

A. Parkinson disease
B. Multisystem atrophy
C. Dopa-responsive dystonia
D. Progressive supranuclear palsy
E. Wilson disease

ANSWER: D

Progressive supranuclear palsy is in the group of neurodegenerative diseases termed *Parkinson-plus diseases* or *atypical parkinsonism*. Patients typically present with symmetric parkinsonism (versus Parkinson disease, which is typically asymmetric), axial rigidity, and vertical gaze palsy. Classically, their postural instability leads to backward falls. Gait is often slightly broad-based, as opposed to the short, shuffling steps seen in Parkinson disease. Cognitive impairment tends to be frontal/subcortical; in this case, difficulty with puzzles may be an example of executive dysfunction.

REFERENCE

Stamelou, M., & Bhatia, K. P. (2014). Atypical parkinsonism: Diagnosis and treatment. *Neurologic Clinics, 33*, 39–56.

48. A 79-year-old woman is diagnosed with major neurocognitive disorder due to Alzheimer disease. Her

primary care doctor is planning to initiate a cholinesterase inhibitor. Which of the following is true about the use of acetylcholinesterase inhibitors in major neurocognitive disorder due to Alzheimer disease?

A. Cholinesterase inhibitors stop cognitive decline but do not reverse existing impairment.
B. Cholinesterase inhibitors both stop and reverse cognitive decline.
C. Galantamine has superior efficacy relative to donepezil.
D. Donepezil has superior efficacy relative to galantamine.
E. Cognitive decline will continue despite cholinesterase inhibitor initiation.

ANSWER: E

Although there are small treatment effects in cognitive function observed among patients diagnosed with major neurocognitive disorder due to Alzheimer disease who take cholinesterase inhibitors, these medications neither stop nor reverse cognitive decline. Cognitive decline should be expected to continue, though the medications may attenuate this progression. There are no differences with respect to efficacy among the three cholinesterase inhibitors approved for treatment of major neurocognitive disorder due to Alzheimer disease (galantamine, donepezil, and rivastigmine).

REFERENCE

Birks, J. (2006). Cholinesterase inhibitors for Alzheimer's disease. *Cochrane Database of Systematic Reviews*, *25*, CD005593.

49. A 78-year-old man presents to a psychiatrist with symptoms of depressed mood, low energy, decreased motivation, poor concentration, and decreased appetite. In addition to treating depression, the psychiatrist performs a Mini Mental State Examination. The patient scores 23 out of 30 points. Which of the following statements is true regarding the relationship of depression and major neurocognitive disorders?

A. Depression is a risk factor for and may be early evidence of major neurocognitive disorder.
B. Treatment of depression should reverse cognitive symptoms and reduce the risk of future major neurocognitive disorder.
C. Elderly patients with cognitive symptoms during depression have the same risk for major neurocognitive disorder as those without cognitive symptoms.
D. Depression is a common symptom of major neurocognitive disorder due to Alzheimer disease but not of major vascular neurocognitive disorder.
E. Depression is associated with increased risk of major neurocognitive disorder only among patients younger than 75 years.

ANSWER: A

Depression is a risk factor for and may be an early sign of major neurocognitive disorder. Although treatment of depression may improve some associated cognitive symptoms, there is still increased risk of future neurocognitive decline. Elderly patients with cognitive symptoms during a depressive episode are more likely than depressed patients without cognitive symptoms to develop major neurocognitive disorder. Depression is seen in both major vascular neurocognitive disorder and major neurocognitive disorder due to Alzheimer disease and in fact may be more common in the former. Depression has been shown to be a risk factor for major neurocognitive disorder even among the oldest old.

REFERENCE

Aziz, R., & Steffens, D. C. (2013). What are the causes of late-life depression? *Psychiatry Clinics of North America*, *36*, 497–516.

50. Risk of major neurocognitive disorder due to Alzheimer disease in Down syndrome is linked to having three copies of which gene?

A. Presenilin 1
B. Presenilin 2
C. Amyloid precursor protein
D. Brain-derived neurotrophic factor
E. Apolipoprotein E, epsilon 4 allele

ANSWER: C

Major neurocognitive disorder due to Alzheimer's disease in Down syndrome (trisomy 21) is related to carrying three copies of the amyloid precursor protein gene, which resides on chromosome 21.

REFERENCE

Ness, S., Rafil, M., Aisen, P., Krams, M., Silverman, W., & Manji, H. (2012). Down's syndrome and Alzheimer's disease: Towards secondary prevention. *Nature Reviews Drug Discovery, 11*, 655–656.

QUESTIONS AND ANSWERS

This chapter has accompanying questions and answers which are available to subscribers as part of the Oxford eLearning platform. To access the questions, follow the link below, or go to http://oxford-elearning.oup.com/books.

http://oxford-elearning.oup.com/books/test/67/10.1093/med/9780190265557.003.0010

11.

TREATMENT OF NEUROPSYCHIATRIC DISORDERS

Michael Maksimowski, Rajesh Tampi

1. Which of the following is the mechanism of action of botulinum toxin used to treat focal dystonias?

A. Blocks release of acetylcholine at the neuromuscular junction
B. Depletes norepinephrine
C. Enhances acetylcholine activity
D. Blocks acetylcholine reuptake
E. Blocks serotonin activity

ANSWER: A

Botulinum toxin blocks the release of acetylcholine at the neuromuscular junction.

REFERENCE

Nigam, P. K., & Nigam, A. (2010). Botulinum toxin. *Indian Journal of Dermatology, 55*, 8–14.

2. Capsaicin acts as an analgesic by which of the following mechanisms?

A. Inhibiting the synthesis of arachidonic acid
B. Acting as an agonist at the kappa receptors
C. Defunctionalization of the nociceptor fibers
D. Antagonizing mu receptors
E. Antagonizing delta receptors

ANSWER: C

Capsaicin acts as an analgesic by defunctionalizing the nociceptor fibers. Defunctionalization occurs due to a number of effects, including a temporary loss of membrane potential, inability to transport neurotrophic factors leading to altered phenotype, and reversible retraction of epidermal and dermal nerve fiber terminals.

REFERENCES

Anand, P., & Bley, K. (2011). Topical capsaicin for pain management: Therapeutic potential and mechanisms of action of the new high-concentration capsaicin 8% patch. *Journal of Anesthesia, 107*, 490–502.

3. Which of the following drugs is a monoamine oxidase B (MAO-B) enzyme inhibitor used for treating motor symptoms in individuals with Parkinson's disease (PD)?

A. Selegiline
B. Bromocriptine
C. Pergolide
D. Pramipexole
E. Ropinirole

ANSWER: A

Selegiline is an MAO-B enzyme inhibitor that is used for treating motor symptoms in individuals with PD. It is available orally for management of PD under the trade name Eldepryl but as a patch for management of depression under the trade name Emsam. Bromocriptine, pergolide, pramipexole, and ropinirole are FDA-approved dopamine agonists used for treating motor symptoms in individuals with PD.

REFERENCE

Faulkner, M. A. (2014). Safety overview of FDA-approved medications for the treatment of the motor symptoms of Parkinson's disease. *Expert Opinion on Drug Safety, 13*, 1055–1069.

4. Which of the following drugs is not FDA approved for the treatment of mild Alzheimer's disease (AD)?

A. Donepezil
B. Rivastigmine
C. Galantamine
D. Memantine
E. All of the above

ANSWER: D

The acetylcholinesterase inhibitors: donepezil, rivastigmine, and galantamine are all FDA approved for the treatment of mild to moderate AD. The NMDA antagonist memantine is approved to treat moderate to severe AD only.

REFERENCE

Cummings, J. L., Isaacson, R. S., Schmitt, F A., & Velting, D. M. A practical algorithm for managing Alzheimer's disease: What, when, and why? *Annals of Clinical and Translational Neurology, 2*, 307–323.

5. In a 75-year-old woman with a major neurocognitive disorder due to Alzheimer's disease, mild severity, a trial with an acetylcholinesterase inhibitor is most likely to result in which one of the following adverse effects?

A. Syncope
B. Nausea
C. Diarrhea
D. Vomiting
E. Anorexia

ANSWER: B

Nausea is the most common adverse effect noted with the use of acetylcholinesterase inhibitors. This is followed by vomiting, diarrhea, anorexia, and syncope.

REFERENCE

Mimica, N., & Presecki, P. (2009). Side effects of approved antidementives. *Psychiatria Danubina, 21*, 108–113.

6. Which one of the following disorders is not an indication for treatment with deep brain stimulations (DBS)?

A. Obsessive–compulsive disorder
B. Schizophrenia
C. Parkinson's disease
D. Primary dystonias
E. Essential tremors

ANSWER: B

Schizophrenia is not an indication for DBS.

REFERENCE

Pandey, S., & Sarma, N. (2015). Deep brain stimulation: Current status. *Neurology India, 63*, 9–18.

7. Which of the following statements is TRUE regarding the treatment of tardive dyskinesia (TD)?

A. Resveratrol is FDA approved for the treatment of TD.
B. Ginkgo biloba is FDA approved for the treatment of TD.
C. Botulinum toxin is FDA approved for the treatment of TD.
D. Tetrabenazine is FDA approved for the treatment of TD.
E. Currently there are no FDA-approved treatments for TD.

ANSWER: E

Currently there are no FDA-approved treatments for TD.

REFERENCE

Rana, A. Q., Chaudry, Z. M., & Blanchet, P. J. (2013). New and emerging treatments for symptomatic tardive dyskinesia. *Drug Design Development and Therapy, 6*, 1329–1340.

8. Which of the following is NOT an essential step in the management of individuals with neuroleptic malignant syndrome (NMS)?

A. Stopping the dopamine blocking agent
B. Intravenous fluids
C. External cooling
D. Administration of cyproheptadine
E. Prescription of benzodiazepines to treat agitation

ANSWER: D

The serotonin antagonist cyproheptadine is not beneficial in the management of NMS. The dopamine agonist bromocriptine and dantrolene, which relaxes muscles by preventing calcium release from sarcoplasmic reticulum, may be beneficial in individuals with NMS.

REFERENCE

Musselman, M. E., & Saely, S. (2013). Diagnosis and treatment of drug-induced hyperthermia. *American Journal of Health-System Pharmacy, 70*, 34–42.

9. Which of the following interventions can worsen symptoms in individuals with serotonin syndrome?

A. Stopping the serotonergic agent
B. Intravenous fluids
C. External cooling
D. Administration of cyproheptadine
E. Administration of bromocriptine

ANSWER: E

Bromocriptine administration may worsen symptoms of serotonin syndrome. Cyproheptadine, which is antihistaminic and an antagonist of 5-HT1A and 5-HT2A receptors, or chlorpromazine, a phenothiazine with antagonistic activity at 5-HT2A receptors, may be used to treat serotonin syndrome.

REFERENCE

Musselman, M. E., & Saely, S. (2013). Diagnosis and treatment of drug-induced hyperthermia. *American Journal of Health-System Pharmacy, 70*, 34–42.

10. Which of the following drugs/drug classes is first-line treatment for Parkinson's disease?

A. Amantadine
B. Anticholinergics
C. Beta blockers
D. Levodopa
E. Catechol-O-methyl transferase inhibitors

ANSWER: D

Levodopa, dopamine agonists, and monoamine oxidase B inhibitors are first-line treatments for Parkinson's disease. Treatment options in advanced Parkinson's disease when oral and transdermal therapies are ineffective include catechol-O-methyl transferase inhibitors, deep brain stimulation, apomorphine, and intrajejunal levodopa gel infusion.

REFERENCE

Muzerengi, S., & Clarke, C. E. (2015). Initial drug treatment in Parkinson's disease. *British Medical Journal, 351*, h4669.

11. Which one of the following analgesics is not a Schedule II controlled drug according to the FDA?

A. Diacetylmorphine
B. Hydromorphone
C. Oxycodone
D. Methadone
E. Meperidine

ANSWER: A

All the drugs on the list except diacetylmorphine (i.e., heroin) are Schedule II controlled drugs. Diacetylmorphine is Schedule I drug. Notably, the opioid dihydrocodeine is Schedule III drug.

REFERENCE

Controlled Substances Schedules. Retrieved from http://www.deadiversion.usdoj.gov/schedules/index.html

12. Nephrolithiasis is associated with the use of which of the following antiseizure drugs?

A. Divalproex
B. Gabapentin
C. Carbamazepine
D. Topiramate
E. Lamotrigine

ANSWER: D

Nephrolithiasis is associated with the use of topiramate by way of increasing bicarbonate.

REFERENCE

Dell'Orto, V. G., Belotti, E. A., Goeggel-Simonetti, B., Simonetti, G. D., Ramelli, G. P., Bianchetti, M. G., & Lava, S. A. (2014). Metabolic disturbances and renal stone promotion on treatment with topiramate: A systematic review. *British Journal of Clinical Pharmacology, 77*, 958–964.

13. A 70-year-old man is diagnosed with neuropathic pain. Which one of the following medications is least likely to benefit this individual?

A. Gabapentin
B. Acetaminophen
C. Tricyclic antidepressant
D. Serotonin–norepinephrine reuptake inhibitor
E. Carbamazepine

ANSWER: B

Acetaminophen is least likely to benefit individuals with neuropathic pain.

REFERENCE

Wong, C. S., Hui, G. K., Chung, E. K., & Wong, S. H. (2014). Diagnosis and management of neuropathic pain. *Pain Management, 4*, 221–231.

14. A 45-year-old woman is diagnosed with multiple sclerosis (MS). Which of the following disease-modifying agents are FDA approved for use in this individual?

A. Interferon beta-1a
B. Interferon beta-1b
C. Glatiramer acetate
D. Natalizumab
E. All of the above

ANSWER: E

All of the above-mentioned drugs are FDA approved for use in individuals with MS.

REFERENCE

Tavazzi, E., Rovaris, M., & La Mantia, L. (2014). Drug therapy for multiple sclerosis. *Canadian Medical Association Journal, 186*, 833–840.

15. Which one of the following drugs is most likely to worsen symptoms of restless legs syndrome (RLS)?

A. Aripiprazole
B. Carbidopa/levodopa
C. Ropinirole
D. Rotigotine transdermal patch
E. Gabapentin

ANSWER: A

About a third of patients with aripiprazole develop akathisia according to its package insert, and the "restlessness" in RLS is a form of nocturnal akathisia. Epidemiological evidence remains inconclusive as to whether SSRIs improve or worsen RLS symptoms. All the other drugs that are listed are used to treat individuals with RLS.

REFERENCE

Comella, C. L. (2014). Treatment of restless legs syndrome. *Neurotherapeutics, 11*, 177–187.

EXTRA QUESTION

Which of the following psychotropics may improve symptoms of restless legs syndrome (RLS)?

A. Sertraline
B. Venlafaxine
C. Risperidone
D. Haloperidol
E. Bupropion

ANSWER: E

Bupropion may improve symptoms of RLS while also improving symptoms of depression, likely due to its dopaminergic activity.

REFERENCE

Bayard, M., Bailey, B., Acharya, D., Ambreen, F., Duggal, S., Kaur, T., & Tudiver, F. (2011). Bupropion and restless legs syndrome: A randomized controlled trial. *Journal of the American Board of Family Medicine, 24*, 422–428.

16. Which of the following is not part of the multimodal approach to treating individuals with fibromyalgia?

A. Education
B. Cognitive behavioral therapy
C. Aerobic exercise
D. Pharmacological therapy
E. Electroconvulsive therapy

ANSWER: E

Electroconvulsive therapy is not part of the multimodal approach to treating individuals with fibromyalgia.

REFERENCE

Borchers, A. T., & Gershwin, M. E. (2015). Fibromyalgia: A critical and comprehensive review. *Clinical Reviews in Allergy and Immunology, 49, 100–151.*

17. Which of the following drug classes has not shown benefit in the treatment of individuals with fibromyalgia?

A. Opioids
B. Tricyclic antidepressants
C. Anticonvulsants
D. Muscle relaxants
E. Serotonin–norepinephrine reuptake inhibitors

ANSWER: A

There is no data supporting the use of opioids in individuals with fibromyalgia.

REFERENCE

Borchers, A. T., & Gershwin, M. E. (2015). Fibromyalgia: A critical and comprehensive review. *Clinical Reviews in Allergy and Immunology, 49*, 100–151.

18. Which of the following areas of the brain is a common target for implants in deep brain stimulation (DBS) for individuals with advanced Parkinson's disease?

A. Caudate nucleus
B. Globus pallidus internus (GPi)
C. Putamen
D. Nucleus accumbens
E. Substantia nigra

ANSWER: B

Globus pallidus internus (GPi) and subthalamic nucleus (STN) are two areas in the basal ganglia that are considered common targets for DBS in the treatment of individuals with advanced Parkinson's disease.

REFERENCE

Liu, Y., Li, W., Tan, C., Liu, X., Wang, X., Gui, Y., & Chen, L. (2014). Meta-analysis comparing deep brain stimulation of the globus pallidus and subthalamic nucleus to treat advanced Parkinson disease. *Journal of Neurosurgery, 121*, 709–718.

19. A 60-year-old man with schizophrenia on clozapine 600 mg/day develops generalized seizures. Which one of the following anticonvulsant medications would not be an appropriate medication to treat this individual's seizures?

A. Sodium valproate
B. Carbamazepine
C. Gabapentin
D. Topiramate
E. Lamotrigine

ANSWER: B

Carbamazepine in combination with clozapine may increase the risk for blood dyscrasias, including neutropenia/agranulocytosis, and hence should be avoided in individuals who are being treated with clozapine.

REFERENCE

Caetano, D. (2014). Use of anticonvulsants as prophylaxis for seizures in patients on clozapine. *Australasian Psychiatry, 22*, 78–83.

20. Chronic use of which one of the following anticonvulsants can result in gingival hyperplasia?

A. Vigabatrin
B. Phenytoin
C. Levetiracetam
D. Topiramate
E. Lamotrigine

ANSWER: B

Gingival hyperplasia is common with the chronic use of phenytoin.

REFERENCE

Cornacchio, A. L., Burneo, J. G., & Aragon, C. E. (2011) The effects of antiepileptic drugs on oral health. *Journal of the Canadian Dental Association, 77*, b140.

21. A 50-year-old, recently divorced man presents with recurrent headaches for the past 6 months. He describes these headaches as a feeling of tightness around his head that fluctuates in intensity. He denies a history of aura, photophobia, or phonophobia. Given this patient's history, which one of the following medications would be most appropriate for the treatment for his symptoms?

A. Caffeine
B. Sumatriptan
C. Nonsteroidal anti-inflammatory drugs (NSAIDs)
D. Codeine
E. Ergotamine

ANSWER: C

The patient has symptoms consistent with tension-type headache. NSAIDs and other simple analgesics are indicated for the treatment of this type of headache. Caffeine, sumatriptan, codeine, and ergotamine have the potential for rebound headaches and are not indicated in the treatment of tension-type headaches.

REFERENCE

Beran, R. G. (2014). Management of chronic headache. *Australian Family Physician, 43*, 106–110.

22. Which of the following drugs is considered abortive therapy for migraines?

A. Sumatriptan
B. Amitriptyline
C. Topiramate
D. Propranolol
E. Carbamazepine

ANSWER: A

Sumatriptan, other triptans, and NSAIDs (with or without antiemetics) are abortive therapy for migraine, which means they "abort" an acute migraine. The other options are for migraine prophylaxis.

REFERENCE

Sinclair, A. J., Sturrock, A., Davies, B., & Matharu, M. (2015). Headache management: Pharmacological approaches. *Practical Neurology, 15*, 411–423.

23. Which of the following antidepressants has not been associated with serotonin syndrome when prescribed with tramadol?

A. Mirtazapine
B. Fluoxetine
C. Paroxetine
D. Citalopram
E. Bupropion

ANSWER: E

Among the antidepressants above, only bupropion has not been reported to cause serotonin syndrome when prescribed with tramadol. However, caution should be taken when these two drugs are prescribed together because there is a greater theoretical risk of seizures with the combination treatment.

REFERENCE

Park, S. H., Wackernah, R. C., & Stimmel, G. L. (2014). Serotonin syndrome: Is it a reason to avoid the use of tramadol with antidepressants? *Journal of Pharmacy Practice, 27*, 71–78.

24. Which one of the following is NOT a standard treatment for myasthenia gravis?

A. Botulinum toxin
B. Pyridostigmine
C. Azathioprine
D. Plasma exchange
E. Thymectomy

ANSWER: A

Of these options, only botulinum toxin is not indicated for the treatment of myasthenia gravis.

REFERENCE

Gilhus, N. E., & Verschuuren, J. J. (2015). Myasthenia gravis: Subgroup classification and therapeutic strategies. *Lancet Neurology, 14*, 1023–1036.

25. Which of the following medications may improve survival in amyotrophic lateral sclerosis (ALS) by about 3 to 6 months?

A. Tamoxifen
B. Namenda
C. Riluzole
D. Ropinirole
E. Pyridostigmine

ANSWER: C

Riluzole is a benzothiazole derivative that modulates glutamatergic activity, thereby theoretically reducing excitotoxicity. It may slightly improve the course of ALS and prolong survival by 3 to 6 months.

REFERENCE

Orsini, M., Oliveira, A. B., Nascimento, O. J., Reis, C. H., Leite, M. A., de Souza, J. A., & Smidt, B. (2015). Amyotrophic lateral sclerosis: New perspectives and update. *Neurology International, 24*, 5885.

26. Which of the following antiepileptic medications is emerging as a drug of choice for use in pregnant women?

A. Phenytoin
B. Levetiracetam
C. Topiramate
D. Valproic acid
E. Carbamazepine

ANSWER: B

Levetiracetam appears to be emerging as the antiepileptic drug of choice for use in pregnant women. Valproic acid, lamotrigine, carbamazepine, topiramate, and phenobarbital have all been reported to increase the risk of fetal malformations at higher dosages in pregnant women.

REFERENCE

Eadie, M. J. (2014). Treating epilepsy in pregnant women. *Expert Opinion on Pharmacotherapy, 15*, 841–850.

27. Which one of the following neurosurgical procedures may be effective for obsessive–compulsive disorder (OCD) refractory to pharmacotherapy?

A. Anterior cingulotomy
B. Thalamotomy
C. Pallidotomy
D. Anterior lobotomy
E. Hippocampal resection

ANSWER: A

Anterior cingulotomy (creating a lesion in the dorsal anterior cingulate) and anterior capsulotomy (lesioning the inferior fronto-thalamic connections of the anterior limb of the internal capsule) may be effective for medication-resistant OCD.

REFERENCE

Fineberg, N. A., Reghunandanan, S., Simpson H. B., Phillips, K. A., Richter, M. A., Matthews, K., & Accreditation Task Force of The Canadian Institute for Obsessive Compulsive Disorders. (2015). Obsessive–compulsive disorder (OCD): Practical strategies for pharmacological and somatic treatment in adults. *Psychiatry Research, 227*, 114–125.

28. Which one of the following medications is a first-line agent for the prophylaxis of cluster headaches?

A. 100% oxygen
B. Verapamil
C. Lithium
D. Topiramate
E. Intranasal zolmitriptan

ANSWER: B

Verapamil is a first-line prophylactic agent for cluster headaches. Lithium is a second-line agent, followed by topiramate. Both 100% oxygen and intranasal zolmitriptan are abortive (acute) agents for this condition.

REFERENCE

Becker, W. J., Findlay, T., Moga, C., Scott, N. A., Harstall, C., & Taenzer, P. (2015). Guideline for primary care management of headache in adults. *Canadian Family Physician, 61*, 670–679.

29. Which of the following statements is NOT true of bright light therapy (BLT) for major depressive disorder, recurrent, with seasonal pattern?

A. 10,000 lux is recommended.
B. Thirty minutes a day is recommended.
C. Early morning use is recommended.
D. Onset of therapeutic effect is within 3 to 7 days of initiation.
E. Therapeutic effect is maintained for more than a month after discontinuation.

ANSWER: E

The therapeutic effect of BLT often vanishes shortly after discontinuation of treatment.

REFERENCE

Pail, G., Huf, W., Pjrek, E., Willeit, M., Praschak-Rieder, N., & Kasper, S. (2011). Bright-light therapy in the treatment of mood disorders. *Neuropsychobiology, 2011*, 152–162.

30. Which of the following accurately describes the role of biofeedback in psychiatric disorder?

A. Biofeedback is used mostly for personality disorders.
B. There are standardized protocols for specific psychiatric disorders.
C. Electroencephalographic neurofeedback is the most studied modality.
D. Unimodal biofeedback is the most effective modality for symptom control.
E. A minority of published articles report statistically significant symptom improvement.

ANSWER: C

Electroencephalographic neurofeedback is the most studied form of biofeedback. Standardized protocols for specific conditions do not exist. Biofeedback has been studied most in anxiety disorders. Multimodal biofeedback is considered the most effective modality. A recent systematic review found that 65% of published articles report a statistically significant improvement on standardized measures.

REFERENCE

Schoenberg, P. L., & David, A. S. (2014). Biofeedback for psychiatric disorders: A systematic review. *Applied Psychophysiology and Biofeedback, 39*, 109–135.

31. Which of the following correctly describes the role of electroconvulsive therapy (ECT) in individuals with Parkinson's disease (PD)?

A. ECT has no role.
B. ECT improves mood symptoms without effect on motor symptoms.
C. ECT improves mood symptoms but worsens motor symptoms.
D. ECT improves mood and motor symptoms.
E. ECT worsens both mood and motor symptoms.

ANSWER: D

ECT improves motor and nonmotor symptoms of PD and is well tolerated in those with the condition. In fact, numerous reports document the beneficial effects of ECT in nondepressed patients with PD. However, the duration of benefit with ECT in individuals with PD remains unclear.

REFERENCE

Popeo, D., & Kellner, C. H. (2009). ECT for Parkinson's disease. *Medical Hypotheses, 73*, 468–469.

32. Which of the following is true of chronotherapy in the treatment of psychiatric disorders?

A. Chronotherapy has documented effectiveness in psychotic patients.
B. The clinical improvements produced by chronotherapy persist after treatment.
C. Wake therapy with sleep-phase advance is an approach to chronotherapy.
D. Chronotherapy is not cost-effective in the treatment of psychiatric disorders.
E. All of the above.

ANSWER: C

Chronotherapy has documented, rapid effectiveness in depressed patients. The clinical improvements seen with chronotherapy are generally short-lived unless light therapy or pharmacotherapy is continued. Wake therapy (historically, framed in the negative as partial or total sleep deprivation) is commonly employed with sleep-phase advance chronotherapy. When these two are combined with bright light therapy, this is known as "triple chronotherapy." Additional benefits of chronotherapy include cost-effectiveness, good tolerability and reduced length of inpatient hospital days.

REFERENCE

Casher, M., Schuldt, S., Haq, A., & Burkhead-Weiner, D. (2012). Chronotherapy in treatment-resistant depression. *Psychiatric Annals, 42*, 166–169

33. Which of the following is CORRECT regarding the comparison between repeated transcranial magnetic stimulation (rTMS) and electroconvulsive therapy (ECT) for the treatment of major depressive disorder?

A. rTMS has higher response and remission rates than ECT.
B. The discontinuation rate is greater for ECT than for rTMS.
C. ECT is clearly superior to rTMS in psychotic depression.
D. rTMS causes more cognitive impairment than ECT.
E. All of the above.

ANSWER: C

A recent meta-analysis compared studies of rTMS and ECT for major depression and included data from nine trials. The researchers found ECT is superior to high-frequency rTMS in terms of response and remission rates (p = .006) and that discontinuation rate was not significantly different between the two treatments (p = .80). The superiority of ECT was more apparent in those with psychotic depression, whereas high-frequency rTMS was as effective as ECT in those with nonpsychotic depression. The researchers obtained the same results when comparing ECT with low-frequency rTMS. Both rTMS and ECT were well tolerated, with only minor side effects reported. These studies suggested that specific cognitive domains such as visual memory and verbal fluency were more impaired in patients receiving ECT rather than rTMS.

REFERENCE

Ren, J., Li, H., Palaniyappan, L., Liu, H., Wang, J., Li, C., & Rossini, P. M. (2014). Repetitive transcranial magnetic stimulation versus electroconvulsive therapy for major depression: A systematic review and meta-analysis. *Progress in Neuro-Psychopharmacology and Biological Psychiatry, 51*, 181–189.

34. Which of the following is TRUE of vagal nerve stimulation (VNS)?

A. The main indication for its use is the treatment of refractory schizophrenia.
B. It is ineffective for the treatment of unipolar or bipolar depression.
C. It is ineffective for the treatment of refractory epilepsy.
D. It does not appear to cause cognitive impairment.
E. All of the above.

ANSWER: D

VNS involves the surgical implantation of a pulse generator in the chest that is connected to a stimulating electrode, which is attached to the vagus nerve in the neck. It has been found to be effective for the treatment of refractory epilepsy. VNS reduces seizure frequency but does not usually allow patients to stop anticonvulsant medication treatment. VNS causes an alteration to voice, neck discomfort, cough, dysphagia, and shortness of breath, with the vocal changes potentially persisting over time. However, VNS does not appear to cause cognitive impairment. VNS is also approved by the FDA for the treatment of unipolar or bipolar depression that has not responded to at least four medication trials, though effects are relatively modest.

REFERENCE

Fitzgerald, P. B. (2011). The emerging use of brain stimulation treatments for psychiatric disorders. *Australian and New Zealand Journal of Psychiatry, 45*, 923–938.

35. Which of the following is TRUE regarding ketamine administration for depression?

A. Depressive symptoms improve significantly with ketamine treatment.
B. Ketamine is effective only for unipolar depression, not bipolar depression.
C. Ketamine is effective only in drug-free individuals with depression.
D. Antidepressant effects of ketamine for depression last for at least a month.
E. All of the above.

ANSWER: A

A recent meta-analysis that included data from nine non-ECT studies indicated that depression scores are significantly decreased in the ketamine groups when compared with those in the control groups ($p < .01$). Ketamine's efficacy was confirmed in major depressive disorder (resistant to previous pharmacological treatments or not, $p < .01$), in bipolar depression, in drug-free individuals, and in individuals on antidepressants. The duration of ketamine's effects was assessed in only two non-ECT studies that showed that the effect persists for 2 to 3 days. Three of four studies found significant decrease of suicidal thoughts, and one found no difference between groups. The dose of ketamine used in most studies was 0.5 mg/kg. Transient blood pressure elevation that may require treatment was noted in the studies.

REFERENCE

Fond, G., Loundou, A., Rabu, C., Macgregor, A., Lançon, C., Brittner, M., & Boyer, L. (2014). Ketamine administration in depressive disorders: A systematic review and meta-analysis. *Psychopharmacology (Berlin), 231*, 3663–3676.

36. Which of the following is considered a first-line agent for the management of psychotic symptoms in Parkinson's disease?

A. Clozapine
B. Quetiapine
C. Risperidone
D. Discontinuation of dopaminergics

ANSWER: B

The FDA approved the 5-HT2A receptor inverse agonist pimavanserin (Nuplazid) as first-in-class for hallucinations and delusions associated with Parkinson's disease shortly before this book's printing. The most common cause of psychosis in Parkinson's disease is iatrogenic (medications), but there are multiple risk factors that include older age, disease severity, sleep disturbance, cognitive impairment, dementia, and depression. Whereas discontinuation of dopaminergics such as levodopa may improve psychotic symptoms, it would certainly lead to a return of Parkinson's disease motor symptoms. Quetiapine is widely the first-line medication for use in psychosis related to Parkinson's disease, although clozapine may be considered if quetiapine is ineffective.

REFERENCE

Zahodne, L. B., & Fernandez, H. H. (2008). Pathophysiology and treatment of psychosis in Parkinson's disease. *Drugs and Aging, 25*, 665–682.

37. Which of the following clinical features should be considered a contraindication to using the revised Clinical Institute Withdrawal Assessment for Alcohol (CIWA-Ar) for alcohol detoxification?

A. Concurrent epilepsy diagnosis
B. Alcoholic hallucinosis
C. Mild alcohol symptoms
D. Delirium
E. Cirrhosis

ANSWER: D

CIWA-Ar is a widely used scale for symptom-triggered management of alcohol withdrawal, but its score is invalid in delirium because more than half of its questions require subjective self-report. It should not be used when a patient has delirium tremens, Wernicke's encephalopathy, or delirium of other cause in the context of alcohol withdrawal.

REFERENCE

Sadock, B. J., & Sadock, V. A. (2007). *Kaplan and Sadock's synopsis of psychiatry* (9th ed., p. 398). Philadelphia, PA: Lippincott Williams and Wilkins.

38. Which of the following is the most appropriate initial treatment of primary insomnia?

A. Polysomnography
B. Short-term zolpidem prescription
C. Education on sleep hygiene
D. Trazodone prescription
E. A nightcap

ANSWER: C

Sleep hygiene refers to practices that tend to improve and/or maintain good sleep. These include consistent bedtime and wake time; elimination of alcohol, caffeine, and tobacco; healthy sleep environment; and physical activity during the day. Often subsumed under the category of sleep hygiene is stimulus control therapy, which includes going to bed only when sleepy, reserving the bedroom for sleep (and sex) only, and getting out of bed if awake after 20 minutes. All patients with insomnia should first receive basic counseling on sleep hygiene. Patients who continue to have insomnia after sleep hygiene issues are addressed warrant further interventions, which can include referral for cognitive behavioral therapy for insomnia, polysomnography, and/or medications. A nightcap (alcohol before bedtime) suppresses REM sleep and leads to greater risk of awakening in the second half of the night; it therefore is not recommended.

REFERENCE

Stepanski, E. J., & Wyatt, J. K. (2003). Use of sleep hygiene in the treatment of insomnia. *Sleep Medicine Reviews, 7,* 215–225.

39. Which of the following has NO role in the management of neuroleptic malignant syndrome (NMS)?

A. Lorazepam
B. Amantadine
C. Dantrolene
D. Bromocriptine
E. Lithium

ANSWER: E

NMS is a neurological emergency that warrants immediate clinical intervention once diagnosed. Recommendations for specific treatment in NMS are based primarily on case reports and anecdotal evidence and include dopamine agonists (amantadine, bromocriptine), skeletal muscle relaxants (dantrolene), and benzodiazepines. Concurrent use of lithium with antipsychotics is a risk factor for NMS.

REFERENCE

Sadock, B. J., & Sadock, V. A. (2007). *Kaplan and Sadock's synopsis of psychiatry* (9th ed., pp. 995–996). Philadelphia, PA: Lippincott Williams and Wilkins.

40. A patient with psychotic decompensation receives an intramuscular injection of olanzapine for pharmacological restraint in the emergency room for violent behavior. Which of the following medications should be avoided at this time?

A. Oral olanzapine
B. Intramuscular chlorpromazine
C. Orally disintegrating risperidone
D. Intravenous haloperidol
E. Intramuscular lorazepam

ANSWER: E

Intramuscular olanzapine leads to a maximum serum concentration five times that of its oral formulation and can cause cardiorespiratory failure due to excessive sedation when combined with parenteral benzodiazepines. Per the package insert for injectable olanzapine, "Concomitant administration of intramuscular olanzapine and parenteral benzodiazepine is not recommended due to the potential for excessive sedation and cardiorespiratory depression."

REFERENCE

National Library of Medicine (2015, July 30). *Olanzapine injection, powder, for solution.* Retrieved from https://dailymed.nlm.nih.gov/dailymed

41. What is the most effective treatment for recurrent focal dystonia?

A. Surgical denervation
B. Haloperidol
C. Trihexyphenidyl
D. Botulinum toxin
E. Reserpine

ANSWER: D

Botulinum toxin is an effective treatment in several neurological diseases, including cervical dystonia, blepharospasm, spasmodic dysphonia (laryngeal dystonia), and other focal dystonias. Reserpine, from *Rauwolfia* extract, causes monoamine depletion via VMAT-2 inhibition and is approved for use in hypertension and agitated psychotic states. Haloperidol can cause a dystonic reaction. Trihexyphenidyl may be useful in the treatment of dystonic reactions related to a medication (e.g., antipsychotic) is but not as effective as botulinum toxin. Surgical denervation is an invasive procedure that is used as a last resort for debilitating dystonias.

REFERENCE

Comella, C. L., & Pullman, S. L. (2004). Botulinum toxins in neurological disease. *Muscle and Nerve, 29*, 628–644.

42. Which of the following is the most effective treatment for chorea associated with Huntington's disease?

A. Levodopa
B. Selegiline
C. Clonidine
D. Amantadine
E. Tetrabenazine

ANSWER: E

Tetrabenazine is the only approved medication for dyskinesias in Huntington's disease and is effective at treating chorea, a hyperkinetic disorder due to hypersensitivity and/or hyperactivity of dopamine receptors. Tetrabenazine is a reversible inhibitor of VMAT-2, which leads to depletion of monoamines, including dopamine. Antipsychotic agents may also have some effect in treating chorea.

REFERENCE

Paleacu, D. (2007). Tetrabenazine in the treatment of Huntington's disease. *Neuropsychiatric Disease and Treatment, 3*, 545.

43. Which of the following drugs is a first-line agent in the treatment of absence seizures?

A. Primidone
B. Phenytoin
C. Lamotrigine
D. Ethosuximide
E. Carbamazepine

ANSWER: D

The FDA has approved ethosuximide and valproic acid as the first-line treatment for absence seizures. These two agents are more effective than lamotrigine in treating absence seizures in childhood, and ethosuximide in particular is associated with fewer attentional deficits.

REFERENCE

Glauser, T. A., Cnaan, A., Shinnar, S., Hirtz, D. G., Dlugos, D., Masur, D., et al. (2010). Ethosuximide, valproic acid, and lamotrigine in childhood absence epilepsy. *New England Journal of Medicine, 362*, 790–799.

44. Based on current evidence, thrombolysis for ischemic stroke reduces which of the following?

A. Risk of mortality and disability
B. Risk of mortality only
C. Risk of disability only
D. Risk of nursing home placement only

ANSWER: C

Treatment of strokes with thrombolysis improves chances of absence of disability but not survival.

REFERENCE

Wardlaw, J. M., Murray, V., Berge, E., & del Zoppo, G. J. (2014). Thrombolysis for acute ischaemic stroke. *Cochrane Database of Systematic Reviews, 7*, 1–56 doi:10.1002/14651858.CD000213

45. Which of the following medications is used to treat motor tics?

A. Pemoline
B. Pimozide
C. Paroxetine
D. Chlorpromazine
E. Protriptyline

ANSWER: B

Pimozide is a high-potency typical antipsychotic, more potent than haloperidol. High-potency antipsychotics like pimozide are the mainstay of treatment for motor tics. Pemoline is a stimulant that was used to treat attention deficit hyperactivity disorder (ADHD) but is no longer available in the United States due to risk of liver failure in children. Paroxetine is a selective serotonin reuptake inhibitor. Chlorpromazine is a low-potency antipsychotic and thus not effective in treating motor tics. Protriptyline is a tricyclic antidepressant used to treat depression and ADHD. The alpha-2 agonists clonidine and guanfacine are also among the first-line agents to treat motor tics.

REFERENCE

Eddy, C. M., Rickards, H. E., & Cavanna, A. E. (2011). Treatment strategies for tics in Tourette syndrome. *Therapeutic Advances in Neurological Disorders, 4*, 25–45.

46. A 43-year-old man with a history of stroke presents after his partner reported he was attacking him in his sleep. Upon wakening, the patient was able to vividly recall a dream that he thinks provoked the aggression. What is the treatment of choice?

A. Quetiapine
B. Zolpidem
C. Clonazepam
D. Doxepin
E. Chlordiazepoxide

ANSWER: C

This is a case of REM sleep behavior disorder, which is characterized by complex, occasionally violent behavior that represents the acting out of a dream. It is most commonly seen in elderly men with a history of central nervous system insults and synucleinopathies such as major neurocognitive disorder with Lewy bodies or Parkinson's disease. The most commonly used treatment for this disorder is clonazepam, although carbamazepine has also proved effective.

REFERENCE

Sadock, B. J., & Sadock, V. A. (2007). *Kaplan and Sadock's synopsis of psychiatry* (9th ed., p. 768). Philadelphia, PA: Lippincott Williams and Wilkins.

47. Which of the following drugs is most likely to be effective in the treatment of restless legs syndrome?

A. Gabapentin
B. Trihexyphenidyl
C. Lamotrigine
D. Topiramate
E. Risperidone

ANSWER: A

Restless legs syndrome, elevated to an independent diagnosis in *DSM-5*, is a distressing urge to move one's legs. It is thought to be related to a depletion of dopamine and/or iron in the body. Whereas dopamine agonists such as levodopa, pergolide, and pramipexole have been the treatments of choice, they are known to cause augmentation (i.e., worsening) of symptoms. As a result, the alpha-2 delta calcium channel ligands such as gabapentin have become increasingly considered first-line agents in this condition.

REFERENCE

Rinaldi, F., Galbiati, A., Marelli, S., Strambi, L. F., & Zucconi, M. (2016). Treatment options in intractable restless legs syndrome/Willis-Ekbom disease (RLS/WED). *Current Treatment Options in Neurology, 18*(2), 1–9.

48. What is the suggested mechanism of action of tricyclic antidepressants in relieving neuropathic pain?

A. Peripheral nerve regeneration
B. Dopamine reuptake inhibition in brain reward pathways
C. Modulation of opioid receptors
D. Modulation of GABA receptors
E. Apoptosis of nociceptors

ANSWER: C

Tricyclic antidepressants (TCAs) have serotonergic and noradrenergic properties, which made them particularly useful in the treatment of depression when they were first discovered. Several studies have suggested that TCAs also exhibit direct and indirect actions on opioid receptors and have been effective in the treatment of chronic and neuropathic pain conditions. Other proposed mechanisms of pain modulation involve release of norepinephrine from descending pathways, which suppresses pain perception in peripheral neurons as well as modulation of voltage-gated sodium channels.

REFERENCE

Sawynok, J., Esser, M. J., & Reid, A. R. (2001). Antidepressants as analgesics: An overview of central and peripheral mechanisms of action. *Journal of Psychiatry & Neuroscience, 26*, 21–29.

49. You are seeing a 75-year-old woman with major neurocognitive disorder, diminished reflexes, poor proprioception, dysesthesia, and anemia. Which of the following abnormal lab values is likely to reveal the cause of these symptoms?

A. Elevated methylmalonic acid
B. Elevated cobalamin
C. Reduced niacin
D. Reduced thiamine
E. Reduced pyridoxine

ANSWER: A

Vitamin B12 (cobalamin) deficiency is characterized by cognitive impairment, hyporeflexia, subacute combined degeneration of the spinal cord (leading to limited proprioception), and megaloblastic anemia (with elevated mean corpuscular volume) and in severe cases can mimic dementia. However, elevation in methylmalonic acid levels is more directly correlated with functional B12 deficiency. Vitamin B1 (thiamine) deficiency leads to Wernicke–Korsakoff syndrome, as well as dry beriberi (neuropathy) and wet beriberi (cardiomyopathy). Vitamin B3 (niacin) deficiency is characterized by diarrhea and dermatitis. Vitamin B6 (pyridoxine) deficiency is characterized by seborrheic dermatitis, glossitis, and somnolence. Vitamin C deficiency (scurvy) is characterized by fatigue, easy bruising, bleeding diathesis, and extrapyramidal symptoms. Vitamin E deficiency is rare and characterized by several neurological deficits (retinopathy, dysarthria, loss of deep tendon reflexes, poor proprioception) but does not cause cognitive issues.

REFERENCE

Kaufman, D. M. (2013). *Clinical neurology for psychiatrists* (7th ed., pp. 65–66). Philadelphia, PA: Elsevier Health Sciences.

50. Which of the following is not considered a disease-modifying treatment for multiple sclerosis?

A. Methylprednisolone
B. Beta interferon 1a
C. Glatiramer acetate
D. Beta interferon 1b

ANSWER: A

Multiple sclerosis (MS) is treated both symptomatically and through immunomodulators, otherwise known as disease-modifying agents. High-dose steroids such as methylprednisolone are the mainstay of treatment for MS flares. Immunomodulators such as beta interferon and glatiramer acetate interrupt T cell activity and reduce central nervous system inflammation.

REFERENCE

Kaufman, D. M. (2013). *Clinical neurology for psychiatrists* (7th ed., p. 337). Philadelphia, PA: Elsevier Health Sciences.

QUESTIONS AND ANSWERS

This chapter has accompanying questions and answers which are available to subscribers as part of the Oxford eLearning platform. To access the questions, follow the link below, or go to http://oxford-elearning.oup.com/books.

http://oxford-elearning.oup.com/books/test/67/10.1093/med/9780190265557.003.0011

12.

DIAGNOSTIC AND CLINICAL EVALUATION OF NEUROLOGICAL DISORDERS AND SYNDROMES

Kristina Zdanys, Kamalika Roy, Shirshendu Sinha

1. A 17-year-old female presents to her primary care doctor to evaluate headache. She reports that in the past year she has had six episodes of severe throbbing pain on the left side of her head. She has associated nausea and sensitivity to light. These symptoms are most consistent with which of the following?

A. Migraine headache
B. Cluster headache
C. Temporal arteritis
D. Postherpetic neuralgia
E. Tension-type headache

ANSWER: A

Migraine headache is classified by at least five attacks lasting 4 to 72 hours (untreated) with two of the following: unilateral location, pulsating quality, moderate or severe pain intensity, or aggravation by or avoidance of physical activity; and also with one of the following: nausea/vomiting or photophobia/phonophobia. Symptoms are not better accounted for by another diagnosis.

REFERENCE

Headache Classification Committee of the International Headache Society (IHS). (2013). The International Classification of Headache Disorders, 3rd edition (beta version). *Cephalalgia*, *33*, 629–808.

2. A 30-year-old woman presents to the emergency room for "going blind." She reports that for 30 minutes prior to arrival at the hospital, the center of her vision appeared gray. While the woman was waiting in the emergency room for 15 minutes, the obscured vision resolved, but she develops a unilateral headache on the right side. What most likely accounts for the patient's visual changes?

A. Partial seizure with sensory symptoms
B. Pituitary tumor
C. Cocaine intoxication
D. Migraine aura
E. Retinal detachment

ANSWER: D

Visual auras occur in more than 90% of patients who present with migraine with aura. Characteristic visual changes may include scotoma ("blind spot," as experienced by this patient), zigzag lines with angulated scintillating edges, or a combination. Other changes that may be seen in aura include tactile or olfactory sensations, dysarthria/aphasia, and motor weakness. Symptoms spread gradually, typically last 5 to 60 minutes, and are followed by headache.

REFERENCE

Headache Classification Committee of the International Headache Society (IHS). (2013). The International Classification of Headache Disorders, 3rd edition (beta version). *Cephalalgia*, *33*, 629–808.

3. A 34-year-old man presents to a neurologist requesting disability paperwork for severe headache that causes him to miss work. The headaches, which happen several times per day and last for 1 to 2 hours, occur in the right orbital area. Associated symptoms include tearing of the right eye, nasal congestion, and ptosis. What is the most likely diagnosis?

A. Migraine headache
B. Cluster headache
C. Temporal arteritis
D. Tension-type headache
E. Malingering

ANSWER: B

Cluster headaches are characterized by severe unilateral pain lasting up to 3 hours and occurring in series, from once every other day up to eight times daily. Associated symptoms include "ipsilateral conjunctival injection, lacrimation, nasal congestion, rhinorrhea, forehead/facial sweating, miosis, ptosis, and/or eyelids oedema, and/or with restlessness or agitation."

REFERENCE

Headache Classification Committee of the International Headache Society (IHS). (2013). The International Classification of Headache Disorders, 3rd edition (beta version). *Cephalalgia*, *33*, 629–808.

4. A 20-year-old obese woman presents to the emergency room for headache. On exam, she demonstrates papilledema. A neurologist performs a lumbar puncture and finds the opening pressure to be 285 mm cerebrospinal fluid (CSF) The patient's headache improves after repeated lumbar puncture. Her presentation is most consistent with:

A. Meningococcal meningitis
B. Normal pressure hydrocephalus
C. Idiopathic intracranial hypertension
D. Benign intracranial mass lesion
E. Cluster headache

ANSWER: C

Idiopathic intracranial hypertension (previously known as pseudotumor cerebri) characteristically affects young obese women. Lumbar puncture reveals elevated CSF pressure greater than 250 mm CSF. Headache is associated with increased intracranial pressure in that it develops concurrently with and/or is aggravated by the increased intracranial pressure or is relieved by reducing intracranial pressure.

REFERENCE

Headache Classification Committee of the International Headache Society (IHS). (2013). The International Classification of Headache Disorders, 3rd edition (beta version). *Cephalalgia*, *33*, 629–808.

5. A 63-year-old man presents to his primary care doctor for evaluation of persistent headache. He describes the pain as dull and occurring in his left temple. He also has noticed pain in his jaw that worsens when he chews. The most likely diagnosis is:

A. Temporomandibular joint dysfunction
B. Facial nerve palsy
C. Trigeminal neuralgia
D. Cluster headache
E. Giant cell arteritis

ANSWER: E

Giant cell arteritis (previously known as temporal arteritis) should top the differential diagnosis of persistent headache in patients over age 60. Presentation may include scalp tenderness or jaw claudication. Diagnosis is made on histology by temporal artery sectioning. Pulse steroids are critical to preventing blindness; they should be initiated based on ample clinical suspicion and not delayed for arterial biopsy results.

REFERENCE

Headache Classification Committee of the International Headache Society (IHS). (2013). The International Classification of Headache Disorders, 3rd edition (beta version). *Cephalalgia*, *33*, 629–808.

6. A 9-year-old girl of Ashkenazi Jewish descent is brought to her pediatrician for evaluation of a change in gait. The pediatrician observes torsion of her left foot. Over time, the girl develops dystonia of her other limbs and trunk. The pediatrician diagnoses her with early-onset primary dystonia. The most common abnormality observed in this illness is associated with what gene?

A. Hypoxanthine-guanine phosphoribosyl transferase (HGPRT)
B. DYT-1
C. Huntingtin
D. TSC-1
E. Amyloid precursor protein

ANSWER: E

DYT-1 is associated with early-onset primary dystonia. *TSC-1* is associated with tuberous sclerosis. *Huntingtin* is associated with Huntington disease. *HGPRT* is associated with Lesch–Nyhan syndrome, which may also cause dystonia in early life. Amyloid precursor protein is associated with early-onset Alzheimer disease.

REFERENCE

Robottom, B. J., Weiter, W. J., & Comella, C. L. (2011). Early-onset primary dystonia. *Handbook of Clinical Neurology, 100*, 465–479.

7. A 78-year-old man presents with unilateral hand tremor for 3 months. On exam, he is observed to have a short, shuffling stride and a positive "pull test." His posture is stooped. He is slow to initiate movement. Which of the following symptoms would NOT be expected in someone with his likely diagnosis?

A. Hypophonia
B. Dysphagia
C. Macrographia
D. Masked facies
E. Autonomic dysfunction

ANSWER: C

This patient likely carries a diagnosis of Parkinson disease (historically "paralysis agitans"). Classic presentation includes tremor, rigidity, akinesia/bradykinesia, and postural instability (easily remembered by the acronym TRAP). The "pull test" is a measure of postural instability. Associated symptoms may include micrographia, hypophonia, masked facies, autonomic dysfunction, anosmia, dysphagia, and multiple neuropsychiatric complications (cognitive decline, depression, sleep disorder, or psychosis).

REFERENCE

Jankovic, J. (2008). Parkinson's disease: Clinical features and diagnosis. *Journal of Neurology, Neurosurgery, and Psychiatry, 79*, 368–376.

8. A 62-year-old man presents to a neurologist for frequent falls. Exam is notable for vertical gaze palsy and bradykinesia. The neurologist orders magnetic resonance imaging (MRI), which is notable for dorsal midbrain atrophy. This presentation is most consistent with which diagnosis?

A. Progressive supranuclear palsy
B. Huntington disease
C. Parkinson disease
D. Olivopontocerebellar degeneration
E. Shy–Drager syndrome

ANSWER: A

Progressive supranuclear palsy classically presents with vertical gaze palsy, symmetrical rigidity, bradykinesia, and frequent falls. MRI may demonstrate atrophy of the dorsal midbrain. Patients may also demonstrate dysarthria, dysphagia, and frontal cognitive deficits.

REFERENCE

Golbe, L. I. (2014). Progressive supranuclear palsy. *Seminars in Neurology, 34*, 151–159.

9. A 42-year-old woman presents to her primary care doctor for evaluation of tremor. She notices the tremor in both her hands and that it gets worse when she tries to pick up a fork or a glass. Exam reveals no cogwheeling or rigidity, with normal gait and posture. Which of the following would be UNLIKELY to bring symptomatic improvement?

A. Alcohol
B. Propranolol
C. Primidone
D. Deep brain stimulation
E. Cognitive behavioral therapy

ANSWER: E

This patient most likely suffers from benign essential tremor. These symptoms may improve with alcohol, propranolol, primidone, and deep brain stimulation. There is no evidence that this movement disorder would be treatable with cognitive behavioral therapy (CBT).

REFERENCE

NINDS Essential Tremor Information Page: National Institute of Neurological Disorders and Stroke. http://www.ninds.nih.gov/disorders/essential_tremor/essential_tremor.htm. Last updated April 25, 2013. Accessed April 11, 2015.

10. A 14-year-old child is brought to a psychiatrist for disruptive behavior. The patient states that he has not been sleeping well and has bad headaches. The psychiatrist observes that the patient's muscles appear rigid and

his gait appears ataxic. She asks him to lift up his arms, which demonstrate a tremor. Concerned, she refers him for neurological evaluation. The neurologist observes a brown ring around the periphery of the iris on ophthalmologic exam. This patient's disease is due to insufficient excretion of what mineral?

A. Copper
B. Iron
C. Zinc
D. Manganese
E. Magnesium

ANSWER: A

The patient likely has a diagnosis of Wilson's disease, or hepatolenticular degeneration. Classic features include wing-beating tremor, Kayser–Fleischer ring (dark ring appearing to encircle the iris), rigidity, and akinesia. Patients may also suffer from migraine headaches, insomnia, or seizures. Neuropsychiatric sequelae are common and include depression, psychosis, and personality changes. A notable MRI finding in the midbrain is known as the "panda sign."

REFERENCE

Ala, A., Walker, A. P., Ashkan, K., Dooley, J.S., & Schilsky, M.L. (2007). Wilson's disease. *Lancet, 369*, 397–408.

11. A 38-year-old man presents to a neurologist for evaluation of gait changes because he has had several months of worsening restlessness and incoordination. He is observed to have jerky, random movements of his limbs. His wife reports that he has been more forgetful recently and is having trouble managing his finances. The patient's father developed similar symptoms in his early 40s. What would be expected on MRI?

A. Cerebellar atrophy
B. Putaminal atrophy
C. Frontotemporal atrophy
D. Caudate atrophy
E. Midbrain atrophy

ANSWER: D

The patient likely has Huntington disease, which is characterized by chorea, cognitive decline (particularly with executive function), behavioral abnormalities, psychosis, and depression with high risk of suicide. It is caused by an autosomal dominant mutation of the *Huntingtin* gene, which causes elongation of the trinucleotide CAG repeat on chromosome 4. Each successive generation is affected at a younger age secondary to a process called "anticipation." On MRI, caudate atrophy results in enlargement of the lateral ventricles, sometimes referred to as "boxcar ventricles."

REFERENCE

Roos, R. A. (2010). Huntington's disease: A clinical review. *Orphanet Journal of Rare Diseases, 5*, 40.

12. A 10-year-old girl with a history of rheumatic fever presents to her pediatrician with new-onset rapid, irregular movements of her limbs, trunk, and face. What is the most likely diagnosis?

A. Huntington disease
B. Sydenham chorea
C. Myoclonic epilepsy
D. Pediatric acute-onset neuropsychiatric syndrome
E. Tourette syndrome

ANSWER: B

Sydenham chorea is seen most frequently in girls who have a history of Group A beta-hemolytic streptococcal infection/rheumatic fever and is characterized by irregular movements of the limbs, trunk, and face. Movements occur as a result of autoantibodies attacking the basal ganglia. Most children recover. Pediatric acute-onset neuropsychiatric syndrome (PANS; until recently known as pediatric autoimmune neuropsychiatric disorder associated with streptococcal infection, or PANDAS) is also a disorder associated with Group A beta-hemolytic streptococcal infection; however, PANS is associated with onset of vocal and/or motor tics. Tics in Tourette syndrome can usually be suppressed with effort and are stereotyped rather than irregular.

REFERENCE

NINDS Sydenham Chorea Information Page: National Institute of Neurological Disorders and Stroke. http://www.ninds.nih.gov/disorders/sydenham/sydenham.htm. Last updated February 14, 2007. Last accessed October 29, 2015.

13. Which clinical condition may present with a clinical syndrome indistinguishable from restless legs syndrome (RLS)?

A. Uremia
B. Cirrhosis
C. Heart failure
D. Copper overload
E. Anticholinergic toxidrome

ANSWER: A

Besides iron deficiency, both pregnancy and uremia can present with RLS symptoms. Lifestyle changes that also may improve symptoms include decreased use of caffeine, tobacco, and alcohol.

REFERENCE

NINDS Restless Legs Syndrome Information Page: National Institute of Neurological Disorders and Stroke. http://www.ninds.nih.gov/disorders/restless_legs/restless_legs.htm. Last updated February 23, 2015. Last accessed October 29, 2015.

14. Which of the following is NOT consistent with neuroleptic malignant syndrome (NMS)?

A. Muscular flaccidity
B. Hypertension
C. Delirium
D. Elevated serum creatine kinase
E. Seizures

ANSWER: A

Patients with NMS typically present with muscular rigidity. Other symptoms may include hyperthermia, altered mental status, dysautonomia, tremor, dystonia, chorea, seizures, ataxia, hyporeflexia/extensor plantar reflexes, elevated serum CK, leukocytosis, proteinuria, and rhabdomyolysis. Risk factors include sudden initiation of high-dose antipsychotic (typical or atypical), younger age, male gender, lithium or SSRI use, dehydration, and hyponatremia. Treatment strategies include agents to decrease muscle rigidity such as benzodiazepines or dantrolene and medications to reverse dopamine blockade such as amantadine or bromocriptine.

REFERENCE

Munhoz, R. P., Moscovich, M., Araujo, P. D., et al. (2012). Movement disorders emergencies: A review. *Arq Neuropsiquiatr, 70*, 453–461.

15. Which of the following is TRUE regarding tardive dyskinesia (TD)?

A. Risk decreases with age.
B. Risk decreases with duration of antipsychotic use.
C. It is more likely to occur with atypical antipsychotics than with typical agents.
D. It did not occur prior to the introduction of chlorpromazine.
E. It may be caused by typical and atypical antipsychotics.

ANSWER: D

Although incidence of TD has decreased since the introduction of atypical antipsychotics, patients are still at risk of developing this side effect with first- or second-generation antipsychotics. Risk factors for TD include increasing age and cumulative drug exposure. Interestingly, tardive dyskinesia was reported in patients with psychotic illness in the *preneuroleptic era*.

REFERENCE

Mehta, S. H., Morgan, J. C., & Sethi, K. D. (2015). Drug-induced movement disorders. *Neurologic Clinics, 33*, 153–174.

16. An 8-year-old boy presents to his pediatrician at the prompting of his teacher. The teacher was concerned that the boy repetitively blinks and clears his throat in an exaggerated manner throughout the day, and several classmates have teased him about this. The boy notes that he can stop blinking and clearing his throat if he tries really hard, but he has a persistent urge to blink and cough. What is an accurate prognostic statement for the pediatrician to tell the boy and his parents?

A. Symptoms are expected to worsen in adolescence.
B. About one third of patients will be tic free by adulthood.
C. Motor tics typically persist into adolescence, but vocal tics resolve.
D. Vocal tics typically persist into adolescence, but motor tics resolve.
E. Medication is ineffective for tics.

ANSWER: B

This patient presents with motor and vocal tics, and as illustrated here typically present in early childhood. Symptoms often improve by adolescence, and about one third of patients will be tic free by adulthood. Treatment may include pharmacological and nonpharmacological approaches. Medications used to treat symptoms of tics include antipsychotics and alpha-2 agonists. Of note, diagnosis of Tourette syndrome requires *both* vocal *and* motor tics for more than a year, and if the patient had symptoms suggestive of strep throat this should raise suspicion for an autoimmune cause (PANS, historically known as PANDAS).

REFERENCES

Bloch, M. H., & Leckman, J. F. (2009). Clinical course of Tourette syndrome. *Journal of Psychosomatic Research, 67*, 497–501.

Bloch, M. H., State, M., & Pittenger, C. (2011). Recent advances in Tourette syndrome. *Current Opinion in Neurology, 24*, 119–125.

17. A 21-year-old college senior presents to the student health center for 2 days of severe headache and fever. Physical exam reveals nuchal rigidity. The patient has no history of trauma or chronic infectious disease. His physician is concerned that he may have bacterial meningitis and performs blood work and lumbar puncture. Which of the following patterns of laboratory tests would be consistent with bacterial meningitis?

A. Total protein 250 mg/dl, total WBC 1,000 cells/μl, 90% neutrophils
B. Total protein 75 mg/dl, total WBC 98 cells/μl, 37% neutrophils
C. Total protein 195 mg/dl, total WBC 300 cells/μl, 37% neutrophils
D. Total protein 90 mg/dl, total WBC 53 cells/μl, <20% neutrophils
E. Total protein 250 mg/dl, total WBC 53 cells/μl, 37% neutrophils

ANSWER: A

Protein, total WBC, and neutrophils are elevated in bacterial meningitis. Choice B is consistent with aseptic meningitis. Choice C is consistent with tuberculous meningitis. Choice D is consistent with cryptococcal meningitis. Choice E is a distractor.

REFERENCE

Bahr, N. C., & Boulware, D. R. (2014). Methods of rapid diagnosis for the etiology of meningitis in adults. *Biomarkers in Medicine, 8*, 1085–1103.

18. Which of the following bacterial causes of meningitis is a gram-negative diplococcus?

A. *Streptococcus pneumoniae*
B. *Neisseria meningitidis*
C. *Haemophilus influenzae*
D. *Listeria monocytogenes*
E. *Escherichia coli*

ANSWER: B

Neisseria meningitidis is a gram-negative diplococcus.

REFERENCE

Bahr, N. C., & Boulware, D. R. (2014). Methods of rapid diagnosis for the etiology of meningitis in adults. *Biomarkers in Medicine, 8*, 1085–1103.

19. An 18-year-old woman has a 24-hour history of headache, fever, and vomiting. Her roommate brings her to the emergency room after she has a seizure. T2-weighted magnetic resonance imaging (MRI) reveals hyperintensity of the temporal and inferior frontal lobes with a mass-like effect. Which of the following is the likely diagnosis?

A. *Streptococcus pneumoniae meningitis*
B. *Neisseria meningitidis meningitis*
C. Herpes simplex virus encephalitis
D. Subarachnoid hemorrhage
E. Idiopathic intracranial hypertension

ANSWER: C

Hyperintensity of the temporal and inferior frontal lobes is seen in herpes simplex virus (HSV) encephalitis.

REFERENCE

Sabah, M., Mulcahy, J., & Zeman A. (2012). Herpes simplex encephalitis. *British Medical Journal, 344*, e3166.

20. Which of the following is expected in the cerebrospinal fluid (CSF) in a patient with herpes simplex virus (HSV) encephalitis?

A. Decreased protein level with red blood cells
B. Elevated glucose with red blood cells
C. Elevated lymphocyte count with red blood cells
D. Elevated glucose and elevated lymphocyte count
E. Elevated protein level and elevated glucose

ANSWER: C

In aseptic encephalitis, CSF reveals increased lymphocyte count, often with red blood cells with or without xanthochromia. The prefix "xantho" means yellow, and this color is due to breakdown of red blood cells in CSF. Protein levels may be mildly raised, and glucose will be normal or mildly decreased.

REFERENCE

Sabah, M., Mulcahy, J., & Zeman, A. (2012). Herpes simplex encephalitis. *British Medical Journal, 344*, e3166.

21. A 35-year-old woman was treated for multiple sclerosis with the monoclonal antibody natalizumab. She develops behavioral changes, cognitive impairment, and hemisensory loss. T2 magnetic resonance imaging (MRI) is notable for hyperintensities in the frontal and parieto-occipital regions. The patient's neurologist diagnoses her with progressive multifocal leukoencephalopathy (PML). What virus most likely would be detected in CSF?

A. Herpes simplex virus
B. Epstein–Barr virus
C. Human T-lymphotropic virus type I
D. Coxsackievirus
E. JC virus

ANSWER: E

JC virus is implicated in PML. Before the era of combined antiretroviral therapy (cART; historically HAART) for HIV, PML was seen commonly in more advanced stages of AIDS. Decreasing in frequency among HIV-positive patients, PML may be seen in other immunosuppressed states, including in patients on monoclonal antibodies such as natalizumab.

REFERENCE

Chalky, J. J., & Berger, J. R. (2013). Progressive multifocal leukoencephalopathy in multiple sclerosis. *Current Neurology and Neuroscience Reports, 13*, 408.

Ataxia: 1 question

22. A 14-year-old boy presents to a pediatric neurologist for difficulty walking. His speech is dysarthric. Gait examination is notable for incoordination of lower limbs. Motor examination reveals weakness in the boy's feet and legs, and sensory examination reveals decreased sensation in his feet. His feet also appear deformed, with fixed plantar flexion and high arch, and he has mild scoliosis. The neurologist suspects an inherited ataxia, and genetic testing is consistent with an autosomal recessive disorder related to triplet repeat expansions of the *Frataxin* gene. What is the most likely diagnosis?

A. Duchenne muscular dystrophy
B. Myotonic dystrophy
C. Neurofibromatosis
D. Friedreich ataxia
E. Sturge–Weber syndrome

ANSWER: D

Friedreich ataxia is an autosomal recessive disorder related to triplet repeat expansions of the *Frataxin* gene. It is the most common inherited ataxia and affects most patients starting in early adolescence. Clinical presentation includes ataxic gait, dysarthria, limb weakness, sensory loss, peripheral neuropathy, scoliosis, and bilateral pes cavus (foot deformity). More than 75% of patients will live more than 34 years after disease onset.

REFERENCE

Collins, A. (2013). Clinical neurogenetics: Friedreich ataxia. *Neurologic Clinics, 31*, 1095–1120.

23. A 79-year-old man with atrial fibrillation and mild neurocognitive disorder falls down several stairs and hits his head. He does not lose consciousness but sustains a laceration on the occiput. He is taken to the emergency room for evaluation and treatment of the laceration. Neurological exam and computerized tomography (CT) scan of the brain are within normal limits. He is discharged home. Two weeks later he begins to experience headache and confusion that worsens over several days. His primary care doctor sends him to the emergency room for immediate evaluation. Should head CT be repeated at this time?

A. No, because a head CT 2 weeks ago revealed no acute findings.
B. No, because subdural hematoma would have been detected on initial imaging.
C. No, because the patient's confusion is likely to cause significant motion artifact.
D. Yes, but only after thorough serological evaluation has been performed.
E. Yes, urgently, because the patient is at risk for interval subdural hematoma development.

ANSWER: E

Older adults are at risk of subacute subdural hematoma, and the worsening headache and confusion should raise concern for increasing intracranial pressure. Expedient head CT is important to prevent further increase in intracranial pressure as decompression may be indicated. This type of hematoma often develops several weeks after a trauma to the head, which may be anywhere from minor in severity to a cause of brain herniation. The patient's advanced age and attendant cerebral atrophy, recent fall, and use of anticoagulants place him at risk. Cerebral atrophy causes the bridging veins to stretch, increasing the likelihood of bleed.

REFERENCE

Adhiyaman, V., Asghar, M., Ganeshram, K.N., & Bhowmick, B.K. (2002). Chronic subdural haematoma in the elderly. *Postgraduate Medical Journal, 78*, 71–75.

24. A 15-year-old male with a history of diarrheal illness develops progressive bilateral weakness of the lower limbs over several days. Neurological exam is notable for areflexia. As the leg weakness worsens, the patient is unable to ambulate and is admitted to the hospital for monitoring of respiratory status. What bacterium is most frequently associated with this illness?

A. *Staphylococcus aureus*
B. *Escherichia coli*
C. *Campylobacter jejuni*
D. *Salmonella*
E. *Clostridium difficile*

ANSWER: C

This patient most likely has Guillain–Barré syndrome (GBS), which worldwide is the most common cause of acute flaccid paralysis. GBS is divided into the demyelinating form, acute inflammatory demyelinating polyneuropathy (AIDP), and the axonal forms, acute motor-sensory axonal neuropathy (AMSAN) and acute motor axonal neuropathy (AMAN). AIDP is the most common form in North America. As the disease progresses, patients may require mechanical ventilation due to respiratory muscle involvement. The bacterial infection most commonly associated with this illness is *Campylobacter jejuni.*

REFERENCE

Nachamkin, I., Allos, B. M., & Ho, T. (1998). Campylobacter species and Guillain–Barré Syndrome. *Clinical Microbiology Reviews, 11*, 555–567.

25. A 54-year-old man presents to a neurologist for evaluation of weakness. The neurologist observes muscle fasciculation and atrophy. Exam is notable for brisk deep tendon reflexes and positive Babinski sign. Electromyography shows fibrillation potentials and positive sharp waves. Which of the following agents is approved by the FDA for this illness?

A. Donepezil
B. Prednisone
C. Intravenous immunoglobulin
D. Riluzole
E. Ropinirole

ANSWER: D

This patient likely has amyotrophic lateral sclerosis (ALS), as evidenced by presentation of upper motor neuron signs (e.g., brisk deep tendon reflexes, positive Babinski sign) and lower motor neuron signs (e.g., muscle fasciculation, positive sharp waves/fibrillation potentials on electromyography). Riluzole is an inhibitor of glutamate release and is used for treatment of ALS, increasing life expectancy by 3 to 6 months.

REFERENCE

Kiernan, M. C., Vucic, S., Cheah, B.C., Turner, M.R., Eisen, A., Hardiman, O., Burrell, J.R., & Zoing, M.C. (2011). Amyotrophic lateral sclerosis. *Lancet, 377*, 942–955.

26. All of the following are risk factors for ischemic stroke EXCEPT:

A. Hypertension
B. Alcohol use disorder

C. Prior transient ischemic attack (TIA)
D. Age greater than 65
E. Caucasian race

ANSWER: E

Hypertension, alcohol use disorder, previous TIA, and age greater than 65 are risk factors for ischemic stroke. Other risk factors include heart disease, atrial fibrillation, diabetes mellitus, tobacco use, substance use disorders, and atherosclerosis. Caucasian race is not a risk for stroke, with African Americans more than twice as likely as Caucasians to die of stroke.

REFERENCE

Sacco, R. L. (1997). Risk factors, outcomes, and stroke subtypes for ischemic stroke. *Neurology, 49*(5 suppl. 4), S39–S44.

27. Which of the following is a contraindication for thrombolysis for ischemic stroke?

A. Systolic blood pressure >185 mm Hg
B. History of myocardial infarction in previous 3 months
C. History of intracranial hemorrhage
D. Seizure with postictal residual neurological impairment
E. All of the above

ANSWER: E

The first and most important feature is duration of symptoms. Current guidelines allow for use of IV thrombolysis up to 4.5 hours after symptom onset, though for those in whom thrombolysis is considered with symptoms of 3 to 4.5 hours in duration there are additional warnings. All of the options listed here are contraindications for use of IV thrombolysis. Other contraindications would include intracranial hemorrhage on CT or MRI, gastrointestinal or urinary tract hemorrhage, major surgery in the 14 days prior, evidence of acute bleeding or trauma, use of oral anticoagulants and international normalized ration (INR) greater than 1.7, use of heparin in the previous 48 hours and currently prolonged activated partial thromboplastin time (aPTT), platelet count less than 100,000 per cubic millimeter, and blood glucose level less than 50 mg/dl.

REFERENCE

van der Worp, H. B., & van Gijn, J. (2007). Acute ischemic stroke. *New England Journal of Medicine, 357,* 572–579.

28. A 46-year-old woman treated with phenelzine for depression calls 911 after sudden onset of the "worst headache of her life." She stated it started following a cocktail party where she sampled several cheeses, among other appetizers. What would be expected on computerized tomography (CT) of the head?

A. Blood in the subdural space
B. Blood in the subarachnoid space
C. Blood in the epidural space
D. Blood in the lateral ventricles
E. No bleeding on CT scan

ANSWER: B

This woman likely ruptured a cerebral aneurysm during hypertensive crisis following exposure to tyramine-containing food. This type of hemorrhage, subarachnoid hemorrhage, causes blood to fill the subarachnoid space. Tyramine is found in several foods, including aged cheeses (cottage cheese and cream cheese are safe) and aged meats.

REFERENCES

Kundhal, P. S., Sockalingam, S., Krishnadev, N., et al. (2004). Monoamine oxidase inhibitors and subarachnoid hemorrhage. *Canadian Journal of Psychiatry, 49,* 573–574.
Vermeulen, M., & van Gijn, J. (1990). The diagnosis of subarachnoid haemorrhage. *Journal of Neurology, Neurosurgery, and Psychiatry, 53,* 365–372.

29. A 9-year-old girl presents to the emergency room for acute headache and confusion. Exam is notable for vision loss and motor weakness. The girl has a history of recurrent headaches, recurrent vomiting, and seizures. Brain magnetic resonance imaging (MRI) is within normal limits. Based on history and presentation, which of the following would explain her presentation?

A. Acute ischemic stroke
B. Acute hemorrhagic stroke
C. Mitochondrial encephalomyopathy, lactic acidosis, and stroke-like episodes (MELAS) syndrome
D. Myoclonic epilepsy with ragged red fibers
E. Psychogenic seizure

ANSWER: C

MELAS syndrome is a maternally inherited mitochondrial disorder. Manifestations may include "stroke-like episodes, dementia, epilepsy, lactic acidemia, myopathy, recurrent headaches, hearing impairment, diabetes, and short stature" (El-Hattab et al. 2015). Workup reveals lactic acidemia and ragged red fibers on muscle biopsy. Management is primarily symptomatic.

REFERENCE

El-Hattab, A. W., Adesina, A. M., Jones, J., et al. (2015). MELAS syndrome: Clinical manifestations, pathogenesis, and treatment options. *Molecular Genetics and Metabolism, 116*, 4–12

30. A 72-year-old woman with hypertension and hyperlipidemia is brought to the emergency room for evaluation of the sensation of the "room spinning." She has difficulty sitting unsupported and leans to one side. Her symptoms began suddenly. Exam is notable for left-sided ptosis and miosis, and decreased pain and temperature sensation on her left face and right trunk and limbs. What is the most likely diagnosis?

A. Benign paroxysmal positional vertigo
B. Basilar artery transient ischemic attack
C. Anterior cerebral artery infarct
D. Posterior cerebral artery transient ischemic attack
E. Lateral medullary infarct

ANSWER: E

Lateral medullary infarct (Wallenberg syndrome) presents with dizziness/vertigo, facial pain, difficulty sitting without support, hoarseness, and dysphagia. Exam may be notable for Horner syndrome, limb ataxia, laryngeal paralysis, and pharyngeal paralysis. Classic for this type of stroke is ipsilateral decreased pain and temperature sensation on the face and contralateral decreased pain and temperature sensation in the trunk and limbs.

REFERENCE

Savitz, S. I., & Caplan, L. R. (2005). Vertebrobasilar disease. *New England Journal of Medicine, 352*, 2618–2626.

31. A 68-year-old man with hypertension presents with weakness of all limbs. He is mute though apparently alert and consistently moves his eyes vertically on command. On examination he is unable to move his eyes laterally. An electroencephalogram reveals normal wakefulness. Which area of the brain is damaged?

A. Dorsal pons
B. Ventral pons
C. Thalamus
D. Midbrain
E. Tegmentum of pons

ANSWER: B

In basilar artery occlusion causing infarction of the ventral pons, patients develop quadriplegia, but consciousness is retained. They can move their eyes vertically and follow commands. This is described as locked-in syndrome. Patients with this condition have normal EEG.

REFERENCE

Simon, R., & Greenberg, D. (2012). Stroke. In *Clinical neurology* (8th ed., p. 393). New York, NY: Lange Medical Books/McGraw-Hill.

32. A 45-year-old man presents with headaches, irritability, and aggressiveness for a few months along with recent-onset weakness of the left lower extremity. On examination, he has loss of vibration sense in the left lower extremity and loss of pain and temperature in the right lower extremity. He walks with an ataxic gait. Magnetic resonance imaging (MRI) of the thoracic spinal cord is normal, but brain MRI reveals punctate areas of infarction in deep white matter in the frontal lobe. Which of the following would be an appropriate next step in investigating the cause?

A. CBC
B. MRI with contrast of brain
C. Vitamin B12 in serum
D. CSF examination and VDRL
E. Serum VDRL

ANSWER: D

The patient presents with features suspicious for syphilitic arteritis resulting from meningovascular syphilis (MVS). MVS occurs usually within 5 years of initial infection. It presents with subacute headache, behavioral changes (frontal lobe involvement), and spinal cord involvement. The progressive form may present with stroke-like symptoms, with clinical features reflecting the specific affected blood-supply region. Acute spinal cord infarcts may present with myelopathy, hemiplegic symptoms (Brown–Sequard syndrome), or transverse myelitis. Medium-sized penetrating arteries are most commonly involved, causing punctate deep white matter lesions on MRI of the brain. MRI of the spinal cord could be normal or show T2 hyperintensities.

REFERENCES

Behrouz, R. (2011, August). Meningo-vascular syphilis: Revisiting an old adversary. *Practical Neurology*, 32–37. Retrieved from http://practicalneurology.com/pdfs/PN0811_MVS Feature.pdf

Simon, R., & Greenberg, D. (2012). Stroke. In *Clinical neurology* (8th ed., p. 393). New York, NY: Lange Medical Books/McGraw-Hill.

33. A 51-year-old woman with diabetes mellitus and atrial fibrillation presents to the emergency room with double vision and right sided ataxia. Examination reveals ptosis of the left eye and right-sided hyperactive deep tendon reflex. Pupils are equal in size and normally reactive to light. Which of the flowing is the likely cause?

A. Left middle cerebral artery lesion affecting optic radiation
B. Posterior cerebral artery stenosis and midbrain infarct
C. Posterior cerebral artery stenosis causing occipital lobe infarct
D. Posterior cerebral artery causing thalamus lesion
E. Vertebral artery causing cerebellar lesion

ANSWER: B

The above vignette describes a case of posterior cerebral artery occlusion affecting the midbrain blood supply. Midbrain lesions may cause oculomotor nerve palsy and spare the pupil. Diabetic microvascular third nerve palsy is also usually pupil sparing. The hallmarks of posterior circulation stroke are crossed findings in which the cranial nerve signs are on the same side of the lesion, and motor and sensory signs are on the opposite side of the lesion. Ataxia, tremors, and hemiplegia are seen ipsilateral to cranial nerve involvement. Diabetes and atrial fibrillation are risk factors for posterior circulation stroke.

REFERENCES

Chugh, J. (2012). Third nerve palsy: An overview. *Indian Journal of Clinical Practice, 22*, 17–20.

Lewandowski, C. (n.d.). Posterior circulation stroke. Retrieved October 25, 2015, from https://www.uic.edu/com/ferne/pdf/posterior0501.pdf

34. Which of the following features differentiates central vertigo from peripheral vertigo?

A. Central vertigo presents with horizontal nystagmus.
B. Central vertigo is often associated with tinnitus.
C. There is a time lag between movement of the head and the beginning of symptoms in central vertigo.
D. Central vertigo is most often caused by a middle cerebral artery lesion.
E. Visual fixation does not obliterate central vertigo.

ANSWER: E

Central vertigo is more commonly seen in posterior circulation stroke. Unlike peripheral vertigo, central vertigo is rarely associated with tinnitus. It starts immediately, without any time lag between head movement and onset of symptoms. It is rarely associated with horizontal nystagmus. The nystagmus does not go away with visual fixation.

REFERENCE

Lewandowski, C. (n.d.). Posterior circulation stroke. Retrieved October 25, 2015, from https://www.uic.edu/com/ferne/pdf/posterior0501.pdf.

35. Impaired blood supply of which anatomical structure is involved in the following type of visual field defect (Figure 12.1)?

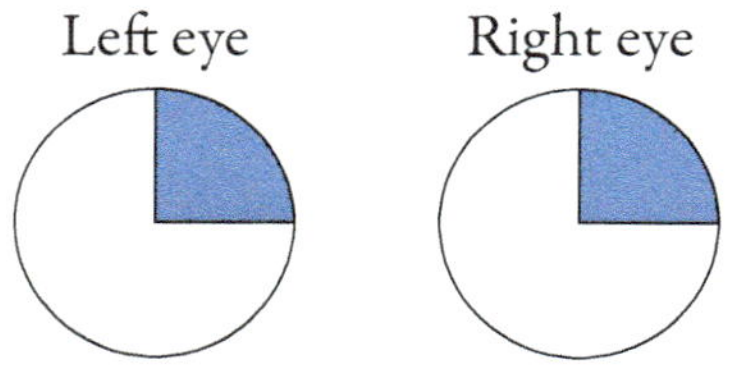

Figure 12.1. Visual field defect

A. Left lateral geniculate nucleus
B. Right lateral geniculate nucleus
C. Left parietal lobe
D. Right parietal lobe
E. Right occipital lobe

ANSWER: A

Right superior homonymous quadrantopia (a "pie-in-the-sky" field deficit) is seen in lesions involving the left hemispheric lateral geniculate nucleus (LGN) or of Myer's loop, the optic radiations that course through the temporal lobe just lateral to the temporal horn of the lateral ventricle. The most common cause of LGN or Meyer's loop lesion is ischemia.

REFERENCE

Disorders of the outer visual field. (n.d.). Retrieved October 26, 2015, from http://nawrot.psych.ndsu.nodak.edu/Courses/465Projects10/VisualDisorders/homosq.html

36. A 50-year-old man presents to the emergency department with a 1-day history of left-sided weakness and left arm spasticity. He visited his chiropractor for neck pain 1 day ago. The symptoms started after his last visit, where a "thrust" was used as part of treatment. On examination, he had loss of pain and temperature sensation in his right foot, leg and arm with loss of vibration sense in his left arm. What was the cause of his symptoms?

A. Anterior spinal artery lesion
B. Posterior cord syndrome
C. Cord hemisection
D. Transverse myelitis
E. Spinal epidural abscess

ANSWER: C

The above case is a typical presentation of spinal cord hemisection or Brown–Sequard syndrome. Below the lesion, there are ipsilateral pyramidal deficits and ipsilateral loss of posterior cord functions (vibration, joint position sensation), with contralateral loss of pain and temperature sensation two or three segments below the lesion. It is most commonly caused by penetrating trauma. Case reports document spinal cord hemisection due to chiropractor-induced trauma generating a blunt force from the flexion extension maneuver.

REFERENCE

Lipper, M. (1998). Brown–Sequard syndrome of the cervical spinal cord after chiropractic manipulation. *American Journal of Neuroradiology, 19,* 1349–1352.

37. A 24-year-old woman presents with paresthesia, headaches, and double vision. She has ataxic gait with weakness of her left lower extremity. She has had similar attacks of double vision twice in the past year and carries a diagnosis of relapsing–remitting multiple sclerosis. She also has major depressive disorder and nonadherence with antidepressant medication. Which of the following is the most suitable treatment to delay disability for this patient?

A. Interferon beta
B. Glatiramer acetate
C. Intravenous steroid
D. Plasmapheresis
E. Mechanical ventilation

ANSWER: B

Multiple sclerosis (MS) is an autoimmune disorder, where antibodies are produced against myelin epitopes. These antibodies cross the blood–brain barrier to produce neurological symptoms. Relapsing–remitting type is the most common type of MS, accounting for 85% of cases. Both interferon beta and glatiramer acetate are FDA-approved pharmacotherapies for relapsing–remitting disease; however, glatiramer acetate would likely be preferred over interferon in this patient because interferon can worsen depression and precipitate suicidal ideation.

REFERENCE

Simon, R., & Greenberg, D. (2012). Motor disorders. In *Clinical neurology* (8th ed., p. 235–238). New York, NY: Lange Medical Books/McGraw-Hill.

38. Which medication has the strongest evidence in support of its ability to reduce the relapse rate of relapsing–remitting multiple sclerosis?

A. Intravenous immunoglobulin
B. Interferon beta 1A
C. Natalizumab
D. Intravenous steroid
E. Interferon beta 1B

ANSWER: C

Natalizumab is an alpha-4 integrin antibody, used in treatment of relapsing–remitting multiple sclerosis. Rarely it can cause progressive multifocal leukoencephalopathy. Its use is limited to relapsing-remitting patients who responded poorly to interferon and/or glatiramer acetate or relapsing-remitting patients with severe initial course. Intravenous immunoglobulin might reduce relapse rate, but there is no clear evidence for this. Intravenous steroid is used to help faster recovery, but the extent of recovery and the effect on relapse rate are unchanged.

REFERENCE

Simon, R., & Greenberg, D. (2012). Motor disorders. In *Clinical neurology* (8th ed., p. 235–238). New York, NY: Lange Medical Books/McGraw-Hill.

39. A 59-year-old HIV-positive patient with documented cognitive decline presents with left leg weakness. On examination, the patient has paresthesias bilaterally over his lower extremities, increased deep tendon reflexes, and spasticity. He also has urinary incontinence. Brain MRI shows moderate cortical and subcortical atrophy, but spinal cord MRI is unrevealing. Which of the following is the likely pathology in this patient's spinal cord?

A. Transverse myelitis at thoracic level
B. Vacuolar myelopathy of the lateral column
C. Vertebral compression
D. Spinal epidural abscess
E. Demyelination of the spinal cord

ANSWER: B

The above case describes HIV myelopathy, which is characterized by a vacuolar myelopathy. This presents gradually, often with concurrent mild or major neurocognitive disorder due to HIV infection (itself newly added to the *DSM-5*). Bilateral or unilateral sensory, motor, and autonomic involvement is present without a discrete sensory level. Lateral and posterior spinal columns are principally affected. MRI of the spinal cord is typically normal. In the above case, MRI of the brain shows cortical and subcortical atrophy, characteristic of neurocognitive disorders due to HIV infection. The case is not of transverse myelitis, which usually has bilateral presentation and a defined sensory level.

REFERENCE

Simon, R., & Greenberg, D. (2012). Motor disorders. In *Clinical neurology* (8th ed., p. 241). New York, NY: Lange Medical Books/McGraw-Hill.

40. Which one of the following consistently differentiates Lambert–Eaton myasthenic syndrome (LEMS) from myasthenia gravis?

A. Ptosis is an invariant feature of myasthenia gravis.
B. Repeated stimulation of motor neurons in myasthenia gravis yields decreasing motor responses.
C. Younger patients typically present with LEMS.
D. Muscle power increases with sustained contraction in myasthenia gravis.
E. Unlike myasthenia gravis, LEMS is often associated with a tumor.

ANSWER: B

Myasthenia gravis presents with ptosis in 25% of cases. In 80% of cases, there is antibody against skeletal muscle nicotinic acetylcholine receptor. The disease has gradual onset with progressive course and can present at any age. It is associated with thymic tumor, thyrotoxicosis, rheumatoid arthritis, and systemic lupus erythematosus. Sustained contraction of the affected muscle leads to temporary weakness. LEMS, on the other hand, is a paraneoplastic syndrome and has an association with autoimmune conditions such as pernicious anemia. Proximal muscles are involved; extraocular muscles are spared. Muscle power steadily increases with sustained contraction. The cause is attributed to an antibody that cross-reacts with tumor antigens and voltage-gated calcium channels involved in acetylcholine release. This, in turn, leads to presynaptic neuromuscular transmission. On electromyogram, muscle responses decrease in response to repeated stimulation in myasthenia gravis but increase in LEMS.

REFERENCE

Simon, R., & Greenberg, D. (2012). Motor disorders. In *Clinical neurology* (8th ed., p. 259–261). New York, NY: Lange Medical Books/McGraw-Hill.

41. A 15-year-old male with a learning disorder develops gradual frontal baldness and generalized stiffness of distal muscles. On examination, he has persistent contraction after percussion in his hand and leg muscles. He is not able to relax his hands after a sustained grip. Genetic testing revealed 40 repeats of CTG trinucleotide. What is the diagnosis?

A. Myotonic dystrophy
B. Duchenne dystrophy
C. Polymyositis

D. Motor neuron disease
E. Myasthenia gravis

ANSWER: A

Myotonic dystrophy is an autosomal dominant disease, caused by expansion of a CTG trinucleotide repeat in the noncoding region of *DMPK*. This condition usually presents in the third or fourth decade but can affect younger adults as well. Distal muscles are most involved, and patients develop frontal baldness. Patients may also have facial muscle weakness, cataracts, testicular atrophy, diabetes mellitus, and cardiac abnormality. Low IQ is often seen in this condition.

REFERENCE

Simon, R., & Greenberg, D. (2012). Motor disorders. In *Clinical neurology* (8th ed., p. 264–266). New York, NY: Lange Medical Books/McGraw-Hill.

42. A 65-year-old man complains of gradual-onset weakness of both thighs with unclear duration. He has had weakness of bilateral forearm for 3 years. There is no pain associated with weakness. Neurological examination is consistent with reduced bilateral knee reflexes, severe leg muscle weakness, and moderate weakness of thigh muscles. There is low muscle power of forearm flexors and extensors. Serum creatinine level is mildly elevated. What is the most likely diagnosis?

A. Polymyositis
B. Dermatomyositis
C. Inclusion body myositis
D. Muscle-wasting syndrome
E. Mitochondrial myopathy

ANSWER: C

Inclusion body myositis is a T cell–mediated myotoxicity in which weakness in the lower extremity develops prior to in the upper extremity. The onset is insidious and sometimes ill-defined by the patient. It is most common in men over 50 years of age. It typically involves quadriceps and forearm flexors and extensors. Polymyositis usually develops within weeks to months and involves proximal more than distal muscles. Dermatomyositis is a microangiopathy affecting skin and muscle. It presents with characteristic eyelid and extensor surface rash called heliotrope rash as well as the shawl sign. A quarter of patients with adult-onset dermatomyositis have an associated malignancy of ovary, lung, or gastrointestinal tract. Muscle-wasting syndrome is seen in patients with HIV disease and usually presents with proximal muscle-wasting and cachexia.

REFERENCE

Simon, R., & Greenberg, D. (2012). Motor disorders. In *Clinical neurology* (8th ed., p. 267–268, Table 9-16). New York, NY: Lange Medical Books/McGraw-Hill.

43. A 20-year-old Asian man presents with episodic muscle paralysis, only after exercise, lasting for 20 to 30 minutes. He has an uncle with similar symptoms. His serum potassium level is 6 meq/L. He was treated with acetazolamide daily, and the episodes reduced in frequency. Which of the following structures is implicated in this patient's weakness?

A. Calcium channel
B. Sodium channel
C. Potassium channel
D. GABA A receptor
E. Chloride channel

ANSWER: B

Hyperkalemic periodic paralysis, a familial disease with dominant inheritance, presents with episodic muscle flaccidity with preserved ventilation. As its name suggests, serum potassium level is high during episodes. The flaccid episodes occur after exercise and last for less than 1 hour. Between episodes, muscle power is normal. It is believed to be caused by a mutation in the gene encoding the alpha subunit of voltage-gated sodium channels.

REFERENCE

Simon, R., & Greenberg, D. (2012). Motor disorders. In *Clinical neurology* (8th ed., p. 270). New York, NY: Lange Medical Books/McGraw-Hill.

44. A 25-year-old man presents with bilateral thigh weakness for 1 week and inability to walk for a day. He had an episode of gastroenteritis 1 month ago. He reports racing heart and sweating. On examination, knee and ankle reflexes are diminished on both of the lower extremities. Both thighs are weak, and he has hypoesthesia over his legs. CSF examination shows

increased albumin and normal cell count. Which of the following correlates with muscle-wasting and hence poor prognosis?

A. Demyelination
B. Axonal loss
C. Sensory loss
D. Cognitive impairment
E. None of the above

ANSWER: B

The above clinical picture is of acute idiopathic polyneuropathy or Guillain–Barré syndrome (GBS), which occurs in two forms: demyelinating variant (common in the United States) and axonal variant (common in China). The disease usually presents with symmetric ascending paralysis, more pronounced in proximal lower extremity muscles. Deep tendon reflexes are typically absent. Affected individuals may also experience symptoms of autonomic dysfunction such as sweating or palpitations (cardiac arrhythmia). The disease is often preceded by recent infection or surgery. CSF classically shows elevated albumin level and a normal or near-normal cell count (so-called cytoalbuminologic dissociation). Electromyography reveals motor and sensory conduction slowing suggestive of demyelination or axonal loss. Muscle-wasting typically develops when axonal degeneration has occurred. Overall, 70% of the cases resolve completely, 25% of affected patients are left with residual paralysis, and 5% die, largely due to respiratory muscle involvement. Symptoms usually decrease and disappear by the 4th weak into the illness. Advanced age, *Campylobacter jejuni* infection, acute onset of symptoms, and axonal degeneration are poor prognostic factors.

REFERENCE

Simon, R., & Greenberg, D. (2012). Sensory disorders. In *Clinical neurology* (8th ed., pp. 295–296). New York, NY: Lange Medical Books/McGraw-Hill.

45. A 51-year-old white man with previous cervical spinal arthritis complains of increasing pain in the neck and bilateral shoulders. Three months ago he was in an automobile accident in which he was a restrained passenger, and immediate cervical spine MRI at the time revealed no changes from his previous study. On examination, he has deltoid wasting bilaterally and reduced pinprick and temperature sensation over both shoulders and neck. Sensation to light touch is preserved. A repeat MRI of the cervical spine at this time is likely to reveal which of the following conditions?

A. Cervical spondylitis
B. Cervical radiculopathy
C. Syringomyelia
D. C6 herniation
E. Transverse myelitis

ANSWER: C

The above case describes presentation consistent with syringomyelia developing a few months after a traumatic injury. Syringomyelia can also develop several years after the initial trauma. It presents with impaired pinprick and temperature sensation with preserved light touch sensation in a "cape-like" fashion over neck and shoulders. Affected individuals often report diffuse neck pain and radicular pain in both arms. MRI of the cervical spine shows focal spinal cord enlargement at the level of the lesion in traumatic cases.

REFERENCE

Simon, R., & Greenberg, D. (2012). Sensory disorders. In *Clinical neurology* (8th ed., p. 307). New York, NY: Lange Medical Books/McGraw-Hill

46. A 25-year-old immigrant from Southeast Asia was brought in by family members with a history of recurrent bouts of twisting, limb thrusting, and grimacing movements with screaming during sleep. This has been happening for the past few weeks. The patient recently broke up with her boyfriend of 3 years. Family reports that her eyes are open at times during the episodes, but she does not respond to questions. Video EEG during one such episode is negative for epileptic correlate. Her mother had similar episodes treated with carbamazepine. What is the most likely diagnosis?

A. Pseudoseizure
B. Temporal lobe epilepsy
C. Frontal lobe epilepsy
D. Generalized tonic–clonic seizure
E. Absence seizure

ANSWER: C

The above case describes the semiology of a frontal lobe seizure, which typically presents as a partial seizure with possible secondary generalization. It typically occurs during non-REM sleep and is characterized by thrusting ("fencing") limb movements, grimacing, and screaming. A patient's eyes may be open, and he or she can appear awake but be unable to respond to questions. Seizures usually last less than a few minutes. A familial version has been described (autosomal dominant nocturnal frontal lobe epilepsy; ADNFLE), and a mutation in the nicotinic acetylcholine receptor genes has been proposed. Encephalitis, arteriovenous malformations, cortical dysplasia, and trauma can also cause similar frontal lobe seizures. The most common differential diagnosis is pseudoseizure (or "conversion disorder with attacks or seizures" per *DSM-5*). An important differentiating feature is nocturnal occurrence of frontal lobe seizures. Diagnosis of frontal lobe seizure is challenging. Continuous video EEG can be normal depending on the location of the source site in the frontal lobe. MRI of brain with gadolinium scan demonstrates the abnormal area in half of cases. PET scan may show areas of interictal hypometabolism in cases with unremarkable MRI. Polysomnography with extended frontal leads may be useful to demonstrate nocturnal disease.

REFERENCE

Simon, R., & Greenberg, D. (2012). Seizures and syncope. In *Clinical neurology* (8th ed., p. 359). New York, NY: Lange Medical Books/McGraw-Hill.

47. Which of the following is commonly seen in patients with temporal lobe epilepsy?

A. Temporal lobe microhemorrhages
B. Hippocampal atrophy
C. Generalized atrophy of frontotemporal region
D.
E. Enlarged sella turcica

ANSWER: B

Hippocampal sclerosis is seen in two thirds of individuals with temporal lobe epilepsy. Cell loss in CA1 and CA2 areas of hippocampus is characteristic of temporal lobe seizure; this is called mesial temporal lobe sclerosis. The lesion is visible on T2-weighted or fluid-attenuated inversion recovery (FLAIR) MRI.

REFERENCE

Berkovic, S.F., Andermann, F., Olivier, A., Ethier, R., Melanson, D., Robitaille, Y., Kuzniecky, R., et al. (1991). Hippocampal sclerosis in temporal lobe epilepsy demonstrated by magnetic resonance imaging. *Annals of Neurology, 29*, 175–82.

48. A 45-year-old man experiences a sudden loss of consciousness while resting on a chair after a workout. He awoke a minute later with a flushed face and a pulse rate of 30 beats per minute. What is the likely cause of syncope?

A. Vasovagal syncope
B. Basilar artery insufficiency
C. Hyperventilation syncope
D. Cardiovascular syncope
E. Migraine

ANSWER: D

This is likely a case of cardiovascular syncope. This happens mostly in patients in a recumbent position after physical exertion. The causes of this condition include brady and tachyarrhythmias, sick sinus syndrome, aortic stenosis, mitral valve prolapse, hypertrophic cardiomyopathy, or pulmonary embolism. A sudden decrease in cardiac output results in cerebral hypoperfusion, which leads to the syncopal event. Vasovagal syncope occurs mostly in a standing or sitting position but very rarely in those lying down. In vasovagal syncope, consciousness is restored upon lying down, allowing for blood return to the brain. A pale, diaphoretic appearance with dilated pupils is common. Consciousness is typically regained in 20 to 30 seconds, but headache, nausea, pallor, and urge to defecate may persist. Yawning, lightheadedness, blurred vision, and tachycardia may serve as prodromal features. Basilar artery insufficiency causes vertigo, diplopia, and occipital headaches, with brief loss of consciousness from seconds to minutes. This characteristically occurs in people in their 60s or older. One fifth of patients will go on to have a cerebrovascular accident. Hyperventilation syncope occurs after sustained hyperventilation due to hypocapnia and is seen mostly in recumbent women. Migraine rarely causes brief syncopal episodes, but it does so in association with headache and upon standing up briskly.

REFERENCE

Simon, R., & Greenberg, D. (2012). Seizures and syncope. In *Clinical neurology* (8th ed., pp. 373–375). New York, NY: Lange Medical Books/McGraw-Hill.

49. Gelastic seizures are commonly associated with:

A. Hypothalamic hamartoma
B. Middle cerebral artery stroke
C. Neurofibromatosis
D. Temporal lobe epilepsy
E. Multiple sclerosis

ANSWER: A

Gelastic seizures are sudden, uncontrollable bouts of laughter without any apparent cause. This condition usually starts insidiously in childhood and increases the risk of learning disability. Gelastic epilepsy has been associated with hypothalamic hamartomas, and when present they can cause precocious puberty in girls due to involvement of the hypothalamo-pituitary axis. Of note, seizures that present with crying as their semiology are known as dacrystic seizures.

REFERENCE

Topff, L., & Gelin, G. (2013). Hypothalamic hamartoma. *Journal of the Belgian Society of Radiology, 96*, 362–364

50. Which one of the following conditions has overlapping features with amyotrophic lateral sclerosis?

A. Neurocognitive disorder with Lewy bodies
B. Neurocognitive disorder due to Alzheimer disease
C. Vascular neurocognitive disorder
D. Frontotemporal neurocognitive disorder
E. Neurocognitive disorder due to Parkinson disease

ANSWER: D

Amyotrophic lateral sclerosis (ALS) and frontotemporal neurocognitive disorder (FTD) have overlapping presentations. Both ALS and FTD patients suffer from executive dysfunction, which is thought due to TAR-DNA-binding protein 43 (TDP-43) inclusions in the hippocampus, amygdala, and spinal cord. TDP-43 burden reflects clinical manifestations. Both conditions may share mechanisms of protein misfolding.

REFERENCES

Achi, E. (2012). ALS and frontotemporal dysfunction: A review. *Neurology Research International,* doi:10.1155/2012/806306
Simon, R., & Greenberg, D. (2012). Motor disorders. In *Clinical neurology* (8th ed., p. 249). New York, NY: Lange Medical Books/McGraw-Hill.

51. A 7-year-old obese boy was brought in by his parents with symptoms suggestive of intellectual disability disorder and relentlessly compulsive eating. What is the likely diagnosis?

A. Angelman syndrome
B. Prader–Willi syndrome
C. Down syndrome
D. Obsessive–compulsive disorder
E. Autism spectrum disorder

ANSWER: B

The child in the above case likely suffers from Prader–Willi syndrome. Approximately 75% of Prader–Willi syndrome cases have paternal inheritance, and the rest are sporadic. This disorder results from a deletion in chromosome 15. Affected children usually have low IQ and behavioral problems, but the most striking characteristic observed is severe hyperphagia and resultant obesity. Patients eat relentlessly and aggressively because they lack the capacity for satiety; families often have to safeguard food in the home, and even then patients with this condition may break locks or doors to access food. The obesity is refractory to behavioral therapy or gastric surgery procedures. Angelman syndrome carries a very closely related microdeletion on the same chromosome 15, inherited from the mother, but has a completely different phenotype.

REFERENCE

Kaufman, D. M. (2013). *Clinical neurology for psychiatrists* (7th ed., pp. 296–297). Philadelphia, PA: Elsevier Health Sciences.

52. A 5-year-old girl with epilepsy and acquired microcephaly displays stereotypies, including incessant movements of her hands as though clapping. The girl's ability to speak and walk have deteriorated considerably over the past 6 months. What is the likely diagnosis?

A. Rett syndrome
B. Angelman syndrome
C. Lesch–Nyhan syndrome
D. Down syndrome
E. Phenylketonuria

ANSWER: A

The girl in the above case likely suffers from Rett syndrome, which is no longer an independent diagnosis in *DSM-5*. The pervasive developmental disorders of *DSM-IV-TR* have been condensed into autism spectrum disorder. Rett syndrome is caused by mutations in the *MECP2* gene and occurs all but exclusively in girls. Development proceeds normally for a few years before symptoms begin. The condition takes a decidedly deteriorating course: the child loses learned motor skills (talking and walking) and progresses to profound intellectual disability. The incidence of seizures in Rett syndrome is 60% to 90%. Two characteristic neurological manifestations include stereotypies and acquired microcephaly. The stereotypies include incessant hand movements such as hand clapping, wringing, flapping or hair pulling. The stereotyped behavior may also manifest by non-hand movements such as bruxism or body twisting. Head circumference is usually normal from birth to about 6 months, after which growth decelerates, and the head becomes relatively small for the body (acquired microcephaly).

REFERENCE

Kaufman, D. M. (2013). *Clinical neurology for psychiatrists* (7th ed., pp. 299–300). Philadelphia, PA: Elsevier Health Sciences.

53. Which of the following chromosomal abnormalities is present in velocardiofacial (VCF) syndrome?

A. Chromosome 21
B. Chromosome 18
C. Chromosome 15
D. Chromosome 22
E. Chromosome 12

ANSWER: D

VCF is an autosomal dominant genetic disorder that results from microdeletion in chromosome 22, and most cases are sporadic. Although VCF's primary manifestations are physical (cleft palate or velopharyngeal dysfunction, congenital ventricular septal defects, and abnormalities in pulmonary artery and aorta), it is associated with significant neuropsychiatric comorbidity. Individuals with VCF have intellectual disability; one third of affected individuals develop features of schizophrenia, and up to 40% develop depression.

REFERENCE

Kaufman, D. M. (2013). *Clinical neurology for psychiatrists* (7th ed., p. 298). Philadelphia, PA: Elsevier Health Sciences.

54. Which of the following is the most common symptom of increased intracranial pressure due to an expanding brain tumor?

A. Headache
B. Nausea
C. Seizure
D. Focal neurological deficit
E. Papilledema

ANSWER: A

Headache is the most common symptom of intracranial pressure. Headache is present in about 50% of patients suffering from brain tumor. By presentation it resembles tension-type headache and is characterized by diffuse, dull, relatively mild pain that initially responds to analgesics such as aspirin. With the increase in intracranial pressure, headaches worsen and begin to wake up patients from sleep. The increased pressure also causes nausea and vomiting. Papilledema, another sign of increased intracranial pressure, happens late, if at all, in the course of the disease.

REFERENCE

Kaufman, D. M. (2013). *Clinical neurology for psychiatrists* (7th ed., p. 457). Philadelphia, PA: Elsevier Health Sciences.

55. Which of the following is least likely to present with apathy, executive dysfunction, and forgetfulness?

A. Frontotemporal neurocognitive disorder
B. Frontal lobe infarction
C. Neurocognitive disorder due to HIV infection
D. Parietal lobe glioblastoma
E. Neurocognitive disorder due to traumatic brain injury

ANSWER: D

Apathy, executive dysfunction, and forgetfulness are suggestive of frontal lobe pathology and would be unlikely in a patient with a parietal lesion.

REFERENCE

Kaufman, D. M. (2013). *Clinical neurology for psychiatrists* (7th ed., p. 458). Philadelphia, PA: Elsevier Health Sciences.

56. An otherwise healthy 60-year-old woman who has been irritable and paranoid over the past week was brought to the emergency room by family after she had a

witnessed seizure. EEG reveals cortical excitability over bilateral temporal lobes. On evaluation, she is unable to remember words for more than 30 seconds. Lumbar puncture reveals very slight lymphocytosis but is negative for herpes simplex virus (HSV). Which of the following is the most likely cause of her presentation?

A. Parasite infection
B. Autoimmunity
C. Thiamine deficiency
D. Endocrinopathy
E. Whipple disease

ANSWER: B

Limbic encephalitis is a clinical term that describes encephalitis with temporal lobe predilection; its classic triad includes anterograde amnesia due to hippocampal dysfunction, temporal lobe seizures due to inflammation, and a host of potential psychiatric symptoms. HSV encephalitis causes a limbic encephalitis, but because this has been ruled out, the next likely etiology is autoimmunity. Several antibodies have been implicated, including anti-Hu, anti–NMDA receptor, anti-LGI-1, and so forth. Identifying the specific antibody will guide management. Autoimmune limbic encephalitis has paraneoplastic and nonparaneoplastic variants. Several antibodies (such as anti-Hu) imply an associated malignancy, whereas others have a fairly weak association with malignancy (such as anti–NMDA receptors in males).

REFERENCE

Kaufman, D. M. (2013). *Clinical neurology for psychiatrists* (7th ed., p. 460). Philadelphia, PA: Elsevier Health Sciences.

57. Which of the following describes ataxic gait?

A. Shuffling, short-stepped gait with stooped posture
B. Limping as though in pain
C. Short-stepped gait with upright stance
D. Broad-based gait
E. Difficulty lifting feet from the ground as though the patient is held by a magnet

ANSWER: D

In ataxic gait, feet are placed widely apart to maintain stability. Because of incoordination, the gait also has an uneven, unsteady, lurching pattern.

REFERENCE

Kaufman, D. M. (2013). *Clinical neurology for psychiatrists* (7th ed., p. 53). Philadelphia, PA: Elsevier Health Sciences.

58. Of the following brain regions that may be injured in a patient with alcohol use disorder, which would account for ataxic gait?

A. Corpus callosum
B. Dorsomedial nucleus of the thalamus
C. Mammillary bodies
D. Cerebellar vermis
E. All of the above

ANSWER: D

Chronic alcoholism can cause atrophy of the cerebellar vermis, which leads to truncal ataxia and an ataxic gait. Damage to the dorsomedial nucleus of the thalamus is the most specific finding associated with Wernicke encephalopathy, though micohemorrhages may also be seen in mammillary bodies. Corpus callosum degeneration in alcohol use disorder is known as Marchiafava–Bignami disease.

REFERENCE

Donnino, M. W., Vega, J., Miller, J., & Walsh, M. (2007). Myths and misconceptions of Wernicke's encephalopathy: What every emergency physician should know. *Annals of Emergency Medicine, 50*, 715–721.

59. A dentist is being evaluated for possible medication diversion and substance use disorder. He presents with cognitive issues and progressively worsening lower extremity weakness, tingling, and numbness. Vibration and touch sense are diminished. A positive Babinski sign is present. Which of the following is the likely cause of this presentation?

A. Nitrous oxide
B. Prescription opioids
C. Cannabis
D. Heroin
E. Cocaine

ANSWER: A

This is likely a case of nitrous oxide toxicity. Nitrous oxide, also known as "laughing gas," is a gaseous anesthetic.

Regular recreational use can lead to vitamin B12 deficiency, which in turn results in cognitive impairment and spinal cord damage (subacute combined degeneration of the spinal cord).

REFERENCE

Kaufman, D. M. (2013). *Clinical neurology for psychiatrists* (7th ed., p. 509). Philadelphia, PA: Elsevier Health Sciences.

60. A 7-year-old boy was brought in by his parents for progressively worsening difficulty in walking and running. When the boy was 5, his parents noticed toe walking. Now, though, when asked to stand up from a seated position, he first pushes his hands against his knees and thighs before reaching a standing position. Which of the following is likely to be absent in biopsies of the muscles of this young boy?

A. Dystrophin
B. Iron channel
C. Acetylcholine
D. Glucose

ANSWER: A

The description in the above case is consistent with Duchenne muscular dystrophy, which is the most common muscular dystrophy in children. This condition is X-linked and presents nearly exclusively in males. Females are carriers. Onset is around age 5 and begins with difficulty walking and running. The affected child uses Gowers' maneuver (using hands to stand up from a sitting position). Muscles are weak due to the absence of dystrophin, a crucial muscle cell membrane protein.

REFERENCE

Kaufman, D. M. (2013). *Clinical neurology for psychiatrists* (7th ed., pp. 87–88). Philadelphia, PA: Elsevier Health Sciences.

61. A 30-year-old woman presents with double vision and nasal speech. On examination she has right-sided ptosis, asymmetric facial muscle weakness, and sagging of the lower lip. Intravenous administration of edrophonium temporarily improves the weakness. What is the likely diagnosis?

A. Myasthenia gravis
B. Lambert–Eaton myasthenic syndrome
C. Myotonic dystrophy
D. Inclusion body myositis
E. Statin myopathy

ANSWER: A

This presentation is consistent with myasthenia gravis, which is due to acetylcholine receptor antibodies that block, impair, or destroy nicotinic acetylcholine receptors at the neuromuscular junction. These antibodies target receptors in the extraocular, facial, neck, and proximal limb muscles. Tensilon (edrophonium) is a cholinesterase inhibitor that prolongs acetylcholine action, thus relieving symptoms temporarily. Edrophonium administration temporarily reverses ocular and facial weakness in an individual suffering from myasthenia gravis.

REFERENCE

Kaufman, D. M. (2013). *Clinical neurology for psychiatrists* (7th ed., pp. 83–85). Philadelphia, PA: Elsevier Health Sciences.

62. Which of the following is NOT caused by the antibodies found in myasthenia gravis?

A. Bulbar palsy
B. Respiratory paralysis
C. Quadriplegia
D. Cognitive impairments
E. Inability to speak

ANSWER: D

Acetylcholine (ACh) receptors at the neuromuscular junction are nicotinic; those in the central nervous system are muscarinic. As such, the nicotinic ACh receptor antibodies found in myasthenia gravis affect only strength, not cognition. Patients with myasthenia gravis do not have cognitive impairment related to the condition—though they certainly may have cognitive impairment of alternate etiology.

REFERENCE

Kaufman, D. M. (2013). *Clinical neurology for psychiatrists* (7th ed., p. 83). Philadelphia, PA: Elsevier Health Sciences.

63. Which of the following remain(s) intact in persistent vegetative states?

A. Sleep–wake cycle
B. Temperature regulation
C. Ability to breathe
D. Enteral digestion
E. All of the above

ANSWER: E

Individuals with persistent vegetative state do open their eyes but are not able to track or interact meaningfully with the people around them. Vital functions such s digestion, breathing, sleeping, and maintaining temperature remain in persistent vegetative state.

REFERENCE

Kaufman, D. M. (2013). *Clinical neurology for psychiatrists* (7th ed., pp. 249–250). Philadelphia, PA: Elsevier Health Sciences.

64. Persistent vegetative state is caused by injuries to which brain region(s)?

A. Brainstem
B. Cerebral cortex
C. Thalamus
D. Cerebellum
E. Ventral tegmentum

ANSWER: B

Extensive damage to the cerebral cortex without brainstem damage can result in persistent vegetative state (PVS). Cerebrocortical damage leads patients with PVS to lack awareness of themselves and their surroundings. They cannot communicate. A functionally intact brainstem continues to perform vital functions such as breathing, digestion, and temperature regulation.

REFERENCE

Kaufman, D. M. (2013). *Clinical neurology for psychiatrists* (7th ed., p. 249). Philadelphia, PA: Elsevier Health Sciences.

65. Which of the following can cause priapism?

A. Treatment with sildenafil
B. Treatment with trazodone
C. Sickle-cell crisis
D. Leukemia
E. All of the above

ANSWER: E

Treatment with medications such as a phosphodiesterase inhibitor or trazodone may produce priapism (a persistent, painful erection) in susceptible males. Other conditions that can cause priapism include sickle-cell crisis, leukemia, vascular abnormalities, and venous thrombosis. All of these can block the venous drainage of the penis and thereby prevent detumescence.

REFERENCE

Kaufman, D. M. (2013). *Clinical neurology for psychiatrists* (7th ed., pp. 356–357). Philadelphia, PA: Elsevier Health Sciences.

66. What is first-line management of priapism?

A. Epinephrine injection
B. Surgical drainage
C. Papaverine injection
D. Stop the offending agent
E. No treatment needed

ANSWER: A

Priapism is an emergency, so simply stopping the offending agent does not address the potential for penile necrosis. Priapism must be treated immediately. The goal is to reduce blood flow, and the first line of treatment is epinephrine injection to produce arterial vasoconstriction. Surgical drainage is considered in cases that remain refractory to epinephrine injection. Intracorporeal papaverine injection is given for erectile dysfunction to induce erection. Thus it will make the priapism worse.

REFERENCE

Kaufman, D. M. (2013). *Clinical neurology for psychiatrists* (7th ed., pp. 354, 356–367). Philadelphia, PA: Elsevier Health Sciences.

67. A 17-year-old male is hit on the left side of his head with a line drive while playing baseball. He collapses

with significant head pain but is able to get up and go home without any discomfort. Over the next hour he becomes more somnolent, and his headache worsens. Which of the following would explain this presentation?

A. Subdural hematoma
B. Epidural hematoma
C. Intraventricular hemorrhage
D. Subarachnoid hemorrhage
E. Concussion

ANSWER: B

The above scenario likely represents a case of epidural hematoma. The epidural hematoma results from temporal bone injury with laceration of the middle meningeal artery. This is essentially a rapidly expanding, high-pressure blood clot, which can compress the underlying brain and produce transtentorial herniation. Individuals with epidural hematoma may regain consciousness for a short while after initial insult before they lapse into coma. This brief period of consciousness is called the lucid interval.

REFERENCE

Kaufman, D. M. (2013). *Clinical neurology for psychiatrists* (7th ed., pp. 354, 528). Philadelphia, PA: Elsevier Health Sciences.

68. Which of the following muscle diseases is caused by an autosomal dominant, trinucleotide repeat on chromosome 19?

A. Steroid myopathy
B. Myotonic dystrophy
C. Duchenne muscular dystrophy
D. Malignant hyperthermia
E. Nemaline myopathy

ANSWER: B

Myotonic dystrophy is caused by excessive CTG repeats. Individuals typically become symptomatic with 50 or more repeats.

REFERENCE

Kaufman, D. M. (2013). *Clinical neurology for psychiatrists* (7th ed., pp. 354, 89–90). Philadelphia, PA: Elsevier Health Sciences.

69. Rates of unintentional overdose on prescription opioids have increased almost fourfold from the year 2000 to 2010, accounting for more than half of all overdose deaths and exceeding overdose deaths attributed to all other illicit drug categories combined. What is the most common factor in prescription opioid-related overdose deaths?

A. Concomitant use of benzodiazepines
B. Male gender
C. Nicotine use
D. Methadone use
E. Higher prescribed opioid dosage

ANSWER: A

Concomitant use of benzodiazepine is the most common factor in prescription opioid overdose deaths. In the United States, deaths from co-prescribed opioids and benzodiazepines increased 14% per year from 2006 to 2010. Potential mechanisms of action in overdose include metabolic drug–drug interactions, genetic differences in sensitivity, changes in drug transport mechanism, muscle relaxant effects in throat/airway, and exacerbation of sleep apnea.

REFERENCES

Brady, K. T., McCauley, J. L., & Back, S. E. (2015). Prescription opioid misuse, abuse, and treatment in the United States: An update. *American Journal of Psychiatry, 173*, 18–26.
Chen LH, Hedegaard H, Warner M. Drug-poisoning deaths involving opioid analgesics: United States, 1999–2011. NCHS Data Brief 2014(166):1–8.

70. Which of the following conditions is characterized by the presence of "K complexes" on electroencephalogram?

A. Coma
B. REM Sleep
C. N2 stage of sleep
D. Hepatic encephalopathy
E. Opioid overdose

ANSWER: C

K complexes along with sleep spindles are required features of the normal N2 stage of sleep, previously known as stage 2 NREM sleep. Of note, NREM sleep phases 3 and 4 have been condensed in the current nomenclature to N3 sleep.

REFERENCE

Kaufman, D. M. (2013). *Clinical neurology for psychiatrists* (7th ed., p. 365). Philadelphia, PA: Elsevier Health Sciences.

QUESTIONS AND ANSWERS

This chapter has accompanying questions and answers which are available to subscribers as part of the Oxford eLearning platform. To access the questions, follow the link below, or go to http://oxford-elearning.oup.com/books.

http://oxford-elearning.oup.com/books/test/67/10.1093/med/9780190265557.003.0012

13.

MANAGEMENT AND TREATMENT OF NEUROLOGICAL DISORDERS

Tatjana Barisic-Dujmovic

1. A 40-year-old woman with migraines presents with symptoms of unilateral throbbing pain, nausea, tinnitus, and ataxia. You suspect basilar-type migraine. What is the recommended abortive treatment of headaches in this case?

A. Sumatriptan
B. Dihydroergotamine
C. Ibuprofen
D. Verapamil
E. Topiramate

ANSWER: C

Basilar migraine is a rare type of migraine that presents with brainstem-related aura symptoms without accompanying weakness. Aura is typically manifested by brainstem symptoms, including dysarthria, vertigo, diplopia, tinnitus, and ataxia. Whereas multiple disorders can resemble basilar migraine, the most important differential diagnoses include brainstem transient ischemic attack (TIA) or stroke. In the case of basilar migraine, triptans are contraindicated. Current recommendations suggest avoiding sympathomimetics such as triptans and ergotamine derivatives due to concerns for cerebral vasoconstriction. Ibuprofen can be used for abortive treatment. The other agents listed, verapamil and topiramate, are effective for basilar migraine prevention.

REFERENCES

Headache Classification Committee of the International Headache Society (IHS). (2013). The International Classification of Headache Disorders, 3rd edition (beta version). *Cephalalgia, 33*, 629–808.

Kaniecki, R. G. (2009). Basilar-type migraine. *Current Pain and Headache Reports, 13*, 217–220.

2. A 28-year-old adopted male with major depression and history of two serious suicide attempts is ultimately diagnosed with Huntington's disease after he developed clumsiness, falls, and athetotic movements. He presents to the clinic for worsening choreiform movements. He is currently euthymic on fluoxetine. Which of the following is critical that the patient knows before starting tetrabenazine?

A. It is available under a humanitarian use exemption by the FDA.
B. Its use is off-label for Huntington's disease.
C. It may be more effective for athetosis than for choreiform movements.
D. It carries a black box warning for risk of depression and suicidality.

ANSWER: D

Tetrabenazine is the only FDA-approved medication for Huntington's disease, specifically for chorea. It is recommended as first-line treatment for Huntington's chorea. It does carry a black box warning for worsening depression and suicidality because it depletes monoamines. Other agents, including antipsychotics (some evidence for olanzapine, risperidone, and aripiprazole), amantadine, and riluzole, may be considered if tetrabenazine is ineffective or contraindicated. Tetrabenazine is metabolized via 2D6, and patients requiring doses more than 50 mg/day should be genotyped for *CYP2D6*.

REFERENCE

Armstrong, M. J., Miyasaki, J. M., & American Academy of Neurology. (2012). Evidence-based guideline: Pharmacologic treatment of chorea in Huntington disease: Report of the Guideline Development

Subcommittee of the American Academy of Neurology. *Neurology, 79*, 597.

3. A 57-year-old woman with no known medical history presents with new-onset, dull, moderate, unilateral pain over the left side of her head and behind the left eye. She reports no history of headaches but has been experiencing fatigue and weight loss for several weeks. Pain has been so unbearable that she has not been able to comb her hair. The patient came urgently to see you after she experienced a brief period of transient vision loss. What is the next step in the management of this patient?

A. MRI angiography
B. Arterial biopsy
C. Erythrocyte sedimentation rate
D. Glucocorticoid treatment
E. Doppler ultrasound

ANSWER: D

The vignette describes a likely case of giant cell arteritis. The condition is rare in individuals younger than 50 years old. Temporal artery biopsy is the gold standard for diagnosis of giant cell arteritis; however, treatment with glucocorticoids should not be delayed for biopsy results. This is especially the case when the patient already presents with visual loss and where intravenous methylprednisone is indicated. Other diagnostic tests including ESR, CRP, MRI, and ultrasound are useful but not required before treatment initiation.

REFERENCE

Hunder, G. G., Bloch, D. A., Michel, B. A., Stevens, M. B., Arend, W. P., Calabrese, L. H., ... & Lightfoot, R. W. (1990). The American College of Rheumatology 1990 criteria for the classification of giant cell arteritis. *Arthritis & Rheumatism, 33*(8), 1122–1128.

4. You are evaluating an 18-year-old female patient with worsening academic performance, depression, and irritability. On interview you note dysarthria, drooling, and wing-beating tremor. What would be the next best step in the management of this patient?

A. Start SSRI because the patient is depressed.
B. Pursue CT scan of the brain.
C. Start stimulant for attention deficit hyperactivity disorder.
D. Refer for neuropsychological testing.
E. Pursue laboratory work and refer the patient to ophthalmology for slit-lamp examination.

ANSWER: E

Wilson's disease is suspected when a young patient presents with a variety of neurological and psychiatric symptoms. Wilson's disease is inherited in an autosomal recessive manner, so obtaining a family history is helpful. This is specifically the case in the beginning of the illness when liver failure is not apparent. Symptoms of Wilson's disease include liver disease (most often with elevated aminotransferase levels, jaundice, and abdominal pain), as well as neurological (dysarthria, dysphagia, tremors, dystonia) and psychiatric (depression, personality change, irritability) symptoms. Among all the symptoms described above, presence of *wing-beating tremor* is specific for Wilson's disease. Finally, given suspicion of Wilson's disease, the next step in management should be referral for ophthalmologic exam (Kayser–Fleischer rings) and labs (serum ceruloplasmin, 24-hour urinary copper excretion, liver function tests).

REFERENCES

Lorincz, M. T. (2010). Neurologic Wilson's disease. Lorincz MT. *Annals of the New York Academy of Sciences, 1184*, 173–187.
Manolaki, N., Nikolopoulou, G., Daikos, G. L., Panagiotakaki, E., Tzetis, M., Roma, E., ... & Syriopoulou, V. P. (2009). Wilson disease in children: Analysis of 57 cases. *Journal of Pediatric Gastroenterology and Nutrition, 48*, 72–77.
Roberts, E. A., Schilsky, M. L., & American Association for Study of Liver Diseases (AASLD). (2008). Diagnosis and treatment of Wilson disease: An update. *Hepatology, 47*, 2089.

5. An elderly man presents with difficulty walking and has been tripping and falling at home. On neurological examination your findings are consistent with the symptoms of both upper and lower motor involvement. What is the proposed mechanism of action of the FDA-approved drug for this condition?

A. NMDA agonism
B. NMDA antagonism
C. Dopamine agonism
D. Dopamine antagonism

ANSWER: B

Medications available as disease-modifying agents for amyotrophic lateral sclerosis (ALS) are limited. Riluzole is the only medication shown to have a major impact on survival of patients with ALS. Its mechanism of action involves noncompetitive block of NMDA receptors. It is postulated that overactivity of NMDA receptors leads to excitotoxicity through increased influx of calcium ions into the cells. Calcium influx into the cells leads to mitochondrial damage and cell death. Additional mechanisms of action include inhibition of glutamate release and direct action on voltage-gated sodium channels. Other agents with a similar mechanism of action (NMDA antagonism) include ketamine, PCP, dextromethorphan, memantine, and amantadine. Riluzole does not directly affect dopamine receptors.

REFERENCES

Blasco, H., Mavel, S., Corcia, P., & Gordon, P. H. (2014). The glutamate hypothesis in ALS: Pathophysiology and drug development. *Current Medicinal Chemistry, 21*, 3551–3575.

Dutta, A., McKie, S., & Deakin, J. F. (2015). Ketamine and other potential glutamate antidepressants. *Psychiatry Research, 225*, 1–13.

Miller, R. G., Mitchell, J. D., & Moore, D. H. (2012). Riluzole for amyotrophic lateral sclerosis (ALS)/motor neuron disease (MND). *Cochrane Database of Systematic Reviews, 3*, CD001447

6. A young, healthy woman presents with mental status changes, including confusion, autonomic instability, choreathetoid movements, seizures, agitation, and bizarre hallucinations. Routine medical workup including CSF examination is significant for lymphocytic pleocytosis, and a brain MRI reveals no acute findings. Viral and bacterial cultures are negative. A few days after the patient has been admitted to the ICU, you are informed that CSF assay for anti–NMDA receptor antibodies returned positive. Which of the following will determine the overall prognosis of this condition is good?

A. Early tumor detection, removal, and immunosuppression
B. Acyclovir treatment
C. Seizure control with antiepileptic agent
D. Treatment of hallucinations
E. Treatment of chorea

ANSWER: A

The above case describes the clinical presentation of anti–NMDA receptor encephalitis. This condition belongs to a group of autoimmune encephalitides. When this condition is associated with teratoma, early detection and removal of the tumor and treatment with immunosuppressants portend a favorable outcome. In many cases of anti-NMDA receptor encephalitis, no tumor can be found. As these antibodies are directly pathogenic by activating NMDA receptors, immunosuppression is first-line management. Other autoimmune encephalitides, such as paraneoplastic meningoencephalitis associated with anti-Hu antibodies, have unfavorable outcomes both because of the associated malignancy and because immunosuppression is largely ineffective. Antibodies such as anti-Hu target *intracellular* epitopes, and neurological symptoms are due principally to cytotoxic (T8) cell effects.

REFERENCES

Dalmau, J., Tüzün, E., Wu, H. Y., Masjuan, J., Rossi, J. E., Voloschin, A., ... & Mason, W. (2007). Paraneoplastic anti-N-methyl-D-aspartate receptor encephalitis associated with ovarian teratoma. *Annals of Neurology, 61*, 25–36.

Vitaliani, R., Mason, W., Ances, B., Zwerdling, T., Jiang, Z., & Dalmau, J. (2005). Paraneoplastic encephalitis, psychiatric symptoms, and hypoventilation in ovarian teratoma. *Annals of Neurology, 58*, 594–604.

7. A 38-year-old man presents with subacute onset of lower extremity weakness accompanied by a "pins and needles" sensation. He reported that 2 weeks ago he experienced abdominal cramping, periumbilical pain, and diarrhea. He has no significant prior medical history. On physical examination there was diffuse muscle weakness in all four extremities with distal weakness greater than proximal. Muscle tone was decreased, and reflexes were absent. Which of the following is first-line management?

A. Oral glucocorticoids
B. Intravenous immune globulin
C. Intravenous glucocorticoids
D. Vitamin B12
E. Pyridostigmine

ANSWER: B

Weakness with loss of reflexes is suggestive of lower motor neuron lesion. Guillain–Barré syndrome is an acute illness that usually follows an infection. Plasmapheresis and intravenous immune globulin are effective by eliminating antimyelin and antiaxonal antibodies. Immunomodulatory agents, as well as supportive care including respiratory and cardiovascular management, are mainstays of treatment. Corticosteroids are typically not beneficial and so are not generally recommended.

REFERENCES

Guillain–Barré Syndrome Steroid Trial Group. (1993). Double-blind trial of intravenous methylprednisolone in Guillain-Barré syndrome. *Lancet, 341*, 586.

Osterman, P. O., Lundemo, G., Pirskanen, R., Fagius, J., Pihlstedt, P., Sidén, Å., & Säfwenberg, J. (1984). Beneficial effects of plasma exchange in acute inflammatory polyradiculoneuropathy. *Lancet, 324*(8415), 1296–1299.

8. A 7-year-old boy presents with recurrent 10- to 20-second episodes of staring and unresponsiveness, at times accompanied by chewing motions and lip smacking. Electroencephalography shows 3-Hz spike and wave discharges. A trial of ethosuximide causes frightening auditory hallucinations. What medication may be used as an alternative to ethosuximide for this condition?

A. Lamotrigine
B. Valproic acid
C. Phenytoin
D. Carbamazepine
E. Levetiracetam

ANSWER: B

Absence seizures present with brief loss of awareness without loss of muscle tone and is often accompanied by automatisms as noted in this vignette. There is no prodromal aura or postictal confusion. EEG is specific for 3-Hz spike wave discharge but can vary from 2.5 to 5 Hz. Ethosuximide is often the first-line treatment for absence seizures, but it may cause psychosis and parkinsonism. Valproic acid is a good alternative without a risk of causing psychosis.

REFERENCE

Glauser, T. A., Cnaan, A., Shinnar, S., Hirtz, D. G., Dlugos, D., Masur, D., ... & Adamson, P. C. (2010). Ethosuximide, valproic acid, and lamotrigine in childhood absence epilepsy. *New England Journal of Medicine, 362*(9), 790–799.

9. An HIV-positive, 45-year-old man presents with fever, headache, speech difficulties, and right hemiparesis. The patient reports that symptoms have been progressively worsening over the past few weeks. He is nonadherent with antiretroviral therapy. CD4 count is 50 cells/µl. Magnetic resonance imaging (MRI) reveals multiple ring-enhancing regions in the left basal ganglia and frontal cortex. Single photon emission computed tomography (SPECT) scan demonstrates decreased uptake of thallium in these lesions. What is the best initial treatment?

A. Sulfadiazine and pyrimethamine
B. Acyclovir
C. Ganciclovir
D. High-dose methotrexate
E. Vancomycin and ceftriaxone

ANSWER: A

Cerebral toxoplasmosis is the leading cause of central nervous system (CNS) infection in acquired immunodeficiency syndrome (AIDS) that usually occurs with CD4 count less than 100 cells/µl. Standard treatment includes a combination of sulfadiazine and pyrimethamine. Differential diagnosis includes CNS lymphoma, mycobacterial infection, bacterial abscess, progressive multifocal leukoencephalopathy (PML), and others. While awaiting serology results, one can make a presumptive diagnosis of toxoplasmosis based on the clinical presentation and imaging results. In contrast to brain lymphoma, lesions in toxoplasmosis will have decreased thallium uptake on SPECT. Acyclovir and ganciclovir are used for herpes simplex encephalitis. High-dose methotrexate is effective treatment of CNS lymphoma. Finally, vancomycin and ceftriaxone are empirical treatments when bacterial meningitis is suspected.

REFERENCES

Nath, A., & Sinai, A. P. (2003). Cerebral toxoplasmosis. *Current Treatment Options in Neurology, 5*, 3.

Skiest, D. J., Erdman, W., Chang, W. E., Oz, O. K., Ware, A., & Fleckenstein, J. (2000). SPECT thallium-201 combined with toxoplasma serology for the presumptive diagnosis of focal central nervous system mass lesions in patients with AIDS. *Journal of Infection, 40*(3), 274–281.

10. Deep brain stimulation of which brain region is effective for medication-refractory essential tremor?

A. Subthalamic nucleus
B. Nucleus accumbens
C. Inferior thalamic peduncle
D. Globus pallidus interna
E. Ventral intermediate nucleus of thalamus

ANSWER: E

Deep brain stimulation (DBS) is a neurosurgical treatment found to be effective for treatment of Parkinson's disease, essential tremor, dystonias, unipolar depression, obsessive–compulsive disorder, and Tourette's disorder. Stimulation of ventral intermediate nucleus of thalamus has been found to be effective for treatment of essential tremor. In patient's with Parkinson's disease, subthalamic nucleus and globus pallidus interna are stimulated. Stimulation of multiple areas of brain, including nucleus accumbens and inferior thalamic peduncle, has been targeted for treatment of obsessive–compulsive disorder and Tourette's disorder.

REFERENCE

Zesiewicz, T. A., Elble, R., Louis, E. D., Hauser, R. A., Sullivan, K. L., Dewey, R. B., ... & Weiner, W. J. (2005). Practice parameter: Therapies for essential tremor: Report of the Quality Standards Subcommittee of the American Academy of Neurology. *Neurology, 64*(12), 2008–2020.

11. A college student presents with severe headache, nausea, vomiting, and delirium. CSF examination reveals 68 WBC/ml with lymphocyte predominance, protein of 89 mg/dl, and glucose 60 mg/dl. T2-weighted MRI is significant for hyperintensity in the medial temporal lobes. Which of the following medications could reduce mortality and morbidity in this patient?

A. Sulfadiazine and pyrimethamine
B. Dexamethasone
C. Acyclovir
D. Cyclophosphamide
E. Penicillin

ANSWER: C

The above case describes clinical presentation of viral encephalitis with lymphocytic pleocytosis, increased protein, and normal glucose in CSF. The MRI findings are highly suggestive of HSV encephalitis and correspond to early edematous changes in temporal lobes. Although definitive diagnosis is made with HSV-PCR, the clinical presentation and supportive findings warrant immediate treatment because untreated HSV encephalitis is usually fatal. Empirical treatment with acyclovir should begin while awaiting PCR results. Sulfadiazine and pyrimethamine are initial treatments for cerebral toxoplasmosis. Adjunctive dexamethasone reduces cerebral edema. Immunosuppressive agents like cyclophosphamide are the treatment of choice for paraneoplastic and nonparaneoplastic autoimmune encephalitis.

REFERENCES

Levitz, R. E. (1998). Herpes simplex encephalitis: A review. *Heart and Lung, 27*, 209.

Whitley, R. J., Alford, C. A., Hirsch, M. S., Schooley, R. T., Luby, J. P., Aoki, F. Y., ... & Soong, S. J. (1986). Vidarabine versus acyclovir therapy in herpes simplex encephalitis. *New England Journal of Medicine, 314*(3), 144–149.

12. Preventive therapy for cluster headache includes verapamil or which of the following?

A. Sumatriptan
B. 100% oxygen at 10 to 12 L via face mask
C. Naproxen
D. Metoclopramide
E. Lithium

ANSWER: E

Verapamil and lithium are commonly used as preventive agents for cluster headache. In fact, unlike in migraine, cluster headaches are commonly headache free with prophylaxis.

REFERENCE

Loder, E. W. (2015). Diagnosis and treatment of headache. In B. S. Fogel & D. B. Greenberg (Eds.), *Psychiatric care of the medical patient* (3rd ed., pp. 963–983). New York, NY: Oxford University Press.

13. Which of the following medications used for treatment of multiple sclerosis (MS) has been associated with reactivation of JC virus?

A. Glatiramer acetate
B. Natalizumab
C. Interferon beta
D. Glucocorticoids
E. Cyclophosphamide

ANSWER: B

Progressive multifocal leukoencephalopathy (PML) is a severe, fatal demyelinating brain disease caused by the polyoma JC virus. Infection with JC virus is very common in the general population, but progression to PML occurs almost exclusively with immunosuppression. It can occur in advanced HIV disease, especially when the CD4 count is less than 200. Similarly, it can present with the use of immunosuppressive agents used for treatment, such as for lymphomas and leukemias. Natalizumab, a monoclonal antibody that targets alpha-4 integrins and indicated for remitting-relapsing MS, has been associated with JC virus reactivation.

REFERENCES

Kappos, L., Bates, D., Edan, G., Eraksoy, M., Garcia-Merino, A., Grigoriadis, N., ... & Kremenchutzky, M. Natalizumab treatment for multiple sclerosis: Updated recommendations for patient selection and monitoring. *Lancet Neurology, 10*(8), 745–758.

Tan, C. S., & Koralnik, I. J. (2010). Progressive multifocal leukoencephalopathy and other disorders caused by JC virus: Clinical features and pathogenesis. *Lancet Neurology, 9*, 425.

14. A previously healthy 26-year-old female presents with worsening low back pain for the past 2 weeks. She is also reporting significant heaviness, numbness, and tingling in both legs and has been stumbling while walking. Further history elicits two recent episodes of urinary incontinence. MRI of the spine is negative for cord compression but suggests cord inflammation. What is the treatment for this condition?

A. Penicillin
B. Vitamin B12
C. Methylprednisolone
D. Acyclovir
E. NSAIDs

ANSWER: C

Transverse myelitis usually presents with back pain and numbness and tingling in the lower extremities, accompanied by leg weakness and symptoms of bladder dysfunction (incontinence, incomplete bladder emptying) and/or bowel dysfunction (incontinence, constipation). Primary transverse myelitis is thought to be autoimmune, but its precise cause remains unknown. Secondary causes infections due to varicella zoster, cytomegalovirus, herpes simplex virus, Epstein–Barr virus, West Nile virus, HIV, *Mycoplasma*, and syphilis. It can also be the initial presentation in multiple sclerosis. Intravenous glucocorticoids are effective, including other immunomodulating therapy (plasmapheresis or cyclophosphamide).

REFERENCES

Beh, S. C., Greenberg, B. M., Frohman, T., & Frohman, E. M. (2013). Transverse myelitis. *Neurologic Clinics, 31*(1), 79–138.

Krishnan, C., Kaplin, A. I., Pardo, C. A., Kerr, D. A., & Keswani, S. C. (2006). Demyelinating disorders: Update on transverse myelitis. *Current Neurology and Neuroscience Reports, 6*(3), 236.

Scott, T. F., Frohman, E. M., De Seze, J., Gronseth, G. S., & Weinshenker, B. G. (2011). Evidence-based guideline: Clinical evaluation and treatment of transverse myelitis: Report of the Therapeutics and Technology Assessment Subcommittee of the American Academy of Neurology. *Neurology, 77*(24), 2128.

15. Baclofen is an effective agent in the treatment of spasticity associated with multiple sclerosis. What is its mechanism of action?

A. Agonism at alpha-2 adrenoreceptors
B. Agonism at GABA A receptors
C. Antagonism at GABA A receptors
D. Agonism at GABA B receptors
E. Antagonism at GABA B receptors

ANSWER: D

Baclofen treats spasticity in multiple sclerosis and is usually given up to 120 mg daily in divided doses. Intrathecal baclofen is also available in the form of a "baclofen pump." Baclofen is an agonist at postsynaptic GABA B receptors.

REFERENCE

Chou, R., Peterson, K., & Helfand, M. (2004). Comparative efficacy and safety of skeletal muscle relaxants for spasticity and musculoskeletal conditions: A systematic review. *Journal of Pain and Symptom Management, 28*, 140.

16. A 19-year-old man presents with intermittent episodes of muscle weakness, especially during rest periods after strenuous exercise or a high carbohydrate meal. He tells you that his father also suffers from similar symptoms and has been diagnosed with hypokalemic periodic paralysis. Which of the following medications can be used to prevent these attacks?

A. Propranolol
B. Thiazide diuretic
C. Pyridostigmine
D. Prednisone
E. Potassium-sparing diuretic

ANSWER: E

Hypokalemic periodic paralysis is a rare autosomal dominant condition characterized by episodes of muscle weakness that coincide with the lowering of blood potassium levels. Between episodes, muscle strength is normal. Weakness is rare during exercise, but it is triggered by resting after exercise. This condition is caused by a hereditary defect in muscle ion channels. Attacks are usually aborted with potassium chloride treatment orally. Preventive strategy includes treatment with potassium-sparing diuretic.

REFERENCE

Miller, T. M., Da Silva, M. D., Miller, H. A., Kwiecinski, H., Mendell, J. R., Tawil, R., ... & Petajan, J. (2004). Correlating phenotype and genotype in the periodic paralyses. *Neurology, 63*(9), 1647–1655.

17. A 65-year-old man has recent onset of moderately severe headaches that have been bothering him at night to the point that he awakens due to the pain. His headaches occur at least twice a week without any specific precipitant. The pain is usually dull and bilateral, without ptosis, miosis, lacrimation, or conjunctival injection. What is the best treatment?

A. Lithium carbonate
B. Oxygen
C. Sumatriptan
D. Valproate
E. Acetaminophen

ANSWER: A

Hypnic headaches often occur in individuals who are older than 50. Recommended treatment includes a low dose of lithium carbonate, usually 300 to 600 mg at bedtime. Alternatives include caffeine at bedtime, indomethacin, or verapamil. Typical clinical features include nocturnal onset of headaches that awaken the person from sleep. Clinical presentation can vary, but usually the individual presents with dull, bilateral (but sometimes unilateral) pain without significant associated autonomic features. Diagnosis is clinical, but neuroimaging should be performed to rule out structural causes.

REFERENCE

Newman, L. C., Lipton, R. B., & Solomon, S. (1990). The hypnic headache syndrome: A benign headache disorder of the elderly. *Neurology, 40*, 1904.

18. Which of the following medications is approved by the FDA for the treatment of recurrent glioblastoma multiforme?

A. Temozolomide
B. Methotrexate
C. Vincristine
D. Cisplatin
E. Bevacizumab

ANSWER: E

Bevacizumab is a recombinant monoclonal antibody directed against vascular endothelial growth factor A (VEGF-A). It is FDA approved for the treatment of recurrent glioblastoma multiforme. For newly diagnosed glioblastoma multiforme, radiation with concurrent temozolomide followed by monthly temozolomide is the standard of care. High-dose methotrexate is indicated for treatment of CNS lymphoma.

REFERENCES

Friedman, H. S., Prados, M. D., Wen, P. Y., Mikkelsen, T., Schiff, D., Abrey, L. E., ... & Vredenburgh, J. (2009). Bevacizumab alone and in combination with irinotecan in recurrent glioblastoma. *Journal of Clinical Oncology, 27*(28), 4733–4740.
Stupp, R., Hegi, M. E., Mason, W. P., van den Bent, M. J., Taphoorn, M. J., Janzer, R. C., ... & Hau, P. (2009). Effects of radiotherapy with concomitant and adjuvant temozolomide versus radiotherapy alone on survival in glioblastoma in a randomised phase III study: 5-year analysis of the EORTC-NCIC trial. *Lancet Oncology, 10*(5), 459–466.

19. A patient on a stable dose of phenytoin develops horizontal nystagmus, unsteady gait, and slurred speech. Which of the following medications, if recently started in this patient, would account for these symptoms?

A. St. John's wort
B. Carbamazepine
C. Rifampin
D. Cimetidine
E. Phenobarbital

ANSWER: D

Phenytoin is a CYP2C9 and 2C19 substrate and is sensitive to drug interactions involving CYP450. Cimetidine is a known inhibitor of many CYP450 enzymes and increases phenytoin levels, leading to phenytoin toxicity. Early symptoms associated with the mild increase in phenytoin level include horizontal nystagmus and unsteady gait. With increased phenytoin plasma level, lethargy, nausea, vomiting, and even coma can occur. Other medications listed here will increase phenytoin metabolism via p450 induction.

REFERENCE

Brodie, M. J., Mintzer, S., Pack, A. M., Gidal, B. E., Vecht, C. J., & Schmidt, D. (2013). Enzyme induction with antiepileptic drugs: Cause for concern? *Epilepsia, 54*(1), 11–27.

20. A 9-year-old child develops worsening headache, especially in the morning, accompanied by vomiting without nausea. MRI with gadolinium reveals enhancing tumor within the fourth ventricle. Microscopic examination reveals the presence of dense, round blue cells. What is the best treatment for this condition?

A. Surgery
B. Radiation therapy
C. Chemotherapy
D. Combination of surgery, radiation therapy, and chemotherapy
E. Glucocorticoids

ANSWER: D

Medulloblastoma accounts for 30% of pediatric brain tumors and is the most common malignant brain tumor in children. Initial symptoms are caused by increased intracranial pressure, and children usually experience headache upon awakening and progressive vomiting without nausea. Hypercellularity and round blue cells on histologic examination are diagnostic. A combination of surgery, radiation, and chemotherapy offers the best outcome. The 5-year survival rate for children with average-risk disease is 70% to 80%.

REFERENCES

Eberhart, C. G., Kepner, J. L., Goldthwaite, P. T., Kun, L. E., Duffner, P. K., Friedman, H. S., ... & Burger, P. C. (2002). Histopathologic grading of medulloblastomas: A Pediatric Oncology Group study. *Cancer, 94*(2), 552–560.

Taylor, R. E., Bailey, C. C., Robinson, K., Weston, C. L., Ellison, D., Ironside, J., ... & Pizer, B. L. (2003). Results of a randomized study of preradiation chemotherapy versus radiotherapy alone for nonmetastatic medulloblastoma: The International Society of Paediatric Oncology/United Kingdom Children's Cancer Study Group PNET-3 Study. *Journal of Clinical Oncology, 21*(8), 1581–1591.

21. A 47-year-old woman who recently moved from South China has been diagnosed with trigeminal neuralgia. She was found to be positive for HLA-B*1502 allele. Which of the following medications preferred for the treatment of her condition?

A. Gabapentin
B. Carbamazepine
C. Oxcarbazepine
D. Lamotrigine
E. Phenytoin

ANSWER: A

Prevalence of HLA-B*1502 allele is low in the general population, but it can be around 10% to 15% in some parts of China, Thailand, Malaysia, Indonesia, the Philippines, and Taiwan. Screening for HLA-B*1502 allele is recommended in all Asian patients; if results are positive, carbamazepine should be avoided to minimize the risk of Stevens–Johnson syndrome. Some studies have suggested avoiding oxcarbazepine, phenytoin, and lamotrigine as well. No such association has been found with the use of gabapentin.

REFERENCES

Chen, P., Lin, J. J., Lu, C. S., Ong, C. T., Hsieh, P. F., Yang, C. C., ... & Yu, H. Y. (2011). Carbamazepine-induced toxic effects and HLA-B*1502 screening in Taiwan. *New England Journal of Medicine, 364*(12), 1126–1133.

Khan, O. A. (1998). Gabapentin relieves trigeminal neuralgia in multiple sclerosis patients. *Neurology, 51*, 611.

22. Which of the following medications improve muscle strength and pulmonary function in patients with Duchenne muscle dystrophy?

A. Cyclosporine
B. Prednisone
C. Azathioprine
D. Statins
E. Zidovudine

ANSWER: B

While gene therapy research is underway, several randomized controlled studies have suggested that prednisone has been associated with a 11% increase in muscle strength compared with placebo in Duchenne muscle dystrophy. Urine creatinine excretion, which is an indirect measure of muscle mass, is increased with prednisone treatment. Forced vital capacity (FVC) also improves significantly after 6 months of therapy with prednisone when compared with placebo. Immunosuppressant medications, including cyclosporine and azathioprine, do not improve muscle strength. Statins and zidovudine cause drug-induced myopathies and have no benefit in improving muscle strength in Duchenne muscle dystrophy.

REFERENCES

Mendell, J. R., Moxley, R. T., Griggs, R. C., Brooke, M. H., Fenichel, G. M., Miller, J. P., ... & Schierbecker, J. (1989). Randomized, double-blind six-month trial of prednisone in Duchenne's muscular dystrophy. *New England Journal of Medicine, 320*(24), 1592–1597.

Moxley, R. T., Ashwal, S., Pandya, S., Connolly, A., Florence, J., Mathews, K., ... & Wade, C. (2005). Practice parameter: Corticosteroid treatment of Duchenne dystrophy: Report of the Quality Standards Subcommittee of the American Academy of Neurology and the Practice Committee of the Child Neurology Society. *Neurology, 64* (1), 13–20.

23. A 12-year-old girl has had difficulty walking since the age of 3 years. She also has gait abnormalities due to leg stiffness. Her symptoms are less prominent in the morning but worsen progressively as the day passes. She will most likely respond to which of the following medications?

A. Baclofen
B. Low dose of L-dopa
C. Tetrabenazine
D. Trihexyphenidyl
E. Botulinum toxin injections

ANSWER: B

Dopa-responsive dystonia (Segawa disease) usually presents in early childhood with symptoms of generalized dystonia and symptoms starting in one leg. Children with this condition are frequently misdiagnosed as having cerebral palsy. The key clinical feature is that the symptoms improve with sleep and worsen as the day progresses. Dopa-responsive dystonia responds dramatically with a low dose of L-dopa. Other agents listed here have been studied for the treatment of various other types of dystonias. Botulinum toxin injection is beneficial with localized types of dystonia such as cervical dystonia and blepharospasm.

REFERENCES

Nygaard, T. G., Trugman, J. M., de Yebenes, J. G., & Fahn, S. (1990). Dopa-responsive dystonia: The spectrum of clinical manifestations in a large North American family. *Neurology, 40*(1), 66–66.

Segawa, M., Hosaka, A., Miyagawa, F., Nomura, Y., & Imai, H. (1976). Hereditary progressive dystonia with marked diurnal fluctuation. *Advances in Neurology, 14*, 215–233.

24. A 68-year-old man with an extensive smoking history presents with severe low back pain, numbness and weakness in the lower extremities, and urinary incontinence. In addition, he reports weight loss and hoarseness of voice. What is the next best step in the management?

A. Bed rest
B. High dose of dexamethasone
C. An MRI in 1 week
D. Surgery
E. External beam radiotherapy

ANSWER: B

The above case suggests the clinical presentation of epidural cord compression in the context of likely lung malignancy. In 20% of cases, epidural cord compression is the initial presenting symptom of the malignancy. The most important prognostic factors are early diagnosis and early therapeutic intervention. MRI imaging is superior over CT when epidural cord compression is suspected. When cord compression is suspected and MRI is not available, glucocorticoids should be initiated, especially with severe symptom presentation. Early administration of glucocorticoids may increase the likelihood that a patient will be ambulatory at the end of treatment and at 6-month follow up. Other modalities, including surgery and external beam radiotherapy, have a role in treatment of cord compression after dexamethasone treatment.

REFERENCES

Loblaw, D. A., Mitera, G., Ford, M., & Laperriere, N. J. (2012). 2011 updated systematic review and clinical practice guideline for the management of malignant extradural spinal cord compression. *International Journal of Radiation Oncology*Biology*Physics, 84*, 312–317.

Sørensen, P. S., Helweg-Larsen, S., Mouridsen, H., & Hansen, H. H. (1994). Effect of high-dose dexamethasone in carcinomatous metastatic spinal cord compression treated with radiotherapy: A randomised trial. *European Journal of Cancer, 30*(1), 22–27.

25. A 25-year-old female, G2P2, who is 10 days postpartum presents to the emergency room with severe left-sided headache with blurred vision. While in the emergency room, she has a general tonic–clonic seizure. Initial head CT scan shows no acute findings, but MR venogram shows absent flow in the right transverse sinus, sigmoid sinus, and internal jugular vein. What is the appropriate treatment for this condition?

A. Sumatriptan
B. Valproate
C. Aspirin
D. Heparin
E. Mannitol

ANSWER: D

Cerebral venous thrombosis is frequently missed and misdiagnosed because it is considered to be a rare clinical entity. It has been associated with hypercoagulable states as in pregnancy or postpartum or with the use of oral contraceptives. Although variable in presentation, it commonly presents with severe headaches, delirium, and seizures. Laboratory tests, including coagulation labs, can be useful, but definite diagnosis requires neuroimaging. Head CT scan can be normal in up to 30% of cases. MRI in conjunction with MR venography is highly sensitive and specific for this diagnosis. Treatment includes use of anticoagulants based on current guidelines. Mannitol can be useful for the management of intracranial pressure as needed. Valproate can be used for seizure prophylaxis.

REFERENCES

Coutinho, J. M., & Stam, J. (2010). How to treat cerebral venous and sinus thrombosis. *Journal of Thrombosis and Haemostasis, 8*(5), 877–883.

26. A migraineur presents to the emergency room with severe headache, photophobia, and blurry vision in both eyes. Intraocular pressure was elevated at 72/67 mm Hg in both eyes. Which medication is the likely cause of this presentation?

A. Sumatriptan
B. Ibuprofen
C. Valproate
D. Gabapentin
E. Topiramate

ANSWER: E

Topiramate is indicated for epilepsy and migraine treatment (prophylaxis). However, it has many off-label indications, including treatment of alcohol use disorder, binge eating disorder, post-traumatic stress disorder, essential tremor, and weight loss. Topiramate is the only anticonvulsant that can cause angle-closure glaucoma. Typical onset of glaucoma occurs within a month of topiramate initiation. Patients should be educated to discontinue topiramate in the case of decreased visual acuity and ocular pain. Other medications that can cause this presentation include anticholinergics, antihistamines, diuretics, and tricyclic antidepressants. Sumatriptan can cause visual disturbances but not acute angle-closure glaucoma.

REFERENCES

Aminlari, A., East, M., & Wei, W. (2008). Topiramate induced acute angle closure glaucoma. *Open Ophthalmology Journal, 2*, 46–47.
Lachkar, Y., & Bouassida, W. (2007). Drug induced angle closure glaucoma. *Current Opinion in Ophthalmology, 18*, 129–133.

27. A 29-year-old immigrant from Great Britain began to experience rapidly progressive neurocognitive decline accompanied by hallucinations over the past 3 months. He now presents with clumsiness, sudden jerking movements, and difficulty speaking. Family history is negative for a similar presentation. What is the most effective treatment for his condition?

A. Tetrabenazine
B. Donepezil
C. L-dopa
D. Deep brain stimulation
E. No known effective treatment

ANSWER: E

Variant Creutzfeldt–Jakob disease is a progressive neurodegenerative disease caused by prions that has been linked to bovine spongiform encephalopathy. Usually, the initial presentation includes psychiatric symptoms, including depression, dementia, hallucinations, and anxiety. As the disease progresses, neurological symptoms appear and include ataxia, myoclonus, dysarthria, and invalidism. One would expect a positive family history if this were a case of Huntington's disease. Variant Creutzfeldt–Jakob disease is relentlessly progressive and fatal because no treatment has been found to be effective.

REFERENCES

Heath, C. A., Cooper, S. A., Murray, K., Lowman, A., Henry, C., MacLeod, M. A., ... & Will, R. G. (2011). Diagnosing variant Creutzfeldt–Jakob disease: A retrospective analysis of the first 150 cases in the UK. *Journal of Neurology, Neurosurgery and Psychiatry, 82*, 646.
Will, R. G., Ironside, J. W., Zeidler, M., Estibeiro, K., Cousens, S. N., Smith, P. G., ... & Hofman, A. (1996). A new variant of Creutzfeldt–Jakob disease in the UK. *Lancet, 347*, 921.

28. A 40-year-old man with acquired immune deficiency syndrome (AIDS) due to failed treatment with antiretroviral therapy presents with acute central vision loss accompanied by floaters in his right eye. He denies eye pain but does have a headache. Ophthalmoscopy was suggestive of retinal atrophy in a "brush-fire" pattern. What is the treatment?

A. Ganciclovir
B. Acyclovir
C. Ribavirin
D. Interferon
E. Oseltamivir

ANSWER: A

Cytomegalovirus (CMV) encephalitis and retinitis had a higher incidence in the era before antiretrovirals. CMV retinitis is still considered the most serious ocular complications of AIDS. When diagnosed, it is usually associated with either medication nonadherence or failed antiretroviral therapy. The presence of floaters is highly suggestive of CMV infection and is a good predictor of CMV retinitis. Clinical presentation and ophthalmoscopy are sufficient for diagnosis. Ganciclovir or its prodrug valganciclovir constitutes effective treatment for CMV encephalitis and retinitis.

REFERENCE

Martin, D. F., Sierra-Madero, J., Walmsley, S., Wolitz, R. A., Macey, K., Georgiou, P., ... & Stempien, M. J. (2002). A controlled trial of valganciclovir as induction therapy for cytomegalovirus retinitis. *New England Journal of Medicine, 346*, 1119–1126.

29. Exclusion criteria for the treatment of acute ischemic stroke with tissue plasminogen activator include all of the following EXCEPT:

A. Systolic blood pressure more than 185 mmHg
B. History of intracranial hemorrhage 10 years earlier
C. INR > 1.7
D. Blood glucose of 55 mg/dl
E. Significant head trauma within past 3 months

ANSWER: D

Blood glucose lower than 50 mg/dl is an exclusion criterion for tPA administration. This is important because hypoglycemia can mimic acute stroke or symptoms of transient ischemic attack (TIA). During early management of stroke, hypoglycemia should be corrected diligently. The other choices (A, B, C, and E) are exclusion criteria for tPA administration.

REFERENCES

Jauch, E. C., Saver, J. L., Adams, H. P., Bruno, A., Demaerschalk, B. M., Khatri, P., ... & Summers, D. R. (2013). Guidelines for the early management of patients with acute ischemic stroke: A guideline for healthcare professionals from the American Heart Association/American Stroke Association. *Stroke, 44*(3), 870–947.

Wallis, W. E., Donaldson, I., Scott, R. S., & Wilson, J. (1985). Hypoglycemia masquerading as cerebrovascular disease (hypoglycemic hemiplegia). *Annals of Neurology, 18*(4), 510–512.

30. Tuberous sclerosis may present with subependymal tumors. Which of the following medications has the FDA recently approved for the management of subependymal giant cell tumors not suitable for surgical resection?

A. Oxcarbazepine
B. Everolimus
C. Temozolomide
D. Bevacizumab
E. High-dose methotrexate

ANSWER: B

Everolimus is an immunosuppressant that inhibits mTOR and is used to prevent organ rejection after renal transplant. It was recently approved by the FDA for the management of subependymal giant cell tumors in patients who are not suitable for surgical resection. Oxcarbazepine can be useful for management of simple partial or complex partial seizures associated with tuberous sclerosis. Temozolomide and bevacizumab are indicated for treatment of glioblastoma multiforme.

REFERENCES

Curatolo, P., Bombardieri, R., & Jozwiak, S. (2008). Tuberous sclerosis. *Lancet, 372*, 657.

Krueger, D. A., Care, M. M., Holland, K., Agricola, K., Tudor, C., Mangeshkar, P., ... & Franz, D. N. (2010), Everolimus for subependymal giant-cell astrocytomas in tuberous sclerosis. *New England Journal of Medicine, 363*(19), 1801–1811.

Tee, A. R., Fingar, D. C., Manning, B. D., Kwiatkowski, D. J., Cantley, L. C., & Blenis, J. (2002). Tuberous sclerosis complex-1 and -2 gene products function together to inhibit mammalian target of rapamycin (mTOR)-mediated downstream signaling. *Proceedings of the National Academy of Sciences*, *99*(21), 13571–13576.

QUESTIONS AND ANSWERS

This chapter has accompanying questions and answers which are available to subscribers as part of the Oxford eLearning platform. To access the questions, follow the link below, or go to http://oxford-elearning.oup.com/books.

http://oxford-elearning.oup.com/books/test/67/10.1093/med/9780190265557.003.0013

PART III

CLINICAL PSYCHIATRY

Edited by Rajiv Radharkrishnan, Lily Arora

14.

CHILDHOOD-ONSET DISORDERS

Waqar Rizvi

1. Which of the following stages of sleep demonstrates abnormality on EEG confirming the diagnosis of somnambulism?

A. N1 (old NREM 1)
B. N2 (old NREM 2)
C. N3 (old NREM 3 and NREM 4)
D. REM stage

ANSWER: C

Somnambulism, more commonly known as sleepwalking is commonly seen in children aged 5 to 12. Sleepwalking and night terrors occur during N3 sleep (also called slow-wave sleep). The modern model of sleep architecture has relabeled NREM 1 as N1, and NREM 2 as N2; NREM 3 and 4 have been condensed to N3.

REFERENCE

Sadock, B. J., & Sadock, V. A. (2015). *Kaplan and Sadock's synopsis of psychiatry* (11th ed.). Philadelphia, PA: Lippincott Williams and Wilkins.

2. A 13-year-old girl with bulimia is admitted to the pediatric service for an eating disorder. She admits to using ipecac to induce vomiting multiple times daily. With which of the following medical issues should the primary care team be most concerned about this time?

A. Refeeding syndrome
B. Blunting of the villi in the small intestine
C. Cardiomyopathy
D. Acute liver toxicity
E. Leukopenia

ANSWER: C

Ipecac is a commonly used emetic agent. Abuse of ipecac on a regular basis increases the likelihood of dangerous cardiac effects, including cardiomyopathy, cardiomegaly, prolonged QTc interval, increased cardiac enzymes, and dysrhythmia. Other effects include leukopenia and increased liver function tests, but the cardiac effects would warrant immediate investigation.

REFERENCE

Sadock, B. J., Sadock, V. A., & Ruiz, P. (Eds.). (2009). *Kaplan and Sadock's comprehensive textbook of psychiatry* (9th ed.). Philadelphia, PA: Wolters Kluwer Health/Lippincott Williams and Wilkins.

3. Which of the following HLA haplotypes is MOST often noted to be positive in patients with narcolepsy?

A. HLA-A
B. HLA-B
C. HLA-B2
D. HLA-C
E. HLA-DQ

ANSWER: E

HLA-DQ and HLA-DR are two alleles that are found in about 85% of patients with narcolepsy. These alleles are found in 15% to 35% of the general population.

REFERENCE

Martin, A., & Volkmar, F. R. (2007). *Lewis' child and adolescent psychiatry* (4th ed.). Philadelphia, PA: Lippincott Williams and Wilkins.

4. An adolescent male who has no concerns about his marijuana use is brought to the outpatient clinic by his mother for substance abuse treatment. Such a patient is most likely presenting in which of the following stages of change?

A. Precontemplative
B. Contemplative
C. Preparation
D. Action
E. Maintenance

ANSWER: A

The patient is likely in the precontemplative stage. More often than not, it is the caregivers who are concerned about substance abuse in children and adolescents, rather than the patients themselves. Motivational interviewing was designed as a means of motivating patients to make progress across the phases of change. For instance, in the precontemplative phase of change, goals of motivational interviewing include establishment of a healthy alliance and encouragement that the patient at least begin observing potential risks associated with the problem behavior.

REFERENCE

Martin, A., & Volkmar, F. R. (2007). *Lewis' child and adolescent psychiatry* (4th ed.). Philadelphia, PA: Lippincott Williams and Wilkins.

5. Which of the following was the most common comorbid diagnosis seen during the National Institute of Mental Health's screening for childhood-onset schizophrenia?

A. ADHD
B. Obsessive–compulsive disorder
C. Depression
D. Bipolar disorder
E. Marijuana abuse

ANSWER: C

During the National Institute of Mental Health's screening for childhood-onset schizophrenia, the most common comorbid diagnosis was depression.

REFERENCE

Martin, A., & Volkmar, F. R. (2007). *Lewis' child and adolescent psychiatry* (4th ed.). Philadelphia, PA: Lippincott Williams and Wilkins.

6. A 12-year-old girl with attention deficit hyperactivity disorder (ADHD) has been optimized on appropriate dosing with methylphenidate. Although she notes some improvement in her symptoms of impulsivity, she still has significant symptoms of inattention, poor concentration, and some hyperactivity. What would be the next best recommended medication to target her symptoms of ADHD?

A. Dextroamphetamine
B. Guanfacine
C. Clonidine
D. Bupropion
E. Atomoxetine

ANSWER: A

Stimulant medications are the gold standard treatment for ADHD. When methylphenidate is only partially effective at best, the next step is to switch to dextroamphetamine or mixed amphetamine salts. Alpha-2 agonists such as guanfacine and clonidine also are used with good effect and would be the drug of choice either if both methylphenidate and dextroamphetamine were ineffective or if there were any significant contraindications to their use. Bupropion and atomoxetine are used for the treatment of ADHD but generally are considered only after other strategies have failed.

REFERENCE

Sadock, B. J., Sadock, V. A., & Ruiz, P. (Eds.). (2009). *Kaplan and Sadock's comprehensive textbook of psychiatry* (9th ed.). Philadelphia, PA: Wolters Kluwer Health/Lippincott Williams and Wilkins.

7. Which of the following is most often seen in patients with encopresis?

A. ADHD
B. Conduct disorder
C. Oppositional defiant disorder
D. History of sexual abuse
E. History of delayed speech

ANSWER: D

All the answers provided may or may not be present in patients with a diagnosis of encopresis, but a known history of sexual abuse has been seen with much greater frequency in such patients. To a lesser degree, encopresis has also been associated with maternal hostility as well as with punitive or harsh parenting styles.

REFERENCE

Sadock, B. J., Sadock, V. A., & Ruiz, P. (Eds.). (2009). *Kaplan and Sadock's comprehensive textbook of psychiatry* (9th ed.). Philadelphia, PA: Wolters Kluwer Health/Lippincott Williams and Wilkins.

8. A woman brings in her 14-month-old daughter for concerns regarding a change in the child's functioning. The mother reports that the child had normal development until about 6 months of age. Around that time, the child began to lose social engagement with her parents. On exam, she has repetitive wringing of her hands and appears to be psychomotorically slowed. Her head growth circumference shows a decelerated pattern. Which of the following is the most likely diagnosis?

A. Childhood disintegrative disorder
B. Rett syndrome
C. Fragile X syndrome
D. Autism spectrum disorder
E. Asperger disorder

ANSWER: B

Rett syndrome presents with normal development up until about 5 months of age. Between 6 months and 2 years of age, the child exhibits a loss of previously acquired motor, social, and language skills. These patients also show a deceleration of head circumference growth. Rett syndrome is seen exclusively in females. Because Rett syndrome is now known to represent a specific neurogenetic syndrome, it is no longer included in the *DSM-5*. Additionally, pervasive developmental disorders of *DSM-IV-TR* have been combined into autism spectrum disorder in *DSM-5*. Accordingly, childhood disintegrative disorder and Asperger disorder are no longer formally present in the *DSM*. Fragile X syndrome can present with deficits in motor, social, and language skills but not a loss of previously acquired skills.

REFERENCE

Martin, A., & Volkmar, F. R. (2007). *Lewis' child and adolescent psychiatry* (4th ed.). Philadelphia, PA: Lippincott Williams and Wilkins.

9. Which of the following is NOT a typical symptom of narcolepsy?

A. Hypnogogic hallucinations
B. Hypnopompic hallucinations
C. Sleep paralysis
D. Cataplexy
E. Catalepsy

ANSWER: E

Narcolepsy is a sleep disorder characterized by irresistible sleep attacks that occur daily for at least 3 months and includes episodes of sleep paralysis, which often involve hypnogogic and/or hypnopompic hallucinations. Cataplexy, which is defined as the loss of muscle tone during sleep attacks, can also be seen. Catalepsy is a phenomenon seen in patients with catatonia and is often used synonymously with the term *waxy flexibility*.

REFERENCE

Sadock, B. J., & Sadock, V. A. (2015). *Kaplan and Sadock's synopsis of psychiatry* (11th ed.). Philadelphia, PA: Lippincott Williams and Wilkins.

10. A 15-year-old male is brought to the emergency room by ambulance for an acute change in behavior. He was found by his family to be screaming in the garage, and the garage was in complete disarray. In the emergency room, he is belligerent and assaultive at times. On exam, he has nystagmus, blurred vision, slurred speech, a perioral rash, and an unsteady gait. Family reports that he has no past psychiatric history and no such presentations in the past. What is the most likely diagnosis?

A. Bipolar disorder
B. Psychotic disorder
C. Conduct disorder
D. Oppositional defiant disorder
E. Substance intoxication

ANSWER: E

The most likely cause for this patient's presentation is substance intoxication, specifically inhalant abuse. Evidence that points to this includes the acute change in his behavior, the lack of a past similar presentation, and the physical findings of the perioral rash (often referred to as the "huffer's rash"). Neurological findings of inhalant abuse include nystagmus, blurred vision, dizziness, slurred speech, incoordination, tremor, and an unsteady gait. Furthermore, such patients can present with a variety of mood and behavioral symptoms such as lethargy, euphoria, belligerence, and aggression.

REFERENCE

Sadock, B. J., Sadock, V. A., & Ruiz, P. (Eds.). (2009). *Kaplan and Sadock's comprehensive textbook of psychiatry* (9th ed.). Philadelphia, PA: Wolters Kluwer Health/Lippincott Williams and Wilkins.

11. An infant in the specialty clinic has symptoms of multifocal myoclonus and rapid dancing movements of the eyes. Which of the following is the MOST common cause of this movement disorder?

A. In utero exposure to cocaine
B. Premature birth
C. Head trauma
D. Neonatal seizures
E. Neuroblastoma

ANSWER: E

The movement disorder described in the question is opsoclonus–myoclonus, which is a paraneoplastic movement disorder, also referred to as dancing eyes–dancing feet syndrome. It is most often seen in infants between the ages of 6 months and 18 months. More than 50% of the cases are notably due to an infantile neuroblastoma. The disorder can also be seen in adults but with less prevalence. In these cases symptoms can be due to lung cancer, postviral encephalitis, multiple sclerosis, or thalamic hemorrhage.

REFERENCE

Daroff, R. B., Fenichel, G. M., Jankovic, J., & Mazziotta, J. C. (2012). *Bradley's neurology in clinical practice* (6th ed.). Philadelphia, PA: Saunders.

12. When during normal development does the highest rate of synapse formation in the brain occur?

A. Within the second trimester
B. Within the third trimester
C. Between 0 and 6 months of age
D. Around 2 years of age
E. During adolescence

ANSWER: D

Synapse formation occurs at a dramatically high rate from the second trimester until age 10. However, it generally peaks during the toddler period, at around 2 years of age, with as many as 30 million synapses forming per second.

REFERENCE

Daroff, R. B., Fenichel, G. M., Jankovic, J., & Mazziotta, J. C. (2012). *Bradley's neurology in clinical practice* (6th ed.). Philadelphia, PA: Saunders.

13. A 5-year-old child is brought to the clinic by his mother for "not being like other children" at home and school. You find that the child does not make appropriate eye contact with others, including his mother, and also fails to respond to the social cues put forth by his mother. Reports from school describe a lack of the ability for spontaneous make-believe play and a delay in language development. Although there are various toys in the office, the child is fixated on playing with a shiny candy bar wrapper that was in the trash bin. His mother reports that some of these symptoms have been present from around the age of 3, but she thought "he'd grow out of it." What is the most likely diagnosis?

A. Normal child development
B. DiGeorge syndrome
C. Autism spectrum disorder
D. Avoidant personality disorder
E. ADHD

ANSWER: C

This presentation is diagnostic of autism spectrum disorder. Patients with autism have deficient social skills such as a lack of the ability to read or use nonverbal gestures or an inability to engage in emotional reciprocity. They demonstrate communication deficits such as delays in language development or repetitive or idiosyncratic use of language. They do not engage in make-believe play. They also exhibit repetitive or stereotypical patterns of behaviors such as abnormal, persistent preoccupation with areas of interest or parts of objects. Some of the symptoms must be present prior to age 3 years.

REFERENCE

Sadock, B. J., Sadock, V. A., & Ruiz, P. (Eds.). (2009). *Kaplan and Sadock's comprehensive textbook of psychiatry* (9th ed.). Philadelphia, PA: Wolters Kluwer Health/Lippincott Williams and Wilkins.

14. Which of the following would be more likely to be seen in a patient with conduct disorder as opposed to ADHD or a mood disorder?

A. Pattern of irritable mood
B. Excessive activity
C. Impulsive behaviors
D. Recurrent fights
E. Sleep disturbance

ANSWER: D

In conduct disorder, the patient shows a pattern of behaviors that violate societal rules and the rights of others. These behaviors are often exemplified by bullying others, starting fights, using weapons, stealing, setting fires, destroying property, being truant, or running away from home. Although patients with ADHD and mood disorders such as depression and bipolar disorder can have significant behavioral problems, they are usually the result of symptoms of inattention, hyperactivity, impulsivity, low mood, irritability, and even mania. In conduct disorder, the behaviors are typically patterns in which the patient is intentionally or malevolently being violent, destructive, or truant.

REFERENCE

Martin, A., & Volkmar, F. R. (2007). *Lewis' child and adolescent psychiatry* (4th ed.). Philadelphia, PA: Lippincott Williams and Wilkins.

15. A school psychiatrist is consulted on a 9-year-old girl whose mother reports she does not want to go to school and has been refusing to do her homework. The girl's teacher states that her behaviors have been relatively good, but she refuses to read out loud in class. Her parents do not note any other changes in behavior at home. They state that their daughter continues to be active socially outside of school and enjoys visiting friends' homes and spending the night at her grandparents' house without her parents. Testing records indicate that her IQ is average for her age. What is the most likely diagnosis?

A. Reading disorder
B. ADHD
C. Autism
D. Separation anxiety disorder
E. Conduct disorder

ANSWER: A

The child's difficulties are all in the context of situations in which she may be asked to read. Although she is refusing to go to school, she does not appear to have any difficulty separating from her parents, as evidenced by her staying with friends and grandparents overnight. Conduct disorder would present with a pattern of behaviors that violate societal rules and offend the rights of others. Although truancy can be seen in patients with conduct disorder, this child's school refusal would not be sufficient to diagnose her with conduct disorder; moreover, her presentation is more concerning for a learning disorder, such as a reading disorder.

REFERENCE

Sadock, B. J., Sadock, V. A., & Ruiz, P. (Eds.). (2009). *Kaplan and Sadock's comprehensive textbook of psychiatry* (9th ed.). Philadelphia, PA: Wolters Kluwer Health/Lippincott Williams and Wilkins.

16. A 10-year-old boy presents for evaluation of behavioral problems. His parents state that he often fights with both his mother and father, mostly surrounding doing chores and setting limits at home. His teacher tells you that he has relatively good grades in school but that he becomes very rude and dismissive toward her when she asks him to do a particular task, and he often refuses to cooperate with her after his tantrums. Which of the following is the most likely diagnosis?

A. Normal child development
B. ADHD
C. Oppositional defiant disorder
D. Conduct disorder
E. Bipolar disorder

ANSWER: C

In oppositional defiant disorder, children show a pattern of negativistic, hostile, and defiant behavior directed at adults or authority figures, often against parents, teachers, care providers, security guards, and even police officers. These behaviors can include arguing with adults, deliberately defying adults or authority figures, intentionally annoying people, behaving in a spiteful or vindictive manner, and even throwing temper tantrums.

REFERENCE

Martin, A., & Volkmar, F. R. (2007). *Lewis' child and adolescent psychiatry* (4th ed.). Philadelphia, PA: Lippincott Williams and Wilkins.

17. A 6-year-old child has been observed to be sexually provocative with peers, using profane sexual language and exposing his genitals to classmates. He is sexualized in his play while in the office and makes sexual gestures when observed. Which of the following is the most likely cause of this behavior?

A. Normal child development
B. Early-onset puberty
C. Neglect at home
D. Sexual abuse
E. Childhood-onset bipolar disorder

ANSWER: D

The child in question is too young to have such detailed knowledge of sexual acts, gestures, and language in the absence of exposure to these, likely in the form of sexual abuse. In such cases, it is often noted that these young children have either witnessed or participated in sexual behaviors, which are classified as sexual abuse.

REFERENCE

Sadock, B. J., Sadock, V. A., & Ruiz, P. (Eds.). (2009). *Kaplan and Sadock's comprehensive textbook of psychiatry* (9th ed.). Philadelphia, PA: Wolters Kluwer Health/Lippincott Williams and Wilkins.

18. What is the most important step in treating a child with school refusal?

A. Establishing an appropriate home school program
B. Sending the child back to school as soon as possible
C. Prescribing an anxiolytic medication to address the underlying anxiety
D. Prescribing a stimulant medication to address the underlying ADHD
E. Starting family therapy

ANSWER: B

Treatment of children with school refusal should be multimodal and include psychoeducation, individual therapy for the child, family-based therapy, and sending the child back to school as soon as possible. Studies show that the more prolonged the school refusal becomes, the more difficult it becomes to treat overall. Underlying or comorbid anxiety, mood disorders, and ADHD should be evaluated and managed as well, but the single most important remains to return to school as soon as possible.

REFERENCE

Martin, A., & Volkmar, F. R. (2007). *Lewis' child and adolescent psychiatry* (4th ed.). Philadelphia, PA: Lippincott Williams and Wilkins.

19. A mother brings in her 30-month-old child because he has not spoken any words yet. What is the best next step?

A. Reassurance
B. Audiometry
C. Chromosomal analysis
D. Brain MRI
E. Speech therapy

ANSWER: B

By this age, the child should have a vocabulary of anywhere between 270 words (by 2 years of age) and 895 words (by 3 years of age), have some conversations with other children, and have speech that is about 50% to 80% intelligible. The first step is to evaluate for hearing impairment with audiometry. Once structural and neurological problems have been investigated, a diagnosis can be made, and the appropriate intervention can be initiated.

REFERENCE

Sadock, B. J., & Sadock, V. A. (2015). *Kaplan and Sadock's synopsis of psychiatry* (11th ed.). Philadelphia, PA: Lippincott Williams and Wilkins.

20. Tourette's syndrome is often comorbid with which of the following psychiatric illnesses?

A. Separation anxiety disorder
B. Generalized anxiety disorder
C. OCD
D. Major depressive disorder
E. Childhood-onset schizophrenia

ANSWER: C

ADHD, OCD, and conduct disorder are three psychiatric manifestations that are more commonly seen in patients with Tourette's syndrome than are other psychiatric manifestations.

REFERENCE

Martin, A., & Volkmar, F. R. (2007). *Lewis' child and adolescent psychiatry* (4th ed.). Philadelphia, PA: Lippincott Williams and Wilkins.

21. Which of the following is the MOST common symptom seen in patients with narcolepsy?

A. Sleep attacks
B. Cataplexy
C. Sleep paralysis
D. Hypnogogic hallucinations
E. Hypnopompic hallucinations

ANSWER: A

All the choices given are common symptoms of narcolepsy, but the most common symptom is sleep attacks. Another common finding of narcolepsy is the initiation of the REM cycle early in the sleep. Treatment includes taking regularly scheduled naps during the day, as well as the use of stimulants and antidepressants.

REFERENCE

Sadock, B. J., Sadock, V. A., & Ruiz, P. (Eds.). (2009). *Kaplan and Sadock's comprehensive textbook of psychiatry* (9th ed.). Philadelphia, PA: Wolters Kluwer Health/Lippincott Williams and Wilkins.

22. Of the following mechanisms of child abuse, which is the most likely to result in death or long-term sequelae?

A. Cerebral hypoxia from asphyxiation
B. Skull fracture from head trauma
C. Seizures from head trauma
D. Subdural hemorrhages from head trauma
E. Embolic stroke from multiple bone fractures

ANSWER: D

Subdural hemorrhages can occur from head trauma, often due to shaken-baby syndrome, and can be fatal. The constant, violent back-and-forth movements result in cerebral trauma related to vascular shearing and tearing. Retinal hemorrhages are also a common finding in such patients. It has been estimated that 95% of severe intracranial injuries in children 1 year of age or younger are due to child abuse.

REFERENCE

Daroff, R, B, Fenichel, G. M., Jankovic, J., & Mazziotta, J. C. (2012). *Bradley's neurology in clinical practice* (6th ed.). Philadelphia, PA: Saunders.

23. Which of the following is MOST appropriate for a child with aggressive behaviors and a diagnosis of intellectual disability?

A. Lithium
B. Lorazepam
C. Methylphenidate
D. Trazodone
E. Imipramine

ANSWER: A

Lithium is a commonly prescribed medication for aggressive behaviors in a wide array of patients, including those with bipolar disorder, schizophrenia, conduct disorder, and intellectual disability. Other commonly used medications for aggressive behaviors in these patient populations include antipsychotics and anticonvulsants. Of note, benzodiazepines can be disinhibiting in children with intellectual disability and can actually worsen the aggressive behaviors.

REFERENCE

Sadock, B. J., Sadock, V. A., & Ruiz, P. (Eds.). (2009). *Kaplan and Sadock's comprehensive textbook of psychiatry* (9th ed.). Philadelphia, PA: Wolters Kluwer Health/Lippincott Williams and Wilkins.

24. Which of the following is the most widely abused recreational substance among high school students in the United States?

A. Amphetamines
B. Cannabis
C. Cocaine
D. Inhalants
E. Opiates

ANSWER: B

Cannabis is the most widely used recreational substance among high school students in the United States. About 35% of 12th graders have reported using cannabis, compared with about 15% for alcohol. The other options have variable rates of abuse among high school students but do not surpass cannabis use.

REFERENCE

Sadock, B. J., Sadock, V. A., & Ruiz, P. (Eds.). (2009). *Kaplan and Sadock's comprehensive textbook of psychiatry* (9th ed.). Philadelphia, PA: Wolters Kluwer Health/Lippincott Williams and Wilkins.

25. Which of the following medications would be the drug of choice for an adolescent with ADHD, depression, and a seizure disorder?

A. Atomoxetine
B. Bupropion
C. Escitalopram
D. Guanfacine
E. Venlafaxine

ANSWER: A

Atomoxetine is efficacious for ADHD and has modest antidepressant activity. Similarly, many studies have shown efficacy for depressive and ADHD symptoms with the use of bupropion. However, it is known to lower the seizure threshold and as such would not be a recommended drug of choice in a patient with a history of seizure disorder. The other choices do not target both depression and ADHD, but rather just one or the other.

REFERENCE

Martin, A., & Volkmar, F. R. (2007). *Lewis' child and adolescent psychiatry* (4th ed.). Philadelphia, PA: Lippincott Williams and Wilkins.

26. Which of the following is the most accurate measure of depression in adolescents?

A. Interview with the patient's parents
B. Interview with the patient's teachers
C. Interview with the adolescent him- or herself
D. Minnesota Multiphasic Personality Inventory (MMPI)
E. Autism Spectrum Rating Scale (ASRS)

ANSWER: C

A standard psychiatric evaluation of the patient should be conducted directly, although information from the collaterals can often be quite illuminating. The MMPI and ASRS would not be as useful in this situation.

REFERENCE

Sadock, B. J., & Sadock, V. A. (2015). *Kaplan and Sadock's synopsis of psychiatry* (11th ed.). Philadelphia, PA: Lippincott Williams and Wilkins.

27. Lesch–Nyhan syndrome results from a deficiency in which enzyme?

A. Arylsulfatase-A (ASA)
B. Beta-glucosidase
C. Galactocerebroside beta-galactosidase
D. Hexosaminidase A
E. Hypoxanthine-guanine phosphoribosyltransferase

ANSWER: E

Lesch–Nyhan syndrome is an X-linked recessive hereditary disorder that results from a deficiency in hypoxanthine-guanine phosphoribosyltransferase enzyme. Clinical hallmarks of the syndrome include cognitive impairment, developmental delay, self-mutilation behavior, hypertonia, hyperreflexia, dysarthria, and choreoathetotic movements. The other choices are causes of other inborn errors of metabolism.

REFERENCE

Daroff, R. B., Fenichel, G. M., Jankovic, J., & Mazziotta, J. C. (2012). *Bradley's neurology in clinical practice* (6th ed.). Philadelphia, PA: Saunders.

28. Which one of the following is NOT a risk factor for persistence of stuttering?

A. Hesitation with interjection
B. Incomplete sentences with change of focus
C. Repetition of a sound

D. Repetition of a syllable
E. Repetition of a word

ANSWER: E

Many children go through periods of dysfluency through the developmental period, known as "normal dysfluency" or stuttering, which are considered to be a normal phase of language development. These often begin during a child's intensive language-learning years and resolve prior to puberty. "Normal dysfluency" tends to occur in the large linguistic units, such as words, phrases, and even sentences. About 75% of children who stutter as such often get better without any treatment.

REFERENCE

Martin, A., & Volkmar, F. R. (2007). *Lewis' child and adolescent psychiatry* (4th ed.). Philadelphia, PA: Lippincott Williams and Wilkins.

29. How are stereotypies differentiated from tics?

A. Stereotypies tend to be unilateral; tics tend to be bilateral.
B. Stereotypies have an earlier onset than tics.
C. Stereotypy intensity tends to fluctuate; tics tend to be consistent over time.
D. Stereotypies have a later onset than tics.
E. Stereotypies and tics are indistinguishable.

ANSWER: B

Stereotypies and tics are easily confused. Stereotypies usually tend to have an earlier age of onset than do tics (usually at around 2 or 3 years of age), are bilateral, and are consistent throughout time as opposed to the fluctuating patterns of tics.

REFERENCE

Martin, A., & Volkmar, F. R. (2007). *Lewis' child and adolescent psychiatry* (4th ed.). Philadelphia, PA: Lippincott Williams and Wilkins.

30. Which one of the following is not typically an effective and recommended method of treating enuresis in childhood?

A. Bell-and-pad conditioning
B. Desmopressin
C. Amitriptyline
D. Imipramine
E. Risperidone

ANSWER: E

Enuresis should first be treated with behavioral conditioning (such as bell-and-pad conditioning) treatments prior to pharmacological modalities. If symptoms persist, medications such as desmopressin (DDAVP) and TCAs such as amitriptyline and imipramine may be effective. Antipsychotics such as risperidone do not play a role in the treatment of childhood enuresis.

REFERENCE

Sadock, B. J., Sadock, V. A., & Ruiz, P. (Eds.).(2009). *Kaplan and Sadock's comprehensive textbook of psychiatry* (9th ed.). Philadelphia, PA: Wolters Kluwer Health/Lippincott Williams and Wilkins.

QUESTIONS AND ANSWERS

This chapter has accompanying questions and answers which are available to subscribers as part of the Oxford eLearning platform. To access the questions, follow the link below, or go to http://oxford-elearning.oup.com/books.

http://oxford-elearning.oup.com/books/test/67/10.1093/med/9780190265557.003.0014

15.

PSYCHIATRIC PRESENTATIONS DUE TO MEDICAL CONDITIONS

Harvinder Singh, Nery Diaz

1. Which of the following would be safest for acute anxiety caused by acute intermittent porphyria?

A. Phenobarbital
B. Valproic acid
C. Ethanol
D. Carbamazepine
E. Diazepam

ANSWER: E

Diazepam is safest for anxiety caused by acute intermittent porphyria. The other options are porphyrinogenic. Furthermore, ethanol has no medical role whatsoever in managing anxiety.

REFERENCES:

Disler, P. B. (1982). Guidelines for drug prescription in patients with the acute porphyrias. *South African Medical Journal, 61*, 656–660.

Millward, L. M., Kelly, P., King, A., et al. (2005). Anxiety and depression in the acute porphyrias. *Journal of Inherited Metabolic Disease, 28*, 1099–1107.

2. Which of the following features is required for a diagnosis of delirium?

A. Disorganized thoughts
B. Inattention
C. Sedation
D. Hallucinations
E. Agitation

ANSWER: B

Inattention is required for a diagnosis of delirium. *DSM-5* has introduced the specifiers hyperactive, hypoactive, and mixed level of activity, but these are not required for delirium diagnosis.

REFERENCE

American Psychiatric Association. (2013). *Diagnostic and statistical manual of mental disorders* (5th ed.). Arlington, VA: American Psychiatric Publishing.

3. Which neurotransmitter abnormality is identified most consistently in delirium?

A. Increased glutamate
B. Decreased dopamine
C. Increased GABA
D. Decreased acetylcholine
E. Increased serotonin

ANSWER: D

There is evidence that cholinergic deficiency plays a role in delirium. Increased dopaminergic activity may also play a role. The roles of serotonin, glutamate, and GABA in delirium are less well established.

REFERENCE

Solai, L. K. K. (2009). Delirium. In B. J. Sadock, V. A. Sadock & P. Ruiz (Eds.), *Kaplan and Sadock's comprehensive textbook of psychiatry* (9th ed., p. 1157). Philadelphia, PA: Wolters Kluwer Health/Lippincott Williams and Wilkins.

4. Which of the following medications can worsen or cause delirium?

A. Lorazepam
B. Aspirin
C. Hydrochlorothiazide
D. Haloperidol
E. Olanzapine

ANSWER: A

Lorazepam and other benzodiazepines can increase risk of delirium from use as well as from withdrawal.

REFERENCE

Solai, L. K. K. (2009). Delirium. In B. J. Sadock, V. A. Sadock & P. Ruiz (Eds.), *Kaplan and Sadock's comprehensive textbook of psychiatry* (9th ed., pp. 1158–1159). Philadelphia, PA: Wolters Kluwer Health/ Lippincott Williams and Wilkins.

5. Which of the following features best differentiates delirium from major neurocognitive disorder?

A. Amnesia
B. Depression
C. Baseline mental status
D. Inability to copy a picture
E. Inability to do math (acalculia)

ANSWER: C

Delirium indicates an acute change from baseline mental status. The baseline cognition is impaired in major neurocognitive disorder. It is possible to have delirium superimposed on major neurocognitive disorder, and this would be reflected as an acute and fluctuating change from the baseline impairment.

REFERENCE

American Psychiatric Association. (2013). *Diagnostic and statistical manual of mental disorders* (5th ed.). Arlington, VA: American Psychiatric Publishing.

6. Which of the following can be diagnosed during an episode of delirium?

A. Major depressive disorder
B. Bipolar disorder
C. Schizophrenia
D. Panic disorder
E. None of the above

ANSWER: E

The diagnosis for each of these illnesses cannot be made in the context of a delirium, as delirium may present with psychiatric symptoms that resolve when the underlying cause of the delirium resolves.

REFERENCE

American Psychiatric Association. (2013). *Diagnostic and statistical manual of mental disorders* (5th ed.). Arlington, VA: American Psychiatric Publishing.

7. Which of the following psychiatric symptoms is a core diagnostic feature of major neurocognitive disorder with Lewy bodies?

A. Visual hallucinations
B. Auditory hallucinations
C. Delusions
D. Anxiety
E. Depression

ANSWER: A

The core diagnostic features of major neurocognitive disorder with Lewy bodies are (A) fluctuating cognition with pronounced variations in attention and alertness, (B) recurrent visual hallucinations that are well formed and detailed, and (C) spontaneous features of parkinsonism with onset subsequent to the development of cognitive decline.

REFERENCE

American Psychiatric Association. (2013). *Diagnostic and statistical manual of mental disorders* (5th ed.). Arlington, VA: American Psychiatric Publishing.

8. What is the most common neuropsychiatric complication seen in patients with HIV?

A. Cognitive decline
B. Visual hallucinations
C. Insomnia
D. Depression
E. Mania

ANSWER: D

Depression is the most common neuropsychiatric complication in HIV.

REFERENCE

Nanni, M. G., Caruso, R., Mitchell, A. J., et al. (2015). Depression in HIV infected patients: A review. *Current Psychiatry Reports, 17,* 530.

9. Use of which antiepileptic medication is MOST associated with new-onset psychosis?

A. Valproic acid
B. Gabapentin
C. Lamotrigine
D. Phenobarbital
E. Levetiracetam

ANSWER: E

Levetiracetam has been associated with development of psychotic symptoms in 1% to 1.4% of adult patients (and higher rates in children). It also is associated with depression, aggressive behavior, emotional lability, and personality changes.

REFERENCE

Sirsi, D., & Safdieh, J. E. (2007). The safety of levetiracetam. *Expert Opinion on Drug Safety, 6,* 241–250.

10. Which of the following statements is TRUE regarding neuropsychiatric symptoms in Huntington's disease?

A. Psychosis is the most common neuropsychiatric symptom.
B. Irritability and depression may present several years prior to onset of motor symptoms.
C. The suicide rate among patients with Huntington's disease is 25%.
D. Symptoms worsen with duration of the disease.
E. The predominant cognitive symptom is attentional dysfunction.

ANSWER: B

Irritability and depression may present several years before the onset of motor symptoms. The suicide rate among patients with Huntington's disease is around 7%, and suicidal ideation among mutation carriers is around 20%. The most common symptoms are depression, apathy, irritability, and anxiety. Symptoms do not correlate with duration of the disease and can be seen very early in the course of illness.

REFERENCES

Di Maio, L., Squitieri, F., Napolitano, G., et al. (1993). Onset symptoms in 510 patients with Huntington's disease. *Journal of Medical Genetics, 30,* 289.
Di Maio, L., Squitieri, F., Napolitano, G., et al. (1993). Suicide risk in Huntington's disease. *Journal of Medical Genetics, 30,* 293.
Kirkwood, S. C., Su, J. L., Conneally, P., et al. (2001). Progression of symptoms in the early and middle stages of Huntington disease. *Archives of Neurology, 58,* 273.
Paulsen, J. S., Ready, R. E., Hamilton, J. M., et al. (2001). Neuropsychiatric aspects of Huntington's disease. *Journal of Neurology, Neurosurgery and Psychiatry, 71,* 310.
Shiwach, R. (1994). Psychopathology in Huntington's disease patients. *Acta Psychiatrica Scandinavica, 90,* 241.
van Duijn, E., Kingma, E. M., Timman, R., et al. (2008). Cross-sectional study on prevalences of psychiatric disorders in mutation carriers of Huntington's disease compared with mutation-negative first-degree relatives. *Journal of Clinical Psychiatry, 69,* 1804–1810.
van Duijn, E., Kingma, E M., & van der Mast, R. C. (2007). Psychopathology in verified Huntington's disease gene carriers. *Journal of Neuropsychiatry and Clinical Neuroscience, 19,* 441–448.

11. Which of the following diseases of the endocrine system has been associated with onset of depression?

A. Hypothyroidism
B. Hyperthyroidism
C. Diabetes mellitus
D. Cushing's syndrome
E. All of the above

ANSWER: E

All of the above endocrine disorders have been associated with onset of depression.

REFERENCE

Akiskal, H. S. (2009). Mood disorders: Clinical features. In B. J. Sadock, V. A. Sadock, & P. Ruiz (Eds.), *Kaplan and Sadock's comprehensive textbook of psychiatry* (9th ed., p. 1727). Philadelphia, PA: Wolters Kluwer Health/Lippincott Williams and Wilkins.

12. What is the approximate lifetime prevalence of depression among patients with multiple sclerosis?

A. 5%
B. 10%
C. 20%
D. 50%
E. More than 75%

ANSWER: D

Multiple sclerosis patients have an approximate lifetime depression prevalence of 50%.

REFERENCE

Sadovnick, A. D., Remick, J., Allen, E., et al. Depression and multiple sclerosis. *Neurology,* 1996 Mar; *46*(3):628–32.

13. Which of the following statements is TRUE regarding depression in cancer patients?

A. Mortality is unaffected by the presence of depression in cancer patients.
B. Terminally ill cancer patients who wish death would come quickly are no more likely to be depressed than patients who do not wish to die.
C. Depression is an expected reaction to a cancer diagnosis and does not need treatment.
D. Depression in cancer patients is highly correlated with physical functioning.
E. Depression rates are comparable for cancer patients in inpatient and outpatient settings.

ANSWER: D

Patients with cancer who are the most physically disabled have significantly higher rates of major depressive disorder than those who are moderately disabled or in good physical condition. The presence of depression increases mortality in cancer patients. Patients who wish death would come quickly are more likely to be depressed than those who do not wish to die. Not all cancer patients are depressed, and cancer patients should be treated for depression because treatment may improve outcomes. Depression rates are lower among cancer patients in the outpatient treatment setting.

REFERENCE

Blazer, D. G., Steffens, D C., & Koenig, H. G. (2009). Mood disorders. In D. G. Blazer & D. C. Steffens (Eds.), *The American Psychiatric Publishing textbook of geriatric psychiatry* (4th ed., p. 287). Arlington, VA: American Psychiatric Publishing.

14. Which of the following is TRUE regarding sleep in patients with chronic obstructive pulmonary disease (COPD)?

A. The degree of sleep disruption is related to hypoxemia.
B. Daytime sleepiness is associated with COPD.
C. Sleep apnea is more common among patients with COPD than in the general population.
D. Zolpidem adversely affects respiration among patients with COPD.
E. Ramelteon has no adverse effect on respiration in patients with mild to moderate COPD.

ANSWER: E

Ramelteon has not shown adverse effect when used to improve sleep among patients with mild to moderate COPD. Zolpidem does not appear to have an adverse effect on respiration among COPD patients, but benzodiazepines have a negative effect on oxygenation among patients with severe COPD. The degree of sleep disruption does not appear to be related to hypoxemia in COPD. Daytime sleepiness is observed among patients with sleep apnea but not those with COPD. Sleep apnea is no more common among patients with COPD than in the general population.

REFERENCE

Krystal, A. D., Edinger, J. D., & Wohlgemuth, W. K. (2009). Sleep and circadian rhythm disorders. In D. G. Blazer & D. C. Steffens (Eds.), *The American Psychiatric Publishing textbook of geriatric psychiatry* (4th ed., p. 400). Arlington, VA: American Psychiatric Publishing.

15. Decrease in sexual desire (libido) after menopause is primarily related to what hormonal change?

A. Decreased estrogen
B. Increased testosterone
C. Decreased testosterone
D. Increased progesterone
E. Decreased progesterone

ANSWER: C

Sexual desire is governed in both sexes by testosterone. Decreased testosterone levels are seen in women after menopause and contribute to decreased libido.

REFERENCE

Agronin, M. C. (2009). Sexual disorders. In D. G. Blazer & D. C. Steffens (Eds.), *The American Psychiatric Publishing textbook of geriatric psychiatry* (4th ed., pp. 359–360). Arlington, VA: American Psychiatric Publishing.

16. What is TRUE regarding psychosis in major neurocognitive disorder due to Alzheimer's disease?

A. Patients with psychotic symptoms have a faster cognitive decline.
B. Psychotic symptoms are observed in approximately 10% of patients.
C. Prevalence of psychotic symptoms is consistent through the course of the disease.
D. Visual hallucinations are the most common psychotic symptom.
E. Psychotic symptoms are more prevalent than agitation.

ANSWER: A

Patients with major neurocognitive disorder due to Alzheimer's disease with associated psychosis have a faster rate of decline than patients without psychotic symptoms. Median prevalence of psychosis in major neurocognitive disorder due to Alzheimer's disease is approximately 41%, although estimates range from 12.2% to 74.1%. Prevalence of psychotic symptoms increases with duration of illness. Delusions (often persecutory) are more common than hallucinations. Agitation is more prevalent than psychosis.

REFERENCE

Jeste, D. V., Lanouette, N. M., & Vahia, I. V. (2009). Schizophrenia and paranoid disorders. In D. G. Blazer & D. C. Steffens (Eds.), *The American Psychiatric Publishing textbook of geriatric psychiatry* (4th ed., p. 321). Arlington, VA: American Psychiatric Publishing.

17. Which of the following is NOT a common neuropsychiatric feature seen in epilepsy?

A. Personality disorder
B. Changes in sexual behavior
C. Interictal psychosis
D. Ictal violence
E. Episodic mood disorder

ANSWER: D

Ictal violence is extremely rare. Personality disorders are the most frequent neuropsychiatric presentation in epilepsy, with personality changes such as hyper- or hyposexuality and religiosity. Interictal psychosis is more common than ictal psychosis and is schizophrenia-like in presentation. Episodic mood disorders may involve depression or mania and are not as common as interictal psychosis.

REFERENCE

Sadock, B. J., & Sadock, V. A. (2003). *Kaplan and Sadock's synopsis of psychiatry: Behavioral sciences/clinical psychiatry* (9th ed., pp. 358–359). Philadelphia, PA: Lippincott Williams and Wilkins.

18. Strokes in which area of the brain are associated with onset of mania?

A. Left medial temporal lobe
B. Left prefrontal cortex
C. Right thalamus
D. Bilateral occipital lobes
E. Bilateral amygdalae

ANSWER: C

Strokes in the right thalamus, and right hemispheric lesions in general, have been associated with onset of mania.

REFERENCE

Santos, C. O., Caeiro, L., Ferro, J. M., et al. (2011). Mania and stroke: a systematic review. *Cerebrovascular Disease,* 2011; *32*(1):11–21.

19. A 38-year-old woman presents to the emergency room for altered mental status, including disorientation, confusion, and inability to register or recall new information. In the emergency room, she has a seizure. She is admitted to the hospital for workup. Laboratory testing is positive for anti-NMDA receptor antibody. What should be included in the differential diagnosis?

A. Systemic lupus erythematosus
B. Ovarian teratoma
C. Creutzfeldt–Jakob disease
D. Multiple sclerosis
E. Phencyclidine abuse

ANSWER: B

In the past decade, paraneoplastic encephalitis has become better recognized. Anti-NMDA receptor encephalitis is often, but not always, associated with tumors such as ovarian teratoma. The other options are not associated with the anti-NMDA receptor antibody.

REFERENCE

Dalmau, J., Lancaster, E., Martinez-Hernandez, E., Rosenfeld, M. R., Balice-Gordon, R. Clinical experience and laboratory investigations in patients with anti-NMDAR encephalitis. *Lancet Neurology,* 2011 Jan; *10*(1):63–74.

20. Rapid eye movement sleep behavior disorder is a suggestive diagnostic feature for which major neurocognitive disorder?

A. Frontotemporal neurocognitive disorder
B. Neurocognitive disorder due to Alzheimer's disease
C. Major vascular neurocognitive disorder
D. Neurocognitive disorder with Lewy bodies
E. Neurocognitive disorder due to traumatic brain injury

ANSWER: D

Rapid eye movement sleep behavior disorder is a suggestive diagnostic feature for major neurocognitive disorder with Lewy bodies.

REFERENCE

American Psychiatric Association. (2013). *Diagnostic and statistical manual of mental disorders* (5th ed.). Arlington, VA: American Psychiatric Publishing.

QUESTIONS AND ANSWERS

This chapter has accompanying questions and answers which are available to subscribers as part of the Oxford eLearning platform. To access the questions, follow the link below, or go to http://oxford-elearning.oup.com/books.

http://oxford-elearning.oup.com/books/test/67/10.1093/med/9780190265557.003.C015

16.

SUBSTANCE-RELATED DISORDERS

Shirshendu Sinha

1. Which of the following substances fulfills *DSM-5* diagnostic criteria for the three major categories of use disorders, intoxication, and withdrawal?

A. Tobacco
B. Cannabis
C. Inhalants
D. Hallucinogens
E. Caffeine

ANSWER: B

Cannabis fulfills the three major categories of substance use disorders. Tobacco has no clinically significant intoxication syndrome. Hallucinogens and inhalants lack consistent withdrawal syndromes.

REFERENCE

American Psychiatric Association. (2013). *Diagnostic and statistical manual of mental disorders* (5th ed., pp. 503–540, 571–577). Arlington, VA: American Psychiatric Publishing.

2. Which of the following non-substance-related disorders has been included in the substance-related and addictive disorders chapter of *DSM-5*?

A. Food addiction disorder
B. Shopping addiction disorder
C. Sex addiction disorder
D. Internet gambling disorder
E. Gambling disorder

ANSWER: E

In addition to substance-related disorders, the *DSM-5* chapter "Substance-Related and Addictive Disorders" also includes gambling disorder. There is evidence that gambling behavior activates the reward system similarly to the way it is activated by drugs of abuse. Other excessive behavioral patterns like Internet gambling have also been described, but evidence-based research examining these and other behavioral syndromes is limited. There is insufficient peer-reviewed evidence to establish diagnosis of repetitive behavioral patterns such as food addiction, shopping addiction (sometimes called oniomania), or sex addiction.

REFERENCE

American Psychiatric Association. (2013). *Diagnostic and statistical manual of mental disorders* (5th ed., p. 481). Arlington, VA: American Psychiatric Publishing.

3. A 34-year-old man presents for an evaluation of substance use disorder. He works as a radiology technician at a major academic medical center. He reports escalating patterns of marijuana use over the past 4 months. He has been having difficulty with his memory, attention, and concentration, and this has negatively impacted his work performance. He avoids his family and spends much of his free time smoking marijuana. He has difficulty quitting because he becomes irritable when he does not use. He admits driving his car under the influence of marijuana. Which one of the following is the most likely diagnosis?

A. Cannabis abuse
B. Cannabis dependence
C. Cannabis intoxication
D. Cannabis-induced mood disorder
E. Cannabis use disorder

ANSWER: E

In this case the *DSM-5* criteria for cannabis use disorder are reflected by frequent use of marijuana in increasing quantities over a period of 4 months, continued use despite having psychological consequences (impaired cognition), recurrent use resulting in a failure to fulfill requirements at work, important family time given up for use, unsuccessful efforts to stop the use, withdrawal symptoms such as irritability, and use under physically hazardous situations such as driving a motor vehicle under the influence.

REFERENCE

American Psychiatric Association. (2013). *Diagnostic and statistical manual of mental disorders* (5th ed., pp. 509–510). Arlington, VA: American Psychiatric Publishing.

4. Which one of the following disorders has the highest co-occurrence with cannabis use disorder?

A. Major depressive disorder
B. Schizophrenia
C. Anxiety disorders
D. Bipolar II disorder
E. ADHD

ANSWER: C

Individuals with past-year or lifetime diagnosis of cannabis use disorder have a high co-occurrence of anxiety disorders (24%). This is followed by bipolar I disorder (13%) and major depressive disorder (11%).

REFERENCE

American Psychiatric Association. (2013). *Diagnostic and statistical manual of mental disorders* (5th ed., p. 515). Arlington, VA: American Psychiatric Publishing.

5. Which of the following areas of the brain is responsible for executive control over incentive salience?

A. Nucleus accumbens
B. Prefrontal cortex
C. Amygdala
D. Thalamus
E. Anterior cingulate cortex

ANSWER: B

Through its projection to the ventral tegmental area, the prefrontal cortex exerts executive control over incentive salience.

REFERENCE

Kalivas, P. W., & Volkow, N. D. (2005). The neural basis of addiction: A pathology of motivation and choice. *American Journal of Psychiatry, 162*, 1403–1413.

6. Which of the following laboratory tests is the best measure of recent heavy alcohol consumption?

A. Ethyl glucuronide (ETG)
B. Asparate aminotransferase (AST)
C. Gamma-glutamyl transpeptidase (GGT)
D. Carbohydrate-deficient transferrin (CDT)
E. Alanine aminotransferase

ANSWER: D

Both GGT and CDT are laboratory indicators of heavy alcohol consumption, but CDT has higher sensitivity and specificity than GGT.

REFERENCE

American Psychiatric Association. (2013). *Diagnostic and statistical manual of mental disorders* (5th ed., p. 495). Arlington, VA: American Psychiatric Publishing.

7. Which of the following is the most common adverse effect of naltrexone?

A. Nausea
B. Headache
C. Tremor
D. Depression
E. Rash

ANSWER: A

Most of the adverse effects of naltrexone are gastrointestinal, including nausea, vomiting, and abdominal pain or discomfort. They occur early in the course of treatment.

REFERENCE

Anton, R. F. (2008). Naltrexone for the management of alcohol dependence. *New England Journal of Medicine, 359*, 715–721.

8. A 40-year-old man presents for medically supervised detoxification in an inpatient addiction service. He has been using a number of substances prior to coming to the hospital. In the unit he is noted to have poor sleep and reports significant anxiety. He is very restless and has been pacing around the room. On physical examination he has tachycardia, with heart rate of 120 beats per minute, and sweaty palms and forehead. His hands exhibit a coarse tremor bilaterally. Which one of the following is the most likely diagnosis for this patient?

A. Cannabis withdrawal
B. Alcohol withdrawal
C. Opioid withdrawal
D. Cocaine withdrawal
E. Caffeine withdrawal

ANSWER: B

Although anxiety, insomnia, and diaphoresis are nonspecific symptoms, coarse bilateral hand tremors are more specifically suggestive of alcohol withdrawal.

REFERENCE

American Psychiatric Association. (2013). *Diagnostic and statistical manual of mental disorders* (5th ed., pp. 499–500, 506, 517–518, 547–548, 569–570). Arlington, VA: American Psychiatric Publishing.

9. When do withdrawal symptoms emerge after quitting the use of tobacco cigarettes?

A. Within 24 hours
B. After 48 hours
C. After 72 hours
D. After 1 week

ANSWER: A

Tobacco withdrawal symptoms usually begin within 24 hours of stopping or cutting down on tobacco use; they peak at 2 to 3 days after stopping smoking and continue for 2 to 3 weeks. Prolonged symptoms beyond 1 month are uncommon.

REFERENCE

American Psychiatric Association. (2013). *Diagnostic and statistical manual of mental disorders* (5th ed., p. 576). Arlington, VA: American Psychiatric Publishing.

10. Which of the following neurotransmitters is most highly associated with the reinforcing effects of drugs of abuse?

A. GABA
B. Dopamine
C. Acetylcholine
D. Norepinephrine
E. Serotonin

ANSWER: B

The reinforcing effects of drugs of abuse are primarily related to their ability to increase dopamine in the nucleus accumbens.

REFERENCE

Kalivas, P. W., & Volkow, N. D. (2005). The neural basis of addiction: A pathology of motivation and choice. *American Journal of Psychiatry, 2005*, 1403–1413.

11. What is the hallmark symptom of caffeine withdrawal?

A. Headache
B. Nausea
C. Diarrhea
D. Tremor
E. Anxiety

ANSWER: A

Headache is the hallmark symptom of caffeine withdrawal. The onset may be gradual, and the headache can be severe and throbbing.

REFERENCE

American Psychiatric Association. (2013). *Diagnostic and statistical manual of mental disorders* (5th ed., p. 506). Arlington, VA: American Psychiatric Publishing.

12. You are considering medication to reduce heavy drinking in a bipolar patient who is known to be nonadherent with oral medication. He is currently on a long-acting injectable antipsychotic medication. He lives by himself, has a good therapeutic relationship

with his healthcare provider, and shows up for appointments. His liver function tests are within the normal range. What is the best medication option for this patient?

A. Gabapentin
B. Acamprosate
C. Valproic acid
D. Disulfiram
E. Naltrexone

ANSWER: E

This patient has normal liver function tests and so would be a good candidate for long-acting naltrexone (trade name, Vivitrol) injections due to his history of nonadherence with oral medications.

REFERENCE

Garbutt, J. C., Kranzler, H. R., O'Malley, S. S., Gastfriend, D. R., Pettinati, H. M., Silverman, B. L., ..., & Ehrich, E. W. (2005). Efficacy and tolerability of long-acting injectable naltrexone for alcohol dependence: A randomized controlled trial. *JAMA, 293*, 1617–1625.

13. Which one of the following psychotherapeutic modalities is most effective for substance use disorder?

A. Cognitive behavioral therapy
B. Interpersonal therapy
C. Motivational interviewing
D. Psychodynamic psychotherapy
E. Exposure and response prevention

ANSWER: C

Although some of these psychotherapeutic modalities are used in patients with substance use disorders, the most effective modality is motivational interviewing.

REFERENCES

Miller, W. R., & Rollnick, S. (2012). *Motivational interviewing: Helping people change*. New York: Guilford Press.
Work Group on Substance Use Disorders. (2006). *American Psychiatric Association practice guideline for the treatment of patients with substance use disorders* (2nd ed., p. 40). Retrieved from http://psychiatryonline.org/guidelines

14. A 50-year-old male executive presents requesting help with smoking cessation. He has attempted to quit with the help of nicotine gum and a nicotine inhaler but was unable to remain abstinent. Which of the following treatments likely would be the most effective for this patient?

A. Bupropion
B. Fluoxetine
C. Varenicline
D. Nicotine lozenge
E. Nicotine patch

ANSWER: C

Varenicline was approved by the FDA as a first-line agent for smoking cessation in 2007. A meta-analysis indicated that varenicline was the most effective treatment, nearly tripling the likelihood of quitting compared with placebo. Varenicline was found to be more effective than nicotine replacement therapy and bupropion.

REFERENCE

Cahill, K., Stevens, S., Perera, R., & Lancaster, T. (2013). Pharmacological interventions for smoking cessation: An overview and network meta-analysis. *Cochrane Database of Systematic Reviews, 5*, CD009329

15. A 45-year-old female patient with alcoholic cirrhosis has abstained from drinking alcohol over the last month but continues to experience cravings. Her renal function is within the normal range. Which of the following medications would you recommend for her?

A. Acamprosate
B. Naltrexone
C. Disulfiram
D. Valproic acid
E. Gabapentin

ANSWER: A

Acamprosate is excreted by the kidneys and is not metabolized by the liver. It is preferred in patients with liver impairment. Liver disease should not affect its metabolism or blood level concentrations.

REFERENCES

Work Group on Substance Use Disorders. (2006). *American Psychiatric Association practice guideline for the treatment of patients with substance use disorders* (2nd ed., p. 152). Retrieved from http://psychiatryonline.org/guidelines

Bouza, C., Angeles, M., Munoz, A., & Amate, J. M. (2004). Efficacy and safety of naltrexone and acamprosate in the treatment of alcohol dependence: A systematic review. *Addiction, 99*, 811–828.

Vuittonet, C. L., Halse, M., Leggio, L., Fricchione S.B., Brickley, M., Haass-Koffler, C.L....& Kenna, G.A. (2014). Pharmacotherapy for alcoholic patients with alcoholic liver disease. *American Journal of Health-System Pharmacy, 71*, 1265–1276. http://doi.org/10.2146/ajhp140028

16. Which of the following is a *DSM-5* diagnostic criterion for cannabis use disorder?

A. Smoking recreationally
B. Recent ingestion of marijuana
C. Growing marijuana in one's residence
D. Smoking marijuana mixed with tobacco
E. Driving repeatedly while under the influence of marijuana

ANSWER: E

Recurrent use of marijuana in a physically hazardous situation is one of 11 *DSM-5* diagnostic criteria for cannabis use disorder.

REFERENCE

American Psychiatric Association. (2013). *Diagnostic and statistical manual of mental disorders* (5th ed., pp. 509–510). Arlington, VA: American Psychiatric Publishing.

17. Voucher-based contingency management has been found to have the best outcome in patients with which of the following substance use disorders?

A. Cocaine use disorder
B. Alcohol use disorder
C. Cannabis use disorder
D. Tobacco use disorder
E. Opioid use disorder

ANSWER: A

Several psychosocial therapies have been studied in cocaine use disorder, including 12-step facilitation, cognitive behavioral therapy, and contingency management. Voucher-based contingency management has yielded better outcomes in a number of studies in patients with cocaine use disorder. Patients with cocaine use disorder tend to score high on reward dependence, which is thought to mediate a portion of the effectiveness of contingency management.

REFERENCES

Budney, A. J., & Higgins, S. T. (1990). *A community reinforcement plus vouchers approach: Treating cocaine addiction*. Rockville, MD: National Institute on Drug Abuse.

Petry, N. M., Tedford, J., Austin, M., Nich, C., Carroll, K. M., & Rounsaville, B. J. (2004). Prize reinforcement contingency management for treating cocaine users: How low can we go, and with whom? *Addiction, 99*, 349–360.

Work Group on Substance Use Disorders. (2006). *American Psychiatric Association practice guideline for the treatment of patients with substance use disorders* (2nd ed., pp. 161–162). Retrieved from http://psychiatryonline.org/guidelines

18. A 20-year-old male patient was brought to the emergency room after being found unconscious in his dormitory. Physical examination reveals respiratory depression, miosis, coma, and pulmonary edema. What is the most likely diagnosis?

A. Alcohol overdose
B. Opioid overdose
C. Sedative–hypnotics overdose
D. Phencyclidine overdose
E. Cannabis overdose

ANSWER: B

The symptoms described here such as unconsciousness, respiratory depression, and miosis are characteristics of opioid overdose. Pupillary constriction or miosis is one of the most important clinical features of opioid overdose in addition to respiratory depression and coma.

REFERENCE

American Psychiatric Association. (2013). *Diagnostic and statistical manual of mental disorders* (5th ed., pp. 546–547). Arlington, VA: American Psychiatric Publishing.

19. A 60-year-old female patient is being successfully treated with naltrexone for alcohol use disorder. She

requires bilateral knee replacements and will require a short course of opioid analgesia after surgery. How long prior to receiving opioid medication should she stop taking naltrexone?

A. 24 hours
B. 72 hours
C. 5 days
D. 7 days
E. 15 days

ANSWER: B

Naltrexone, an FDA-approved treatment for alcohol use disorder, blocks mu-opioid receptors and must be discontinued 48 to 72 hours prior to receiving opiate analgesia.

REFERENCE

Anton, R. F. (2008). Naltrexone for the management of alcohol dependence. *New England Journal of Medicine, 359*, 715–721.

20. Prenatal exposure to alcohol is most commonly associated with development of which of the following psychiatric disorders?

A. Autism spectrum disorder
B. ADHD
C. Bipolar disorder
D. Intellectual disability disorder
E. Major depressive disorder

ANSWER: B

Psychiatric conditions are common in individuals with histories of significant prenatal exposure to alcohol. The most predominant psychiatric diagnosis is ADHD. Oppositional defiant disorder and conduct disorder are also quite common. The presence of mood disorders has been described, including depression and bipolar disorder. Prenatal exposure to alcohol is a risk factor for subsequent development of tobacco, alcohol, and other substance use disorders.

REFERENCE

American Psychiatric Association. (2013). *Diagnostic and statistical manual of mental disorders* (5th ed., pp. 800–801). Arlington, VA: American Psychiatric Publishing.

21. Opioid withdrawal and sedative–hypnotic withdrawal present similarly. Which of the following would differentiate opioid withdrawal from sedative–hypnotic withdrawal?

A. Anxiety
B. Yawning
C. Nausea or vomiting
D. Insomnia
E. Restlessness

ANSWER: B

Yawning is a characteristic feature of opioid withdrawal.

REFERENCE

American Psychiatric Association. (2013) *Diagnostic and statistical manual of mental disorders* (5th ed., pp. 547–548, 557–558). Arlington, VA: American Psychiatric Publishing.

22. Which of the following *DSM-5* criteria might persist in a patient with substance use disorder who has achieved sustained remission?

A. Important social, occupational, or recreational activities are given up or reduced because of substance use.
B. The substance is often taken in larger amounts or over a longer period of time.
C. Recurrent substance use results in a failure to fulfill major role obligations at work, school, or home.
D. Craving, or a strong desire or urge to use the substances.
E. A great deal of time is spent in activities necessary to obtain the substance, use the substance, or recover from its effects.

ANSWER: D

"Craving, or a strong desire to use a specific substance," is the only option listed that might be present in both early abstinence (for more than 3 months but less than 12 months) and sustained remission (abstinence for 12 months or longer).

REFERENCE

American Psychiatric Association. (2013). *Diagnostic and statistical manual of mental disorders* (5th ed., pp. 483–484). Arlington, VA: American Psychiatric Publishing.

23. A 55-year-old male nurse was referred to an addiction outpatient clinic by his employer after he was caught stealing his patients' prescription opioid medication. Over the past year his use increased from one 10-mg tablet of oxycodone once daily to six times daily. He reports feeling tired and missing work. He has tried to stop using on numerous occasions. He endorses worsening of mood and memory with his escalating pattern of use. His desire to use is intense, and he feels anxious when he attempts to decrease his use. What *DSM-5* diagnosis would you give him?

A. Opioid intoxication
B. Opioid withdrawal
C. Opioid use disorder, mild
D. Opioid use disorder, moderate
E. Opioid use disorder, severe

ANSWER: E

In *DSM-5*, substance use disorders are classified by a range of severity, from mild to severe based on the number of symptom criteria. A mild substance use disorder is suggested by the presence of two or three symptoms, moderate by four or five symptoms, and severe by six or more symptoms. The patient described here meets seven *DSM-5* diagnostic criteria, which is consistent with opioid use disorder, severe.

REFERENCE

American Psychiatric Association. (2013). *Diagnostic and statistical manual of mental disorders* (5th ed., pp. 484, 541–542). Arlington, VA: American Psychiatric Publishing.

24. A 45-year-old male patient receiving treatment in an addiction treatment program reports complete abstinence from alcohol use for 5 months. This has been confirmed by periodic urine toxicology screens and breathalyzers. He is attending Alcoholics Anonymous meetings and has a sponsor. He requests medication that will help mitigate his intermittent cravings. What would be the most appropriate pharmacological intervention for this patient?

A. Acamprosate
B. Gabapentin
C. Disulfiram
D. Topiramate
E. Fluoxetine

ANSWER: A

Acamprosate and disulfiram are FDA-approved drugs for alcohol use disorder. Acamprosate has the best evidence for the maintenance of complete abstinence from alcohol.

REFERENCE

Rosner, S., Hackl-Herrwerth, A., Leucht, S., et al. (2010). Acamprosate for alcohol dependence. *Cochrane Database of Systematic Reviews, 9*, CD004332.

25. Use of which of the following substances is most strongly associated with polysubstance use?

A. 3,4-Methylenedioxymethamphetamine (MDMA/Ecstasy)
B. Tobacco
C. Cocaine
D. Alcohol
E. Phencyclidine

ANSWER: A

Both adults and adolescents who use MDMA are more likely than those who use the other drugs listed to be polysubstance users and to have other substance use disorders.

REFERENCE

American Psychiatric Association. (2013). *Diagnostic and statistical manual of mental disorders* (5th ed., p. 527). Arlington, VA: American Psychiatric Publishing.

26. Among patients seeking treatment for stimulant use disorder, what route of stimulant administration is most common?

A. Snorting
B. Smoking
C. Intravenous
D. Oral
E. Other

ANSWER: B

Smoking (especially crack cocaine) is the most prevalent method of stimulant administration in treatment-seeking individuals. Sixty-six percent of patients in treatment have used stimulants via smoking, 18% use by injection, and 10% snort.

REFERENCE

American Psychiatric Association. (2013). *Diagnostic and statistical manual of mental disorders* (5th ed., p. 565). Arlington, VA: American Psychiatric Publishing.

27. Open-ended questions, affirmations, reflective statements, and summary statements (OARS) are the central components of which of the following therapeutic modalities used in the treatment of substance use disorder?

A. Motivational enhancement therapy
B. Cognitive behavioral therapy
C. Interpersonal therapy
D. Insight-oriented therapy
E. Supportive psychotherapy

ANSWER: A

Some of these techniques are used in a variety of psychotherapeutic treatment modalities, but together they constitute the four essential techniques of motivational enhancement therapy commonly administered in the setting of substance use disorder.

REFERENCE

Miller, W. R., & Rollnick, S. (2012). Motivational interviewing: Helping people change. New York, NY: Guilford Press.

28. Which of the following illicit substance use disorders is most prevalent in the United States?

A. Cocaine use disorder
B. Cannabis use disorder
C. Phencyclidine use disorder
D. Stimulant use disorder
E. Opioid use disorder

ANSWER: B

Cannabinoids, especially cannabis, are the most commonly used illicit psychoactive substances in the United States. The 12-month prevalence of cannabis use disorder is 3.4% among 12- to 17 year-olds and 1.5% among adults aged 18 and older.

REFERENCE

American Psychiatric Association. (2013). *Diagnostic and statistical manual of mental disorders* (5th ed., p. 512). Arlington, VA: American Psychiatric Publishing.

29. Which of the following psychiatric comorbidities is more prevalent in men with substance use disorders than in women?

A. ADHD
B. Anxiety
C. Depression
D. Borderline personality disorder
E. Eating disorder

ANSWER: A

Higher rates of anxiety, depression, eating disorder, and borderline personality disorder are present in women with substance use disorders. Men with substance use disorders have higher rates of antisocial personality disorder and ADHD.

REFERENCE

Kessler, R. C. (2004). The epidemiology of dual diagnosis. *Biological Psychiatry, 56*, 730–737.

30. Which of the following is the most prevalent physical exam finding in men abusing anabolic–androgenic steroids?

A. Hypertension
B. Male-pattern baldness
C. Testicular atrophy
D. Prostatic hypertrophy
E. Hirsutism

ANSWER: C

Testicular atrophy results from negative feedback inhibition of testosterone production when exogenous anabolic–androgenic steroids are administrated in high doses. This can ultimately lead to low or zero sperm count and sterility. The other physical findings described here are possiblybut not reliably associated with the abuse of anabolic–androgenic steroids.

REFERENCES

De Souza, G. L., & Hallak, J. (2011). Anabolic steroids and male infertility: A comprehensive review. *BJU International, 108*, 1860–1865.

Kanayama, G., Brower, K.J., Wood, R.I., Hudson, J.I., & Pope, H.G. (2010). Treatment of anabolic–androgenic steroid dependence: Emerging evidence and its implications. *Drug and Alcohol Dependence, 109*, 6–13.

QUESTIONS AND ANSWERS

This chapter has accompanying questions and answers which are available to subscribers as part of the Oxford eLearning platform. To access the questions, follow the link below, or go to http://oxford-elearning.oup.com/books.

http://oxford-elearning.oup.com/books/test/67/10.1093/med/9780190265557.003.0016

17.

SCHIZOPHRENIA AND OTHER PSYCHOTIC DISORDERS

Harvinder Singh, Aarti Gupta

1. Which of the following symptoms is NOT among criteria for brief psychotic disorder?

A. Hallucinations
B. Disorganized speech
C. Catatonic behavior
D. Negative symptoms
E. Delusions

ANSWER: D

According to *DSM-5*, brief psychotic disorder is characterized by the presence of one or more of the following symptoms: delusions, hallucinations, disorganized speech (e.g., frequent derailment or incoherence), and grossly disorganized or catatonic behavior.

REFERENCE

American Psychiatric Association. (2013). *Diagnostic and statistical manual of mental disorders* (5th ed.). Arlington, VA: American Psychiatric Publishing.

2. Which of the following is NOT a risk factor for schizophrenia?

A. Infections
B. Fetal hypoxia
C. Cannabis use
D. Immigrant population
E. All of the above

ANSWER: E

Several epidemiological findings suggest a role of infectious agents in the development of schizophrenia. Schizophrenia appears to be more prevalent in immigrant populations than in native-born populations. Epidemiological studies suggest that cannabis use is a risk factor for the development of psychosis. Various perinatal problems, grouped together for analysis as "obstetrical complications," increase the risk of later development of schizophrenia twofold. These perinatal problems include hemorrhage, preterm labor, blood group incompatibilities, fetal hypoxia, and maternal infection.

REFERENCES

Kuepper, R., van Os, J., Lieb, R., Wittchen, H. U., Höfler, M., & Henquet, C. (2011). Continued cannabis use and risk of incidence and persistence of psychotic symptoms: 10 year follow-up cohort study. *British Medical Journal, 342*, d738.
Susser, E., Neugebauer, R., Hoek, H. W., Brown, A. S., Lin, S., Labovitz, D., & Gorman, J. M. (1996). Schizophrenia after prenatal famine: Further evidence. *Archives of General Psychiatry, 53*, 25.
Werbeloff, N., Levine, S. Z., & Rabinowitz, J. (2012). Elaboration on the association between immigration and schizophrenia: A population-based national study disaggregating annual trends, country of origin and sex over 15 years. *Social Psychiatry and Psychiatric Epidemiology, 47*, 303.

3. Which of the following features is a good prognostic factor in schizophreniform disorder?

A. Flat affect
B. Poor premorbid social functioning
C. Acute onset of psychotic symptoms
D. Absence of confusion at the height of psychotic episodes

ANSWER: C

The following are considered good prognostic features in schizophreniform disorder: absence of flat or blunted affect; good premorbid social or occupational functioning; acute onset of psychotic symptoms; and presence of confusion or perplexity at the height of psychotic episodes.

REFERENCE

American Psychiatric Association. (2013). *Diagnostic and statistical manual of mental disorders* (5th ed.). Arlington, VA: American Psychiatric Publishing.

4. Which of the following increases the risk of tardive dyskinesia from antipsychotic use?

A. Male sex
B. Old age
C. Hypothyroidism
D. Negative symptoms
E. Postsecondary education

ANSWER: B

Age over 50 increases the risk of tardive dyskinesia. Children are also at high risk. Female sex and comorbid mood disorders are also risk factors.

REFERENCE

Sadock, B. J., & Sadock, V. A. (2003). Biological therapies. In *Kaplan and Sadock's synopsis of psychiatry* (9th ed., p. 1059). Philadelphia, PA: Lippincott Williams and Wilkins.

5. Which of the following neurochemical abnormalities is associated with catatonia?

A. High dopamine activity in basal ganglia
B. Low GABA activity in frontal cortex
C. Low glutamate activity in parietal cortex
D. Low cholinergic activity in the medial temporal lobe

ANSWER: C

Catatonia is associated with low GABA activity in the frontal cortex, high glutamate activity in the parietal cortex, and low dopamine (D2) activity in the basal ganglia. Reduced GABA activity in the frontal cortex is often cited as the reason for benzodiazepine efficacy in catatonia.

REFERENCE

Brendan, T. C., Christopher, T., Kameshwari, J., John, M. H., & Carrie, B. (2005). Treating persistent catatonia when benzodiazepines fail. *Current Psychiatry, 4*(3):56–64

6. Psychosis with peripartum onset is MOST closely related to which class of psychiatric disorders?

A. Mood
B. Psychotic
C. Anxiety
D. Substance use
E. Personality

ANSWER: A

Evidence suggests a relationship between psychosis with peripartum onset and mood disorders, including bipolar disorder and major depressive disorder.

REFERENCE

Sadock, B. J., & Sadock, V. A. (2003). Other psychotic disorders. In *Kaplan and Sadock's synopsis of psychiatry* (9th ed., p. 526). Philadelphia, PA: Lippincott Williams and Wilkins.

7. Which of the following statements is TRUE about schizophrenia with onset in childhood or adolescence?

A. Prognosis is better than in adult-onset schizophrenia.
B. Onset is typically sudden.
C. It is seen exclusively among patients with autism spectrum disorder.
D. Patients with onset before adolescence have poorer medication response.
E. Affect is usually appropriate.

ANSWER: D

Childhood-onset schizophrenia is often chronic and debilitating. Patients with an onset before adolescence appear to have a worse response to medication and a worse prognosis. The prognosis for childhood-onset schizophrenia and adolescent-onset schizophrenia is worse than for adult-onset schizophrenia, with worst prognosis for patients diagnosed before age 10 or with preexisting personality disorders. Onset is insidious. Schizophrenia is distinguished from autism spectrum disorder by later age of onset and generally normal intelligence. Inappropriate or blunted affect is very common.

REFERENCE

Sadock, B. J., & Sadock, V. A. (2003). Early-onset schizophrenia. In *Kaplan and Sadock's synopsis of psychiatry* (pp. 1282–1285). Philadelphia, PA: Lippincott Williams and Wilkins.

8. Family history of which personality disorder has the highest correlation with schizophrenia?

A. Paranoid
B. Schizoid
C. Schizotypal
D. Obsessive–compulsive
E. Dependent

ANSWER: C

Family history of schizotypal personality disorder is most closely correlated with schizophrenia.

REFERENCE

Silverman, J. M., Siever, L. J., Horvath, T. B., Coccaro, E. F., Klar, H., Davidson, M., Pinkham, L., Apter, S. H., Mohs, R. C., Davis, K. L. (1993). Schizophrenia-related and affective personality disorder traits in relatives of probands with schizophrenia and personality disorders. *American Journal of Psychiatry, 150*(3), 435–442.

9. Which of the following is NOT a major feature of metabolic syndrome?

A. Insulin resistance
B. Obesity
C. Dyslipidemia
D. Renal impairment
E. Hypertension

ANSWER: D

The five major features of metabolic syndrome are disturbed insulin metabolism and/or disturbed glucose metabolism; obesity; dyslipidemia; and hypertension. Renal impairment may occur as a complication of diabetes.

REFERENCE

Liese, A. D., Mayer-Davis, E. J., & Haffner, S. M. (1998). Development of the multiple metabolic syndrome: An epidemiologic perspective. *Epidemiologic Reviews, 20*, 157–172.

10. The Clinical Antipsychotic Trials of Intervention Effectiveness (CATIE) Study, funded by the National Institute of Mental Health, was a nationwide public health–focused clinical trial that compared the effectiveness of typical and atypical antipsychotic medications used to treat schizophrenia. What was the most common reason for study discontinuation?

A. Lack of efficacy
B. Weight gain
C. Patient's decision
D. Extrapyramidal symptoms
E. Sedation

ANSWER: C

In the CATIE Study, 30% of discontinuation rate was due to the patient's decision, followed by lack of efficacy (24%) and intolerability due to weight gain, sedation, or extrapyramidal symptoms (16%).

REFERENCE

Lieberman, J. A., Stroup, T. S., McEvoy, J. P., Swartz, M. S., Rosenheck, R. A., Perkins, D. O., Keefe, R. S., Davis, S. M., Davis, C. E., Lebowitz, B. D., Severe, J., Hsiao, J. K. (2005). Clinical Antipsychotic Trials of Intervention Effectiveness (CATIE) Investigators. Effectiveness of antipsychotic drugs in patients with chronic schizophrenia. *New England Journal of Medicine, 353*, 1209–1223.

11. A patient with schizophrenia is in the emergency room. He does not answer any questions and refuses to sit down. He later walks backward to a corner in the corridor and does not move. The family reports that for the past few days he has been isolating himself, has not been eating, and has been sitting on his bed for hours. What is the most probable diagnosis?

A. Schizophrenia, disorganized type
B. Major depressive disorder
C. Schizophrenia with catatonia
D. Schizoaffective disorder
E. Neuroleptic malignant syndrome

ANSWER: B

Schizophrenia subtypes have been removed in *DSM-5*, but "with catatonia" is a possible specifier. Catatonia is diagnosed by the presence of three or more of the following symptoms: stupor (i.e., no psychomotor activity; not actively relating to environment); catalepsy (i.e., passive induction of a posture held against gravity); waxy flexibility (i.e., slight, even resistance to positioning by examiner); mutism (i.e., no, or very little, verbal response [exclude if known aphasia]); negativism (i.e., opposition or no response to instructions or external stimuli); posturing (i.e., spontaneous and active maintenance of a posture against gravity); mannerism (i.e., odd, circumstantial caricature of normal actions); stereotypy (i.e., repetitive, abnormally frequent, non-goal-directed movements); agitation, not influenced by external stimuli; grimacing; echolalia (i.e., mimicking another's speech); or echopraxia (i.e., mimicking another's movements).

The patient in the question above meets criteria for catatonia. Although he could be depressed with catatonic features, given his past diagnosis of schizophrenia, he is more likely to have schizophrenia with catatonia.

REFERENCES

American Psychiatric Association. (2013). *Diagnostic and statistical manual of mental disorders* (5th ed.). Arlington, VA: American Psychiatric Publishing.

Kammen, D. P. v., Hurford, I., & Marder, S. R. (2009). First-generation antipsychotics. In S. E. Howes (Ed.), *Kalpan & Sadock's comprehensive textbook of psychiatry* (vol. 2, p. 3118). Philadelphia, PA: Lippincott Williams and Wilkins.

12. A patient believes aliens are communicating with him through a microchip they inserted in his teeth after abducting him 2 months prior. Despite being reassured there is no microchip, the patient insists that he can "feel it" with his tongue. He denies ever hearing aliens through his ears or seeing them. His thought process is coherent. He denies any such thoughts until 2 months prior. What is the MOST likely diagnosis?

A. Schizophrenia
B. Delusional disorder
C. Schizophreniform disorder
D. Brief psychotic disorder

ANSWER: B

DSM-5 specifies the following criteria for a diagnosis of delusional disorder as the following:

- Presence of one or more delusions with a duration of 1 month or longer.
- Criterion A of schizophrenia is never met.
- Functioning is not markedly impaired.
- If manic or depressive episodes have occurred, these have been brief relative to the delusional periods.
- Presentation is not better explained by another mental illness such as body dysmorphic disorder or obsessive–compulsive disorder.

An important distinction between *DSM-IV* and DSM-5 relevant to this question is that the requirement that delusions be non-bizarre has been removed in *DSM-5*.

REFERENCES

American Psychiatric Association. (2013). *Diagnostic and statistical manual of mental disorders* (5th ed.). Arlington, VA: American Psychiatric Publishing.

13. What is the prognosis for a 24-year-old man diagnosed with schizophrenia who is adherent to antipsychotic medication treatment?

A. His delusions and hallucinations are likely to worsen, but his tendency to isolate and his cognitive abilities may improve.
B. His delusions and hallucinations are likely to worsen, but his tendency to isolate and his cognitive abilities may improve.
C. His delusions and hallucinations may improve, but his tendency to isolate and his cognitive abilities may not.
D. All his symptoms may gradually improve.

ANSWER: C

The course of psychotic symptoms in schizophrenia is variable, but in general positive symptoms (i.e., hallucinations and delusions) are more amenable to treatment with antipsychotics than are negative and cognitive symptoms. Positive symptoms may fluctuate across active-phase psychotic episodes, but negative symptoms and cognitive dysfunction are relatively constant. Furthermore, negative symptoms are more predictive of overall functional status and are associated with poorer prognosis. Cognitive symptoms often precede psychotic symptoms and may predict functional outcome for a patient.

REFERENCE

Tamminga, C. A., Buchanan, R. W., & Gold, J. M. (1998). The role of negative symptoms and cognitive dysfunction in schizophrenia outcome. *International Clinical Psychopharmacology, 13* (suppl. 3), S21–S26.

14. Which of the following are considered good prognostic factors for schizophrenia?

A. Good premorbid functioning, affective symptoms, no precipitating factors, soft neurological signs
B. Later age of onset, good premorbid functioning, family history of mood disorder, positive symptoms
C. Younger age at onset, being single/divorced/widowed, family history of schizophrenia, longer duration of untreated illness
D. History of perinatal trauma, multiple relapses, poor premorbid functioning, acute onset

ANSWER: B

Good prognostic factors for schizophrenia include later age of onset, good premorbid functioning, affective symptoms, family history of mood disorder, acute onset, married, good support system, and positive symptoms. In contrast, poor prognostic factors for schizophrenia include younger age at onset, poor premorbid functioning, no precipitating factors, negative symptoms, being single/divorced/widowed, family history of schizophrenia, soft neurological signs, cognitive symptoms, negative symptoms, history of perinatal trauma, multiple relapses, history of assaultive behavior, and longer duration of untreated illness.

REFERENCE

Sadock, B. J., & Sadock, V. A. (2003). *Kaplan and Sadock's synopsis of psychiatry: Behavioral sciences/clinical psychiatry* (9th ed.). Philadelphia, PA: Lippincott, Williams and Wilkins.

15. What are the most common structural abnormalities revealed by brain MRI in schizophrenia?

A. Corpus callosum abnormalities, reduced cerebellar volume, increased basal ganglia volume
B. Enlarged lateral ventricles, medial temporal volume reduction, enlarged third ventricle
C. Decreased basal ganglia volume, decreased thalamus volume, enlarged cavum septum pellucidum
D. Parietal lobe volume reduction, frontal lobe volume reduction, and occipital lobe volume reduction

ANSWER: B

Enlargement of lateral ventricles is the most replicated brain structural abnormality in MRI studies, although this finding is not specific to schizophrenia. It may be seen, for instance, in other brain disorders such as Alzheimer's disease. The second most common finding is reduction of medial temporal lobe structures and volume reduction, including the amygdala, hippocampus, parahippocampal region, and neocortical temporal regions such as superior temporal gyrus. The third most replicated finding is third ventricle enlargement. In summary, MRI studies confirm structural brain abnormalities in schizophrenia, and the pattern and number of abnormalities are consistent with a disturbance of connectivity within and between brain regions, most likely of neurodevelopmental origin.

REFERENCE

Shenton, M. E., & Kubicki, M. (2009). Structrual brain imaging in schizophrenia. In S. E. Howes (Ed.), *Kalpan & Sadock's comprehensive textbook of psychiatry* (9th ed., pp. 1498–1499). Philadelphia, PA: Lippincott Williams and Wilkins.

16. Which of the following statements is TRUE of the genetics of schizophrenia?

A. Schizophrenia is determined principally by genetic susceptibility loci.
B. Intrauterine factors, rather than genetics, predispose to schizophrenia.
C. No genes have been found to confer risk of schizophrenia.
D. Schizophrenia has both genetic and environmental contributors.

ANSWER: D

Genetic studies have shown that genetic factors contribute significantly to the etiology of schizophrenia, but not exclusively. Heritability in monozygotic twins is shown to be only about 50%, and meta-analysis has demonstrated more than 10% environmental influence on liability to schizophrenia. Schizophrenia has been shown to be polygenic (caused by multiple genes) and pleiotropic (one gene affecting multiple phenotypic traits). Multiple environmental risk factors have been hypothesized as contributing to etiology of schizophrenia, including maternal stress, maternal infections, nutritional deficiencies, intrauterine growth retardation, pregnancy and birth complications, socioeconomic factors, childhood adversity, immigration (both first and second generation), late winter or early spring birth, being born or raised in cities, and having relatively old fathers (aged 40 years or older) or young parents (aged 20 or younger).[3]

REFERENCES

Castellani, C. A., Laufer, B. I., Melka, M. G., Diehl, E. J., O'Reilly, R. L., & Singh, S. M. (2015). DNA methylation differences in monozygotic twin pairs discordant for schizophrenia identifies psychosis related genes and networks. *BMC Med Genomics, 8*, 17.

Sullivan, P. F., Kendler, K. S., & Neale, M. C. (2003). Schizophrenia as a complex trait: Evidence from a meta-analysis of twin studies. *Archives of General Psychiatry, 60*, 1187–1192.

Owen, M. J., Sawa, A., and Mortensen, P. B. (2016). Schizophrenia. *Lancet*. Jul 2; *388*(10039): 86–97.

17. Which of the following statements is TRUE of neurocognitive symptoms in schizophrenia?

A. First-generation antipsychotics are better than second-generation antipsychotics in treating cognitive symptoms secondary to schizophrenia.
B. Neurocognitive deficits may be a part of prodromal symptoms in patients at high risk for schizophrenia.
C. Neurocognitive deficits in schizophrenia are mild and not much different from those in healthy controls.
D. NMDA receptor antagonists are now recommended for treatment of memory deficits in schizophrenia.

ANSWER: B

Neurocognitive impairment is a core feature of schizophrenia and predicts functional outcome. The deficits are significant across a wide range of domains, most notably memory, attention, working memory, problem-solving, processing speed, and social cognition. Neurocognitive deficits may be a part of prodromal symptoms. Currently no effective treatments are identified for treatment of cognitive impairment in schizophrenia, although neurocognitive rehabilitation programs show some promise.

REFERENCES

Keefe, R. S. E., & Eesley, C. E. (2009). Neurocognition in schizophrenia. In S. E. Howes (Ed.), *Kalpan & Sadock's comprehensive textbook of psychiatry* (9th ed., vol. 1, pp. 1531–1541). Philadelphia, PA: Lippincott Williams and Wilkins.

18. Which of the following statements is TRUE regarding mortality in patients with schizophrenia compared with the general population?

A. Patients have the same mortality rate, including suicide rates.
B. Patients have a lower mortality rate, including suicide rates.
C. Patients have an overall higher mortality rate but lower suicide rates.
D. Patients have a higher mortality rate, including suicide rates.

ANSWER: D

Studies have shown that patients with schizophrenia have two to three times increased mortality rate as compared with the general population. Suicide rates are reported as 4% lifetime risk, but rates as high as 10%- to -13% have been reported.

REFERENCES

Hor, K., & Taylor, M. (2010). Suicide and schizophrenia: A systematic review of rates and risk factors. *Journal of Psychopharmacology, 24*(4 suppl.), 81–90.

Saha, S., D. Chant, D., & McGrath, J. (2007). A systematic review of mortality in schizophrenia: Is the differential mortality gap worsening over time? *Archives of General Psychiatry, 64*, 1123–1131.

19. Which of the following antipsychotics is LEAST likely to cause to hyperprolactinemia?

A. Haloperidol
B. Paliperidone
C. Aripiprazole
D. Amisulpride

ANSWER: C

Aripiprazole has some evidence of decreasing prolactin levels due to its partial dopamine agonistic effects and has been suggested as an augmenting agent to antipsychotics that cause hyperprolactinemia. Aripiprazole treatment is also associated with a low incidence of EPS (extra pyramidal symptoms)-related symptoms, QTc interval, and metabolic syndrome.

REFERENCES

Chen, J. X., Su, Y. A., Bian, Q. T., Wei, L. H., Zhang, R. Z., Liu, Y. H., ... & Zhang, X. Y. (2015). Adjunctive aripiprazole in the

treatment of risperidone-induced hyperprolactinemia: A randomized, double-blind, placebo-controlled, dose-response study. *Psychoneuroendocrinology, 58*, 130–140.
Haddad, P. M., & Wieck, A. (2004). Antipsychotic-induced hyperprolactinaemia: Mechanisms, clinical features and management. *Drugs, 64*, 2291–2314.

20. Which of the following is TRUE regarding the risk of agranulocytosis and seizures with use of clozapine?

A. Incidence of agranulocytosis is 1% to 2%, and incidence of seizures is 5% to 10%.
B. Incidence of seizures is 1% to 2%, and incidence of agranulocytosis is 5% to 10%.
C. Both agranulocytosis and seizures have the same incidence rate of 1% to 2%.
D. Both agranulocytosis and seizures have the same incidence rate of 5% to 10%.

ANSWER: A

Use of clozapine is limited by the potentially life-threatening side effect of agranluocytosis, although it has a low incidence rate of 1% to 2%. Agranulocytosis is defined as absolute neutrophil count (ANC) of less than 500/mm^3. Risk is greater in the first 3 months of use, in women, and in the elderly. Seizures occur in 5% to 10% of patients taking clozapine. The risk is higher with rapid escalation of dosage and high clozapine plasma levels.

REFERENCES

Alvir, J. M., J. A. Lieberman, J. A. Safferman, A. Z., Schwimmer, J. L., & Schaaf, J. A. (1993). Clozapine-induced agranulocytosis: Incidence and risk factors in the United States. *New England Journal of Medicine, 329*, 162–167.
Marder, S. R., & Wirshing, D. A. (2009). Clozapine. In *The American Psychiatry Publication Textbook of Psychopharmacology*.

21. Which of the following antipsychotics is preferred for a heavy smoker?

A. Clozapine
B. Olanzapine
C. Haloperidol
D. Risperidone

ANSWER: D

Smoking induces the CYP 1A2 enzyme, impacting the levels of its substrates in the blood. Many psychotropics are metabolized by CYP 1A2, including the antipsychotics chlorpromazine, haloperidol, trifluperazine, clozapine and olanzapine. Antidepressants that are a substrate of CYP 1A2 include amitriptyline, clomipramine, imipramine, and fluvoxamine. When choosing any of the above medications for a patient who is a heavy smoker, higher dosages may be needed to reach a therapeutic level. Conversely, dosages of these medications may need to be lowered in patients who suddenly give up smoking. Risperidone is mostly metabolized by CYP 2C19 and CYP 2D6.

REFERENCE

Desai, H. D., J. Seabolt and M. W. Jann (2001). "Smoking in patients receiving psychotropic medications: a pharmacokinetic perspective." *CNS Drugs, 15*(6): 469–494.

22. A patient with schizophrenia is brought to the emergency room in an acutely agitated state. He is administered haloperidol 5 mg intramuscularly. A few minutes later, the nurse reports that the patient's neck is twisted to one side and his eyes are rolled back. What is the MOST likely diagnosis?

A. Acute dystonia
B. Akathisia
C. Tardive dyskinesia
D. Neuroleptic-induced parkinsonism

ANSWER: A

Neuroleptic-induced acute dystonia includes abnormal positioning of the head and neck (e.g., torticollis); spasm of jaw muscles; impaired swallowing, speaking, or breathing; thickened or slurred speech; tongue protrusion or dysfunction; deviated eyes in any direction (e.g., oculogyric crisis); and abnormal positioning of the limbs or trunk. It may occur within a few minutes of receiving a high-potency typical antipsychotic but generally occurs within days of starting and/or increasing an oral antipsychotic. It often occurs in young African American men. Laryngeal involvement can compromise breathing and can be fatal.

Neuroleptic-induced parkinsonism is characterized by rigidity, bradykinesia, decreased spontaneous motor activity, slowed speech, decreased arm movements during walking, masked facies, and tremor. Neuroleptic-induced acute akathisia includes an inner sense of restlessness and at least one objective, observable movement such as fidgeting or swinging of the legs, rocking from foot to foot while standing, pacing, lifting the feet as if marching in place, crossing and uncrossing the legs when sitting, or the inability to sit or stand in one place for several minutes. Neuroleptic-induced tardive dyskinesia is characterized by involuntary movements of the tongue, jaw, lips, trunk, or extremities.

REFERENCE

Janicak, P. G., & Beedle, D. (2009). Medication-induced movement disorders. In *The American Psychiatry Publication Textbook of Psychopharmacology* (vol. 2, pp. 2997–3003).

23. Which of the following is TRUE regarding late-onset schizophrenia?

A. Schizophrenia is considered late onset after age 65.
B. It is more common in women than in men.
C. It accounts for 10% of schizophrenia cases.
D. Genetic risk is higher than in patients with early-onset schizophrenia.
E. Positive family history is less common than in patients with early-onset schizophrenia.

ANSWER: B

Women are more likely than men to develop late-onset schizophrenia. Schizophrenia is considered late onset after age 40. Twenty-three percent of patients with schizophrenia have late-onset disease. Genetic risk and positive family history are comparable in early-onset and late-onset schizophrenia.

REFERENCE

Vahia, I. V., Lanouette, N. M., & Jeste, D. V. (2014). Schizophrenia and paranoid disorder. In M. E. Thakur, D. G. Blazer, & D. C. Steffens (Eds.), *Clinical manual of geriatric psychiatry* (pp. 159–174). Arlington, VA: American Psychiatric Association.

24. What is the first-line pharmacological treatment recommendation for late-life schizophrenia?

A. Quetiapine
B. Olanzapine
C. Risperidone
D. Haloperidol
E. Chlorpromazine

ANSWER: C

A 2004 consensus survey of 48 American experts concluded that the first-line recommendation for late-life schizophrenia is risperidone, 1.25 to 3 mg daily. Olanzapine, quetiapine, and aripiprazole are considered second-line treatment.

REFERENCE

Alexopoulos GS, Streim J, Carpenter D, Docherty JP (2004). Expert consensus panel for using antipsychotic drugs in older patients: Using antipsychotic agents in older patients. *Journal of Clinical Psychiatry, 65*, 5–99.

25. Who popularized the term *dementia praecox* to describe patients with a generally long-term deteriorating course and symptoms including hallucinations and delusions?

A. Carl Jung
B. Sigmund Freud
C. Melanie Klein
D. Emil Kraepelin
E. Harry Stack Sullivan

ANSWER: D

Emil Kraepelin first popularized the term *dementia praecox* (a cognate with the word *precocious*) to describe the disease that would later come to be known as schizophrenia. The term was first used by Benedict Morel, using the French form *démence précoce*.

REFERENCE

Falkai P, Rossner MJ, Schulze TG, Hasan A, Brzózka MM, Malchow B, Honer WG, Schmitt A. (2015). Kraepelin revisited: Schizophrenia from degeneration to failed regeneration. *Molecular Psychiatry, 20*, 671–676.

26. Which of the following is considered a positive symptom in schizophrenia?

A. Bizarre behavior
B. Poverty of speech
C. Asociality
D. Poor eye contact
E. Social inattentiveness

ANSWER: A

Bizarre behavior is considered a positive symptom in schizophrenia, such as inappropriate clothing, appearance, or social behavior; agitated behavior; or stereotyped behavior.

Other positive symptoms include hallucinations, delusions, and positive formal thought disorder. Negative symptoms include the other options (options B-E), as well as affective flattening, alogia, apathy, and anhedonia.

REFERENCE

Andreasen, N. C. (1987). The diagnosis of schizophrenia. *Schizophrenia Bulletin, 13*, 9.

27. What is the most commonly abused substance among patients with schizophrenia?

A. Alcohol
B. Tobacco
C. Cocaine
D. Cannabis
E. Opioids

ANSWER: B

It is estimated that more than 75% of patients with schizophrenia smoke cigarettes. In addition, 30% to 50% abuse alcohol, 15% to 25% abuse cannabis, and 5% to 10% abuse cocaine.

REFERENCE

Sadock, B. J., & Sadock, V. A. (2003). *Kaplan and Sadock's synopsis of psychiatry: Behavioral sciences/clinical psychiatry* (9th ed.). Philadelphia, PA: Lippincott, Williams and Wilkins.

28. What is the lifetime prevalence of schizophrenia in the United States?

A. 0.05%
B. 0.1%
C. 0.5%
D. 1%
E. 5%

ANSWER: D

The lifetime prevalence of schizophrenia in the United States is approximately 1%.

REFERENCE

Sadock, B. J., & Sadock, V. A. (2003). *Kaplan and Sadock's synopsis of psychiatry: Behavioral sciences/clinical psychiatry* (9th ed.). Philadelphia, PA: Lippincott, Williams and Wilkins.

29. Which of the following factors is correlated with increased risk of schizophrenia?

A. Birth in winter or early spring
B. Birth in late spring or summer
C. Birth in summer or early fall
D. Birth in late fall or early winter

ANSWER: A

Patients with schizophrenia are much more likely to have been born in the winter or early spring. This is true for the northern hemisphere months of January to April and the southern hemisphere months of July to September.

REFERENCE

Sadock, B. J., & Sadock, V. A. (2003). *Kaplan and Sadock's synopsis of psychiatry: Behavioral sciences/clinical psychiatry* (9th ed.). Philadelphia, PA: Lippincott, Williams and Wilkins.

30. Which of the following is NOT a clinical feature of catatonia?

A. Stupor
B. Waxy flexibility
C. Mutism
D. Echolalia
E. Auditory hallucinations

ANSWER: E

Auditory hallucinations are not features of catatonia. The other options all can be seen in catatonia.

REFERENCE

American Psychiatric Association. (2013). *Diagnostic and statistical manual of mental disorders* (5th ed.). Arlington, VA: American Psychiatric Publishing.

QUESTIONS AND ANSWERS

This chapter has accompanying questions and answers which are available to subscribers as part of the Oxford eLearning platform. To access the questions, follow the link below, or go to http://oxford-elearning.oup.com/books.

http://oxford-elearning.oup.com/books/test/67/10.1093/med/9780190265557.003.0017

18.

MOOD DISORDERS

Harvinder Singh, Brian Frankel

1. Which of the following is NOT a risk factor for postpartum mood disorder?

A. Primigravida
B. Single mother
C. Vaginal birth
D. Sexual abuse history
E. Family history of postpartum mood disorder

ANSWER: C

Cesarean section, as well as other perinatal or natal complications, increases risk for postpartum disorders.

REFERENCE

Rai, S., Pathak, A., & Sharma, I. (2015). Postpartum psychiatric disorders: Early diagnosis and management. *Indian Journal of Psychiatry, 57*(suppl. S2), 216–221.

2. A 35-year-old patient is treated for major depressive disorder with an SSRI that is titrated to an adequate dosage. She takes the SSRI as prescribed for 10 weeks without improvement in symptoms. She also does not respond to an adequate therapeutic trial of an SNRI. The patient's prominent symptoms are decreased energy, increased sleep, and increased appetite with weight gain. She reports having a "good day" about once per week if something positive happens to her or her friends. Which treatment is particularly useful in this type of presentation?

A. Amitriptyline
B. Buspirone
C. Mirtazapine
D. Lithium
E. Phenelzine

ANSWER: E

Atypical depression is a specifier defined by *DSM-5* including criteria of mood reactivity (mood brightens in response to actual or potential positive events) and two (or more) of the following symptoms: weight gain or increased appetite, hypersomnia, leaden paralysis, and interpersonal rejection sensitivity. MAOIs (Monoamine Oxidase Inhibitors) (e.g., phenelzine) are useful in treating atypical depression.

REFERENCE

Niciu, M. J., Sinclair, C. M., Zarate, C. A., & Shelton, R. C. (2014). Pharmacological and somatic treatments for major depressive disorder. In G. O. Gabbard (Ed.), *Gabbard's treatments of psychiatric disorders* (5th ed.). Arlington, VA: American Psychiatric Publishing.

3. A patient presents with atypical depression, including increased sleep, increased appetite with weight gain, mood reactivity, and rejection sensitivity. Which of the following attributes of her presentation is most likely to persist throughout life?

A. Hypersomnia
B. Increased appetite
C. Mood reactivity
D. Rejection sensitivity
E. Weight gain

ANSWER: D

Pathological sensitivity to perceived interpersonal rejection is a feature of atypical depression that has an early onset and persists, occurring during periods of depression and euthymia. It may be exacerbated during depressive episodes. The other features of atypical depression (mood reactivity, increased appetite, hypersomnia, leaden paralysis) are more likely to resolve with appropriate treatment.

REFERENCE

McInnis, M. G., Riba, M., & Greden, J. F. (2014). Depressive disorders. In R. E. Hales, S. C. Yudofsky, & L. W. Roberts (Eds.), *The American Psychiatric Publishing textbook of psychiatry* (6th ed.). Arlington, VA: American Psychiatric Publishing.

4. A mother describes her 8-year-old son as chronically irritable and reports that in the last few years he has begun to have frequent behavioral outbursts as well. He yells uncontrollably at his mother several times per week. He is aggressive with classmates and teachers, and school administration is considering a suspension. He was not invited to several friends' birthday parties because he hit a friend's sister during a community barbecue. What primary psychiatric disorder is this patient most likely to develop as an adult?

A. Attention deficit hyperactivity disorder (ADHD)
B. Bipolar disorder
C. Intermittent explosive disorder
D. Major depressive disorder
E. Schizophrenia

ANSWER: D

The patient's presentation fits the diagnosis of disruptive mood dysregulation disorder (DMDD), a new diagnosis in *DSM-5*. Criteria involve recurrent temper outbursts on the background of a chronic irritable or angry mood. This pattern of behavior and temperament predicts emergence of unipolar depressive disorders. Notably, DMDD was introduced to *DSM-5* to prevent overdiagnosis of bipolar disorder in children.

REFERENCE

McInnis, M. G., Riba, M., & Greden, J. F. (2014). Depressive disorders. In R. E. Hales, S. C. Yudofsky, & L. W. Roberts (Eds.), *The American Psychiatric Publishing textbook of psychiatry* (6th ed.). Arlington, VA: American Psychiatric Publishing.

5. Which of the following is observed in the personality trait that best predicts the development of major depressive disorder?

A. Difficulty with self-discipline
B. Low stress tolerance
C. Low concern for other people's well-being
D. Low social engagement and energy level
E. Preference of familiarity over novelty

ANSWER: B

Neuroticism (emotional instability, tendency to experience negative emotions, low stress tolerance) is a well-established risk factor for developing major depressive disorder.

REFERENCE

McInnis, M. G., Riba, M., & Greden, J. F. (2014). Depressive disorders. In R. E. Hales, S. C. Yudofsky, & L. W. Roberts (Eds.), *The American Psychiatric Publishing textbook of psychiatry* (6th ed.). Arlington, VA: American Psychiatric Publishing.

6. In the context of a major loss, which of the following is a symptom that distinguishes major depressive disorder from grief?

A. Insomnia
B. Intense sadness
C. Persistent dysphoria
D. Decreased appetite
E. Weight loss

ANSWER: C

Dysphoria in grief, as opposed to major depressive disorder, often comes in waves ("pangs of grief"). Dysphoria is likely to decrease in days to weeks. Other factors that distinguish grief from major depressive disorder include ability to experience humor and positive emotions, preserved self-esteem, and the focus of any thoughts of death and dying pertaining to "joining" the deceased as opposed to feeling unable to cope with life. Self-derogatory ideations in grief are often specific to feeling one failed the deceased. Insomnia, weight loss and decreased appetite, and intense sadness can apply to both grief and major depressive disorder.

REFERENCE

American Psychiatric Association. (2013). *Diagnostic and statistical manual of mental disorders* (5th ed.). Arlington, VA: American Psychiatric Publishing.

7. For a woman who has had a prior postpartum episode with psychotic features, what is the risk of recurrence with subsequent delivery?

A. 5% to 10%
B. 15% to 25%
C. 30% to 50%
D. 60% to 80%
E. More than 85%

ANSWER: C

A woman who has had a prior postpartum episode with psychotic features has a 30% to 50% risk of recurrence with subsequent delivery.

REFERENCE

American Psychiatric Association. (2013). *Diagnostic and statistical manual of mental disorders* (5th ed.). Arlington, VA: American Psychiatric Publishing.

8. Which of the following symptoms is not a criterion of the "mixed features" specifier for a manic or hypomanic episode?

A. Anhedonia
B. Fatigue
C. Indecisiveness
D. Suicidal thinking
E. Feelings of worthlessness

ANSWER: C

Criterion A of the mixed features specifier for manic or hypomanic episode requires at that least three of the following symptoms be present during the majority of days of the current episode: depressed mood, anhedonia, psychomotor retardation, fatigue, feelings of worthlessness or guilt, and suicidal thinking. Indecisiveness, insomnia/hypersomnia, and psychomotor agitation do not count toward this specifier because these symptoms can occur in either affective pole.

REFERENCE

American Psychiatric Association. (2013). *Diagnostic and statistical manual of mental disorders* (5th ed.). Arlington, VA: American Psychiatric Publishing.

9. Which of the following is an alteration of the hypothalamic–pituitary–adrenal (HPA) axis that occurs in bipolar disorder?

A. Decreased cortisol concentration in cerebrospinal fluid
B. Decreased cortisol concentration in plasma
C. Decreased diurnal variation of cortisol levels
D. Suppression of glucocorticoids following dexamethasone administration
E. All of the above

ANSWER: C

The normal physiological diurnal variation of cortisol is blunted in bipolar disorder. The other answer choices are the opposite of HPA abnormalities that occur in bipolar disorder: increased cortisol concentration in cerebrospinal fluid and plasma and nonsuppression of glucocorticoids in the dexamethasone–CRH test.

REFERENCE

Gillespie, C. F., Garlow, S. J., Binder, E. B., Schatzberg, A. F., & Nemeroff. C. B. (2009). Neurobiology of mood disorders. In A. F. Schatzberg & C. B. Nemeroff (Eds.), *The American Psychiatric Publishing textbook of psychopharmacology* (4th ed.). Arlington, VA: American Psychiatric Publishing.

10. Which of the following brain structures involved in response inhibition is hypoactive in mania, suggesting a link to symptoms of impulsivity (e.g., risk taking and pressured speech)?

A. Amygdala
B. Anterior cingulate cortex
C. Insular cortex
D. Orbitofrontal cortex
E. Thalamus

ANSWER: D

During a no-go task, a test to measure response inhibition, neuroimaging shows hypoactivity in the orbitofrontal cortex in manic patients compared with healthy controls. This finding suggests that problems of impulsivity seen in bipolar disorder are linked to this brain region.

REFERENCE

Stahl, S. M. (2013). *Stahl's essential psychopharmacology: Neuroscientific basis and practical applications* (4th ed., pp. 370–387). Cambridge, UK: Cambridge University Press.

11. Which of the following populations is MOST at risk for developing a secondary mood disorder (i.e., either substance induced or due to another medical condition)?

A. Adolescents
B. The elderly
C. Latinos
D. The impoverished
E. Women

ANSWER: B

The three most at-risk populations for developing a secondary mood disorder are patients with mixed features, patients with frequent episodes, and the elderly. In geriatric populations this is especially important to keep in mind so as to rule out likely medical or organic causes when a new-onset mood disorder is suspected.

REFERENCE

Ketter, T. A., & Chang, K. D. (2014). Bipolar and related disorders. In R. E. Hales, S. C. Yudofsky, & L. W. Roberts (Eds.), *The American Psychiatric Publishing textbook of psychiatry* (6th ed.). Arlington, VA: American Psychiatric Publishing.

12. Which of the following is more common in males with bipolar disorder than in females with bipolar disorder?

A. Co-morbid anxiety
B. Mixed features
C. Rapid cycling
D. Substance use disorder
E. Suicide attempts

ANSWER: D

There are several gender differences related to bipolar disorder, although they are not as well established or heavily investigated as in unipolar depression. Women with bipolar disorder are more likely to have suicide attempts, mixed features, rapid cycling, atypical symptoms during depression, and comorbid anxiety and eating disorders. Comorbid substance use disorders, however, are more common in men with bipolar disorder than in women.

REFERENCE

Stahl, S. M. (2013). *Stahl's essential psychopharmacology: Neuroscientific basis and practical applications* (4th ed., pp. 237–283). Cambridge, UK: Cambridge University Press.

13. A 25-year-old woman reports that for the last several years her mood "never seems to be stable," and this has been impacting her work and relationships negatively. On further interview she endorses periods of feeling elevated and irritable and other times of feeling abnormally sad, but never so much in either direction to feel "out of control." When she is irritable, she often has racing thoughts, and her friends sometimes tell her she is speaking too quickly. When she feels low, she cries more often and feels a sense of worthlessness, but she denies any neurovegetative symptoms or suicidal thoughts. She cannot remember the last time she "felt normal" for more than 2 or 3 weeks in a row. Which of the following is the MOST likely diagnosis?

A. Chronic major depressive disorder with atypical features
B. Cyclothymic disorder
C. Bipolar II disorder with rapid cycling
D. Schizoaffective disorder
E. Unspecified bipolar disorder

ANSWER: B

The following are diagnostic criteria for a diagnosis of cyclothymic disorder: 2 or more years of numerous periods of hypomanic symptoms and periods of depressive symptoms that do not meet criteria for a major mood episode; and symptoms were present for at least half the time, and no period without symptoms was longer than 2 months

REFERENCE

American Psychiatric Association. (2013). *Diagnostic and statistical manual of mental disorders* (5th ed.). Arlington, VA: American Psychiatric Publishing.

14. How many times greater is the lifetime risk of suicide in individuals with bipolar disorder than in the general population?

A. 5 times greater
B. 10 times greater
C. 15 times greater
D. 20 times greater
E. No difference

ANSWER: C

The estimated lifetime suicide risk is 15 times greater for individuals with bipolar disorder than for the general population, and bipolar disorder may account for up to 25% of all completed suicides.

REFERENCE

American Psychiatric Association. (2013). *Diagnostic and statistical manual of mental disorders* (5th ed.). Arlington, VA: American Psychiatric Publishing.

15. In addition to affective and behavioral symptoms, prospective daily ratings are required to make a diagnosis of premenstrual dysphoric disorder. For how many consecutive symptomatic menstrual cycles is the prospective rating required?

A. One
B. Two
C. Three
D. Four
E. 5

ANSWER: B

DSM-5 requires confirmation of at least two cycles of prospective daily ratings to make a diagnosis of premenstrual dysphoric disorder. Otherwise, the diagnosis should be accompanied by a "provisional" suffix.

REFERENCE

American Psychiatric Association. (2013). *Diagnostic and statistical manual of mental disorders* (5th ed.). Arlington, VA: American Psychiatric Publishing.

16. The presence of which of the following symptoms is more consistent with melancholic features of major depressive disorder than atypical features?

A. Hypersomnia
B. Leaden paralysis
C. Lack of mood reactivity
D. Weight gain
E. Interpersonal rejection sensitivity

ANSWER: C

Melancholic features include loss of pleasure in all, or almost all, activities; lack of mood reactivity; depression regularly worse in the morning; early morning awakening (at least 2 hours before usual time of awakening); marked psychomotor retardation or agitation; significant anorexia or weight loss; and excessive or inappropriate guilt. Atypical features include mood reactivity, increased appetite or weight gain, hypersomnia, leaden paralysis, and interpersonal rejection sensitivity.

REFERENCE

McInnis, M. G., Riba, M., & Greden, J. F. (2014). Depressive disorders. In R. E. Hales, S. C. Yudofsky, & L. W. Roberts (Eds.), *The American Psychiatric Publishing textbook of psychiatry* (6th ed.). Arlington, VA: American Psychiatric Publishing.

17. Which of the following is TRUE regarding treatment of premenstrual dysphoric disorder?

A. Cyclic discontinuation of sertraline results in significant adverse effects.
B. Clinical response is seen within 4 to 6 weeks of initiation of sertraline.
C. Evidence does not support the use of continuous administration of sertraline through the menstrual cycle.
D. Intermittent dosing of sertraline during the luteal phase has similar efficacy to continuous administration through the menstrual cycle.
E. Ideal dosing of sertraline for premenstrual dysphoric disorder is 200 mg daily.

ANSWER: D

Intermittent administration and continuous administration of sertraline for treatment of premenstrual dysphoric disorder have similar efficacy. There are no significant adverse effects from cyclic discontinuation. Clinical response is observed within a few days. Sertraline doses of 50 to 150 mg daily are efficacious for treatment of this disorder.

REFERENCE

Halbreich, U., & Kahn, L. S. (2003). Treatment of premenstrual dysphoric disorder with luteal phase dosing of sertraline. *Expert Opinion on Pharmacotherapy, 4,* 2065–2078.

18. In a patient diagnosed with premenstrual dysphoric disorder, symptoms are predominantly present during

the ___a___ phase of the menstrual cycle and disappear by the ___b___ phase of the menstrual cycle.

A. a: Luteal; b: luteal
B. a: Follicular; b: follicular
C. a: Luteal; b: beginning of menses
D. a: Follicular; b: beginning of menses

ANSWER: C

Symptoms are predominantly present during the luteal phrase of the menstrual cycle and disappear by the beginning of menses. Hence, intermittent dosing of an SSRI for treatment of premenstrual dysphoric disorder is given during the luteal phase only.

REFERENCE

Halbreich, U., & Kahn, L. S. (2003). Treatment of premenstrual dysphoric disorder with luteal phase dosing of sertraline. *Expert Opinion on Pharmacotherapy, 4*, 2065–2078.

19. Which of the following sleep changes is commonly observed in patients with major depressive disorder?

A. Decreased REM density
B. Decreased REM latency
C. Increased REM density
D. Increased REM latency
E. No changes in either REM latency or density

ANSWER: B

Decreased REM latency (i.e., the time between onset of sleep and onset of REM sleep) is seen in depression.

REFERENCE

Wang, Y. Q., Li, R., Zhang, M. Q., Zhang, Z., Qu, W. M., Huang, Z. L. (2015). The neurobiological mechanisms and treatments of REM sleep disturbances in depression. *Current Neuropharmacology, 13*, 543–553.

20. Which of the following statements is NOT a feature of the "with seasonal pattern" for bipolar disorder?

A. A temporal relationship is present between the onset of major depressive episode or hypomanic symptoms and the particular time of the year.
B. A temporal relationship is present between the full remission of major depressive episode or hypomanic symptoms and the particular time of the year.
C. In the last 3 years, mood episodes have demonstrated this temporal relationship.
D. No nonseasonal episodes have occurred in the patient's lifetime.

ANSWER: D

Although the lifetime total of seasonal episodes greatly outnumbers nonseasonal episodes, there may be a history of nonseasonal manic, hypomanic, or depressive episodes. No nonseasonal episodes should have occurred during the 2-year period preceding diagnosis.

REFERENCE

American Psychiatric Association. (2013). *Diagnostic and statistical manual of mental disorders* (5th ed.). Arlington, VA: American Psychiatric Publishing.

21. Which of the following statements is FALSE regarding bipolar disorder with rapid cycling?

A. Patients must experience at least four mood episodes in 1 year.
B. Rapid cycling is a risk factor for antidepressant-induced mania
C. Lithium is the treatment of choice.
D. Episodes must meet criteria for major depressive, manic, or hypomanic episode, including episode duration.
E. Rapid cycling is a poor prognostic factor in bipolar disorder.

ANSWER: C

Lithium is less effective for mood stabilization among bipolar disorder patients with rapid cycling than among those who do not have rapid cycling. The other statements are true.

REFERENCES

American Psychiatric Association. (2013). *Diagnostic and statistical manual of mental disorders* (5th ed.). Arlington, VA: American Psychiatric Publishing.
Post, R. M. (2016). Treatment of bipolar depression: Evolving recommendations. *Psychiatry Clinics of North America, 39*, 11–33.

22. Which symptom distinguishes childhood bipolar disorder from ADHD?

A. Irritability
B. Decreased need for sleep
C. Accelerated speech
D. Hyperactivity
E. All of the above are seen in both ADHD and bipolar disorder.

ANSWER: B

The following symptoms are more prominent in children with bipolar disorder than in those with only ADHD: elevated mood, grandiosity, flight of ideas, decreased need for sleep, and hypersexuality. The presence of the following does not differentiate these two disorders: irritability, accelerated speech, and distractibility.

REFERENCES

Geller, B., Williams, M., Zimerman, B., Frazier, J., Beringer, L., Warner, K. L. (1998). Prepubertal and early adolescent bipolarity differentiate from ADHD by manic symptoms, grandiose delusions, ultra-rapid or ultradian cycling. *Journal of Affective Disorders, 51*, 81–91.

Post, R. M. (2014). Differentiating pediatric bipolar disorder from attention-deficit/hyperactivity disorder. *Psychiatric Annals, 44*, 406–408.

23. Which of the following statements is TRUE regarding cognitive symptoms in late-life depression?

A. The neuropsychological profile of depression-associated neurocognitive disorder is indistinguishable from Alzheimer type.
B. There is no increased risk of neurocognitive disorder when depressive symptoms are adequately treated.
C. Late-life depression may be a risk factor for later cognitive decline, even when symptoms remit.
D. Risk of later cognitive decline is significant only in the presence of comorbid neurological illness, such as history of stroke.
E. Cognitive symptoms typically precede depressive symptoms.

ANSWER: C

Late-life depression is a risk factor for later cognitive decline, even if cognitive symptoms initially improve with treatment of depression. Emerging evidence suggests that a good portion of "pseudodementia" cases often involve early neurocognitive impairment at the least and are at elevated risk of neurocognitive decline.

REFERENCES

Steffens, D. C., Otey, E., Alexopoulos, G. S., Butters, M. A., Cuthbert, B., Ganguli, M., Geda, Y. E., Hendrie, H. C., Krishnan, R. R., Kumar, A., Lopez, O. L., Lyketsos, C. G., Mast, B. T., Morris, J. C., Norton, M. C., Peavy, G. M., Petersen, R. C., Reynolds, C. F., Salloway, S., Welsh-Bohmer, K. A., Yesavage, J. (2006). Perspectives on depression, mild cognitive impairment, and cognitive decline. *Archives of General Psychiatry, 63*, 130–138.

Welsh-Bohmer, K. A., & Attix, D. K. (2015). Neuropsychological assessment of late-life cognitive disorders. In D. C. Steffens, D. G. Blazer, & M. E. Thakur (Eds.), *The American Psychiatric Publishing textbook of geriatric psychiatry* (5th ed., pp. 142–144). Washington, DC: American Psychiatric Publishing.

24. What is the approximate rate of depression among patients with Parkinson's disease?

A. 20%
B. 40%
C. 60%
D. 80%
E. More than 85%

ANSWER: B

Depression is seen in up to 40% of patients with Parkinson's disease.

REFERENCE

Kimchi, E. Z., & Lyketsos, C. G. Dementia and mild neurocognitive disorders. In D. C. Steffens, D. G. Blazer, & M. E. Thakur (Eds.), *The American Psychiatric Publishing textbook of geriatric psychiatry* (5th ed., p. 204). Washington, DC: American Psychiatric Publishing.

25. Persistent depressive disorder (dysthymia) requires that symptoms include depressed mood for most of the day, for more days than not, for at least what period of time?

A. 2 weeks
B. 4 weeks
C. 6 months
D. 1 year
E. 2 years

ANSWER: E

DSM-5 criteria for persistent depressive disorder stipulate that depressed mood must be present for most of the day, more days than not, for at least 2 years (in adults).

REFERENCE

American Psychiatric Association. (2013). *Diagnostic and statistical manual of mental disorders* (5th ed.). Arlington, VA: American Psychiatric Publishing.

26. A specifier for depressive disorders in *DSM-5* is "with anxious distress." Which of the following symptoms does NOT support this diagnosis?

A. Feeling keyed up or tense
B. Feeling unusually restless
C. Fear that something awful will happen
D. Difficulty concentrating because of worry
E. Loss of appetite

ANSWER: E

Symptoms consistent with the specifier "with anxious distress" include feeling keyed up or tense, feeling unusually restless, fear that something awful will happen, difficulty concentrating because of worry, and the feeling that the individual might lose control of him- or herself. Loss of appetite may be seen in depressive disorders but is not included in the criteria for this specifier.

REFERENCE

American Psychiatric Association. (2013). *Diagnostic and statistical manual of mental disorders* (5th ed.). Arlington, VA: American Psychiatric Publishing.

27. Which of the following is a risk factor for poststroke depression?

A. Older age
B. Male gender
C. Intact cognition
D. Functional impairment
E. Recurrent stroke

ANSWER: D

Functional impairment (in both activities of daily living and social functioning) is a risk factor for poststroke depression, particularly among men. Younger age and female gender are risk factors. Cognitive impairment is also a risk factor for depression, particularly among women.

REFERENCE

Raskind, M. A. (2008). Diagnosis and treatment of depression comorbid with neurologic disorders. *American Journal of Medicine, 121*, S28–S37.

28. Which of the following is TRUE regarding gender differences in bipolar disorder?

A. Bipolar I disorder is seen more frequently in men.
B. Bipolar II disorder is seen more frequently in men.
C. Bipolar I disorder is seen more frequently in women.
D. Bipolar II disorder is seen more frequently in women.
E. Gender distribution is equal for both bipolar I disorder and bipolar II disorder.

ANSWER: D

Bipolar I disorder affects men and women equally, but bipolar II disorder is seen more frequently in women.

REFERENCES

Grande, I., Berk, M., Birmaher, B., & Vieta, E. (2016). Bipolar disorder. *Lancet, 387*, 1561–1572.
Nivoli, A. M., Pacchiarotti, I., Rosa, A. R., Popovic, D., Murru, A., Valenti, M., Bonnin, C. M., Grande, I., Sanchez-Moreno, J., Vieta, E., & Colom, F. (2011). Gender differences in a cohort study of 604 bipolar patients: The role of predominant polarity. *Journal of Affective Disorders, 133*, 443–449.

29. Which of the following is TRUE regarding suicide in bipolar disorder?

A. People with bipolar disorder account for more than 25% all suicide deaths.
B. Self-poisoning is the most common method.
C. Ten percent of patients with bipolar disorder attempt suicide.
D. Risk of suicide attempt decreases after hospital admission.
E. There is comparable risk of suicide among bipolar disorder patients whether or not they are engaged in treatment.

ANSWER: B

Self-poisoning and hanging are the two most common methods of suicide in individuals with bipolar disorder. Individuals with bipolar disorder account for 3.4% to 14% of all suicide deaths, and 23% to 26% of patients with bipolar disorder attempt suicide. Hospitalization and posthospitalization are considered high-risk periods for suicide among patients with bipolar disorder. Patients who are not in treatment are at higher risk of suicide than those engaged in treatment.

REFERENCE

Schaffer, A., Isometsä, E. T., Tondo, L., Moreno, D. H., Sinyor, M., Kessing, L. V., Turecki, G., Weizman, A., Azorin, J. M., Ha, K., Reis, C., Cassidy, F., Goldstein, T., Rihmer, Z., Beautrais, A., Chou, Y. H., Diazgranados, N., Levitt, A. J., Zarate, C. A. Jr, & Yatham, L. (2015). Epidemiology, neurobiology and pharmacological interventions related to suicide deaths and suicide attempts in bipolar disorder: Part I of a report of the International Society for Bipolar Disorders Task Force on Suicide in Bipolar Disorder. *Australian and New Zealand Journal of Psychiatry, 49*, 785–802.

30. Which of the following is TRUE regarding suicide in adolescents?

A. The highest rates of attempted and completed suicides in adolescents are among Caucasians.
B. Male adolescents have higher rates of suicidal ideation and attempts than do female adolescents.
C. The leading method of completed suicide among US adolescents is by self-poisoning.
D. Suicide is the leading cause of death among adolescents.
E. Adolescents who identify as gay, lesbian, bisexual, or transgender are at higher risk than their peers to attempt suicide.

ANSWER: E

The increased risk of suicide attempts among gay, lesbian, bisexual, or transgender adolescents persists when controlling for other suicide risk factors. The highest rates of attempted and completed suicides among adolescents are in those with American Indian and Alaskan Native background. Female adolescents have higher rates of suicidal ideation and attempts, but males have higher rates of completed suicide. The leading method of completed suicide among adolescents is self-inflicted gunshot wound. Suicide is the third leading cause of death among adolescents.

REFERENCE

Neves, M. G., & Leanza, F. (2014). Mood disorders in adolescents: Diagnosis, treatment, and suicide assessment in the primary care setting. *Primary Care, 41*, 587–606.

QUESTIONS AND ANSWERS

This chapter has accompanying questions and answers which are available to subscribers as part of the Oxford eLearning platform. To access the questions, follow the link below, or go to http://oxford-elearning.oup.com/books.

http://oxford-elearning.oup.com/books/test/67/10.1093/med/9780190265557.003.0018

19.

ANXIETY DISORDERS

Ambreen Ghori, Aarti Gupta

1. Which of the following medication classes is NOT recommended for use in the treatment of generalized anxiety disorder?

A. SSRIs
B. Benzodiazepines
C. Bupropion
D. Buspirone
E. SNRIs

ANSWER: C

Antidepressants, specifically SSRIs and SNRIs, are considered first-line treatment of generalized anxiety disorder based on safety, efficacy, and lack of abuse potential. Benzodiazepines, although not recommended for long-term use in generalized anxiety disorder due to tolerability and safety issues, can be very helpful for acute control of symptoms while SSRIs and SNRIs take effect. Several studies support the use of buspirone for generalized anxiety disorder. Bupropion may exacerbate anxiety symptoms.

REFERENCE

Reinhold, J. A., & Rickels, K. (2015). Pharmacological treatment for generalized anxiety disorder in adults: An update. *Expert Opinion on Pharmacotherapy, 16*, 1669–1681. doi:10.1517/14656566.2015.1059424

2. Which of the following statements is TRUE regarding specific phobia?

A. Specific phobia generally develops in early adulthood.
B. It is more prevalent in men than women.
C. It is commonly comorbid with other anxiety disorders.
D. In vivo exposure therapy should be avoided to prevent traumatization.

ANSWER: B

Specific phobia manifests as marked fear or anxiety associated with a particular situation or object (e.g., fear of flying, sight of blood, spiders). It is not age specific but usually starts in childhood, when it often occurs with other anxiety disorders such as separation anxiety disorder and social phobia. As with most anxiety disorders, females are more frequently affected than males in a ratio of 2:1. There is evidence that supports the efficacy of in vivo exposure therapy, a technique based on concepts of respondent conditioning, extinction, and learning theory, for specific phobia. The patient is exposed to the phobic stimulus in a controlled and systematic fashion.

REFERENCES

American Psychiatric Association. (2013). Specific phobia. In *Diagnostic and statistical manual of mental disorders* (5th ed. pp 197–202). Arlington, VA: American Psychiatric Publishing.

Silverman, W. K., & Moreno, J. (2005). Specific phobia. *Child and Adolescent Psychiatric Clinics of North America, 14*, 819–843. doi:10.1016/j.chc.2005.05.004

3. Which of the following anxiety disorders is most prevalent?

A. Social phobia
B. Specific phobia
C. Generalized anxiety disorder
D. Panic disorder

ANSWER: B

Specific phobia is the most common anxiety disorder, with a 12-month prevalence rate of 7% to 9% in the United States. This statistic often comes as a surprise because individuals with specific phobia often do not seek psychiatric help. Social phobia is also quite prevalent at a 12-month prevalence rate of 7%. Generalized anxiety disorder (0.9%–2.9%) and panic disorder (2%) are not as frequent as some other anxiety disorders.

REFERENCES

American Psychiatric Association (2013). Specific phobia. In *Diagnostic and statistical manual of mental disorders* (5th ed.: pp. 197–202) Arlington, VA: American Psychiatric Publishing.

Bandelow, B., & Michaelis, S. (2015). Epidemiology of anxiety disorders in the 21st century. *Dialogues in Clinical Neuroscience, 17,* 327–335.

4. A patient was stabbed by his coworker at work 15 days ago. After the assault he developed intense anxiety about going back to work. He says he has not been able to sleep well since the attack due to nightmares of the event. He ruminates daily about the assault, often experiencing it as if it were happening again. He is constantly "on edge" about the possibility of strangers attacking him. Which of the following diagnoses is most consistent with his presentation?

A. Acute stress disorder
B. Post-traumatic stress disorder
C. Adjustment disorder
D. Panic disorder
E. Agoraphobia

ANSWER: A

He is suffering from acute stress disorder (ASD), which may remit or progress to post-traumatic stress disorder (PTSD). ASD and PTSD have very similar symptoms, and they are typically best distinguished based on a timeline of symptoms. ASD develops within 3 days to 1 month of the occurrence of the trauma and resolves within a month of the index trauma. If the symptoms persist for more than 1 month, the diagnosis of PTSD is made. Although ASD may remit within a month, it can also progress to PTSD. Half of patients suffering from PTSD report symptoms of ASD preceding PTSD. In the course of PTSD, 50% of patients remit within 3 months, but some patients suffer from the disorder for longer periods of time.

REFERENCES

American Psychiatric Association (2013). Trauma and stress related disorder. In *Diagnostic and statistical manual of mental disorders* (5th ed., pp. 265–290). Arlington, VA: American Psychiatric Publishing.

Elklit, A., & Brink, O. (2004). Acute stress disorder as a predictor of post-traumatic stress disorder in physical assault victims. *Journal of Interpersonal Violence, 19,* 709–726. doi:10.1177/0886260504263872

5. The anxiolytic property of benzodiazepines is related to which of the following receptors?

A. $GABA_B$
B. $GABA_A$
C. NMDA
D. Glycine
E. AMPA

ANSWER: B

GABA is the main inhibitory neurotransmitter in the brain, whereas glutamate is the main excitatory neurotransmitter. Benzodiazepines primarily bind with the $GABA_A$ receptor and enhance the inhibitory effects of GABA, making them a positive allosteric modulator of $GABA_A$ receptors. The $GABA_A$ receptor alpha-1 subunit appears to be involved in sedation, whereas the alpha-2 and/or alpha-3 subunits are involved in effects on anxiety. NMDAR is a glutamate receptor, and it can be activated via glycine-dependent or glycine-independent mechanisms. It is implicated in excitatory synaptic transmission, synaptic plasticity, and memory function. GlyR is a receptor that binds glycine, an inhibitory neurotransmitter, and is implicated in inhibitory synaptic neurotransmission in the brain and spinal cord.

REFERENCES

Atack, J. R. (2005). The benzodiazepine binding site of GABA(A) receptors as a target for the development of novel anxiolytics. *Expert Opinion on Investigational Drugs, 14,* 601–618. doi:10.1517/13543784.14.5.601

Volianskis, A., France, G., Jensen, M. S., Bortolotto, Z. A., Jane, D. E., & Collingridge, G. L. (2015). Long-term potentiation and the role of N-methyl-D-aspartate receptors. *Brain Research, 1621,* 5–16. doi: 10.1016/j.brainres.2015.01.016

6. A 19-year-old man presents to the emergency room in an acutely anxious state. He tells you that he snorted cocaine for the first time with his friends a few hours earlier, after which he started sweating, trembling, and

experiencing chest pain with palpitations. He thought he was about to die, so he called 911. He denies ever experiencing such symptoms in the past. His medical history is significant for treated hypothyroidism and family history of panic disorder in his mother. What is the most likely diagnosis?

A. Panic disorder
B. Substance-induced anxiety disorder
C. Anxiety disorder due to another medical condition
D. Unspecified anxiety disorder

ANSWER: B

The patient has suffered a panic attack induced by cocaine as evidenced by the temporal correlation of symptoms with use. Substance- or medication-induced anxiety disorder is diagnosed when a panic attack or anxiety is the predominant symptom and develops during or soon after substance or medication intoxication or withdrawal. The substance or medication has to be capable of producing the symptom, and the symptom should not be better explained by an anxiety disorder that is not substance induced. Many medical conditions cause anxiety and panic attacks. Examples include endocrine diseases (e.g., hyperthyroidism, pheochromocytoma, hyperadrenocortisolism, hypoglycemia), cardiovascular disorders (e.g., congestive heart failure, pulmonary embolism, arrhythmia), respiratory illness (e.g., chronic obstructive pulmonary disease, asthma, pneumonia), metabolic disturbances (e.g., vitamin B12 deficiency, porphyria), and neurological illness (e.g., neoplasms, vestibular dysfunction, encephalitis, seizure disorders). The other options are less likely given the temporal correlation of the attack with substance use as well as the lack of prior episodes.

REFERENCE

American Psychiatric Association. (2013). Substance/medication induced anxiety disorder. In *Diagnostic and statistical manual of mental disorders* (5th ed., pp.485–490). t. e. Arlington, VA: American Psychiatric Publishing.

7. A 62-year-old woman from Puerto Rico presents for outpatient evaluation. Her husband died unexpectedly 2 months ago. Since then, she has had multiple episodes of extreme rage, yelling and cursing at her family members for no good reason. During those times she feels a surge of heat in her chest rising to her head, feels like she is about to pass out, and is "all nerves." Her heart beats too fast, and she feels like she is trembling. The family is very distressed and thinks she is "possessed." What is the most likely diagnosis?

A. Adjustment disorder
B. ***Susto***
C. ***Ataque de nervios***
D. ***Nervios***
E. Normal grief

ANSWER: C

Culture-bound syndromes are a group of psychiatric symptoms and behaviors that are specific to certain cultures and may not fit the diagnostic criteria of any one *DSM-5* diagnosis, even though they may have overlapping symptoms with different mental disorders. Culture-bound syndromes are categorized under "Other Specified Anxiety Disorder" in *DSM-5*. It is important to understand different culture-bound syndromes to avoid overdiagnosing mental illness and to find therapeutic treatment in cultural context.

Ataque de nervios (attack of nerves) is observed in individuals of Latino descent, particularly Caribbean Hispanics, and characterized by intense emotional upset, including acute anxiety, anger, or grief; screaming and shouting uncontrollably; attacks of crying; trembling; heat in the chest rising into the head; and becoming verbally and physically aggressive. Dissociative experiences, seizure-like or fainting episodes, and suicidal gestures may occur. Attacks are frequently brought on by a stressful event in the family such as a death, accident, or conflict with a family member.

Nervios (nerves) is a common idiom of distress among Latinos in the United States and Latin America; it refers to a general state of vulnerability to life circumstances and stressors. The most common symptoms include headaches, irritability, stomach disturbances, sleep difficulties, nervousness, easy tearfulness, inability to concentrate, trembling, tingling sensations, and *mareos* (dizziness with vertigo-like exacerbations).

Susto (fright) is a cultural explanation for distress and misfortune prevalent among some Latinos in the United States and among people in Mexico, Central America, and South America, but it is not recognized among Caribbean Hispanics. *Susto* is attributed to one's soul leaving the body due to a frightening incident, leading to misery and sickness. In extreme cases, *susto* may result in death. The symptoms resemble those of major depressive disorder and may include appetite and sleep disturbances, feelings of sadness, low self-worth, and lack of motivation. *Susto* may be accompanied by somatic symptoms like headache, stomachache, or muscle aches and pains.

REFERENCES

American Psychiatric Association. (2013). Glossary of cultural concepts of distress. In *Diagnostic and statistical manual of mental disorders* (5th ed., pp. 833–837). Arlington, VA: American Psychiatric Publishing.

Razzouk, D., Nogueira, B., & Mari Jde, J. (2011). The contribution of Latin American and Caribbean countries on culture bound syndromes studies for the ICD-10 revision: Key findings from a working in progress. *Revista Brasileira de Psiquiatria, 33*(suppl. 1), S5–S20.

8. A 14-year-old girl has difficulty socializing with friends. Her mother reports that her daughter has a very difficult time visiting her friends' homes, and while she is there she often calls home to make sure her mother is fine and will be able to pick her up. One week ago she went to a friend's home and began sweating, shaking, crying, and vomiting. She could not be comforted until she was brought back home. Her mother says that when her daughter was 5, she was very clingy and would hit her mother when she dropped her off at school. The patient does not experience these symptoms when her friends come to her home and while her mother is nearby. What is the most likely diagnosis?

A. Dependent personality disorder
B. Oppositional defiant disorder
C. Separation anxiety disorder
D. Social anxiety disorder
E. Borderline personality disorder

ANSWER: C

A characteristic feature of separation anxiety disorder is experiencing anxiety in the context of separation from home or attachment figures. Individuals with separation anxiety disorder refuse to go anywhere that would take them away from attachment figures, and some children may get aggressive if forced to separate. They also worry about something happening to themselves or to the attachment figures when they are not together. They often have difficulty sleeping by themselves and away from parents and may experience nightmares of something bad happening to the parents. Physical symptoms like headaches and gastrointestinal discomfort are common. The disturbance must last for a period of at least 4 weeks in children and adolescents younger than 18 years and is typically 6 months or longer in adults. The patient described above is able to socialize well at her home and is anxious only when she separates from her mother, which makes social anxiety disorder less plausible.

REFERENCES

American Psychiatric Association. (2013). Separation anxiety disorder. In *Diagnostic and statistical manual of mental disorders* (5th ed, pp.190–195). Arlington, VA: American Psychiatric Publishing.

Masi, G., Mucci, M., & Millepiedi, S. (2001). Separation anxiety disorder in children and adolescents: Epidemiology, diagnosis and management. *CNS Drugs, 15*, 93–104.

9. Which of the following medications would NOT be a good choice for treating a 28-year-old woman with obsessive–compulsive disorder (OCD)?

A. Clomipramine
B. Fluoxetine
C. Bupropion
D. Fluvoxamine
E. Sertraline

ANSWER: C

SSRIs are considered first-line agents for the treatment of OCD followed by clomipramine. Bupropion has not shown benefit in the treatment of OCD.

REFERENCE

Marazziti, D., & Consoli, G. (2010). Treatment strategies for obsessive–compulsive disorder. *Expert Opinion on Pharmacotherapy, 11*, 331–343.

10. Which of the following psychological treatment modalities has been found to be MOST effective in the treatment of OCD?

A. Supportive therapy
B. Exposure and response prevention
C. Dialectical behavioral therapy
D. Interpersonal therapy
E. Problem-solving therapy

ANSWER: B

Exposure and response prevention (ERP) is considered the most effective psychological treatment for OCD.

REFERENCE

Marazziti, D., & Consoli, G. (2010). Treatment strategies for obsessive–compulsive disorder. *Expert Opinion on Pharmacotherapy, 11*, 331–343.

11. Which of the following disorders is NOT part of the *DSM-5* classification of anxiety disorders?

A. Separation anxiety disorder
B. Selective mutism
C. OCD
D. Panic disorder
E. Agoraphobia

ANSWER: C

The *DSM-5* chapter on anxiety disorders does not include OCD but instead includes a new chapter titled "Obsessive–Compulsive and Related Disorders." Similarly, the chapter on anxiety disorders does not include PTSD or ASD, which now appear in a new chapter titled "Trauma- and Stressor-Related Disorders." Panic disorder and agoraphobia are now separate disorders in the *DSM-5*, each with its own diagnostic criteria. Separation anxiety disorder and selective mutism are now classified as anxiety disorders.

REFERENCE

Kupfer, D. J. (2015). Anxiety and *DSM-5*. *Dialogues in Clinical Neuroscience, 17*, 245–246.

12. Which of the following drugs has been shown to be INEFFECTIVE in the treatment of individuals with PTSD?

A. Lorazepam
B. Fluoxetine
C. Paroxetine
D. Mirtazapine
E. Imipramine

ANSWER: A

Fluoxetine, paroxetine, and sertraline are noted to be particularly efficacious in the treatment of PTSD. Imipramine, mirtazapine, and amitriptyline have shown benefit in the treatment of individuals with PTSD. Available evidence indicates that benzodiazepines are ineffective for the treatment and prevention of PTSD, and the risks associated with their use tend to outweigh the potential short-term benefits. Additionally, benzodiazepines are associated with specific problems in individuals with PTSD, including worse overall severity of the illness, significantly increased risk of developing PTSD with use after a recent trauma, worse psychotherapy outcomes, worse aggression, worse depression, and greater substance use. Hence benzodiazepines like lorazepam should not be used in the treatment of individuals with PTSD.

REFERENCES

Gu, W., Wang, C., Li, Z., Zhang, X. (2016). Pharmacotherapies for posttraumatic stress disorder: A meta-analysis. *Journal of Nervous and Mental Disease, 205*, 331–338.

Guina, J., Rossetter, S. R., DeRhodes, B. J, Nahhas, R.W and Welton, R.S. (2015). Benzodiazepines for PTSD: A systematic review and meta-analysis. *Journal of Psychiatric Practice, 21*, 281–303.

13. A 75-year-old man developed left hemiplegia secondary to a cerebrovascular accident. He was unable to successfully complete the course of rehabilitation and needed to be placed at a skilled nursing facility for long-term care. He walks very slowly with a walker and is incontinent of urine. He has been at the skilled nursing facility for the past 7 months. Since his admission to the facility, he has been fearful of scrutiny by others and avoids coming out of his room. He requests that visitors stay out of his room as much as possible. He has not participated in any social activities since his admission to the facility. He does not appear to be sad and is eating and sleeping well. There are no active medical issues or cognitive impairment noted at this time. Based on the available information, which of the following would be the most appropriate diagnosis for this individual?

A. Agoraphobia
B. Social anxiety disorder
C. Generalized anxiety disorder
D. Specific phobia
E. Major depressive disorder

ANSWER: B

Based on the available evidence, the most appropriate diagnosis for this man would be social anxiety disorder. He appears to have marked fear of coming out of his room because he thinks he would be exposed to possible scrutiny by others. The very thought of leaving his room provokes fear, and he has avoided coming out of his room for over 6 months. This avoidance has caused significant impairment in his social functioning. Additionally, there are no other known medical or psychiatric causes for his symptoms.

REFERENCE

American Psychiatric Association. (2013). *Desk reference to the diagnostic criteria from* DSM-5 (pp. 115–128). Arlington, VA: American Psychiatric Publishing.

14. Which of the following statements is CORRECT regarding the efficacy of sertraline, venlafaxine, mirtazapine, and nefazodone for the treatment of social anxiety disorder among adults?

A. No one drug has shown greater efficacy over the others.
B. Sertraline has shown the greatest efficacy.
C. Venlafaxine has shown the greatest efficacy.
D. Mirtazapine has shown the greatest efficacy.
E. Nefazodone has shown the greatest efficacy.

ANSWER: A

A meta-analysis of second-generation antidepressants indicated that these medications are efficacious in the treatment of social anxiety disorder among adults. The data did not suggest any difference in efficacy among the various drugs.

REFERENCE

de Menezes, G. B., Coutinho, E. S., Fontenelle, L. F.,Vigne, P., Figueira, I and Versiani, M. (2011). Second-generation antidepressants in social anxiety disorder: Meta-analysis of controlled clinical trials. *Psychopharmacology (Berlin)*, *215*, 1–11.

15. Which of the following therapies has the LEAST evidence for the treatment of panic disorder?

A. Cognitive therapy
B. Interpersonal therapy
C. Exposure therapy
D. Relaxation training
E. Breathing retraining

ANSWER: B

Among these therapies, interpersonal therapy has the least evidence for the treatment of individuals with panic disorder.

REFERENCE

Sánchez-Meca, J., Rosa-Alcázar, A. I., Marín-Martínez, F., & Gomez-Conesa, A. (2010). Psychological treatment of panic disorder with or without agoraphobia: A meta-analysis. *Clinical Psychology Review, 30*, 37–50.

16. Which of the following mental health disorders is the MOST prevalent in the general population?

A. Developmental disorders
B. Anxiety disorders
C. Mood disorders
D. Psychotic disorders
E. Substance use disorders

ANSWER: B

Anxiety disorders are the most prevalent class of mental health disorders.

REFERENCE

Merikangas, K. R., & Kalaydjian, A. E. (2009). Anxiety disorders. In B. J. Sadock, V. A. Sadock, P. Ruiz, & H. I. Kaplan (Eds.), *Kaplan and Sadock's comprehensive textbook of psychiatry* (9th ed., p. 1856). Philadelphia, PA: Wolters Kluwer Health/Lippincott Williams and Wilkins.

17. Which of the following statements about gender differences in anxiety is TRUE?

A. Women are twice as likely as men to have anxiety disorders.
B. Women and men are at equal risk of having anxiety disorders.
C. Men are twice as likely as women to have anxiety disorders.
D. Men have higher rates of anxiety before age 20 and lower rates of anxiety after age 40.

ANSWER: A

Women are twice as likely as men to have anxiety disorders.

REFERENCE

Merikangas, K. R., & Kalaydjian, A. E. (2009). Anxiety disorders. In B. J. Sadock, V. A. Sadock, P. Ruiz, & H. I. Kaplan (Eds.), *Kaplan and Sadock's comprehensive textbook of psychiatry* (9th ed., p. 1860). Philadelphia, PA: Wolters Kluwer Health/Lippincott Williams and Wilkins.

18. A 14-year-old girl has constant and recurrent distress when her mother goes to work in the morning. She worries that her mother will die during her commute or never return home. The girl worries that when she is not under her mother's supervision she may be harmed or the house may be robbed. These thoughts have impaired her daily activities. She hides her mother's car keys most days, making her mother late for work. She also refuses to go to school. These symptoms started 12 weeks ago. The girl's presentation is MOST consistent with which diagnosis?

A. Generalized anxiety disorder
B. Specific phobia
C. Separation anxiety disorder
D. Social phobia
E. Panic disorder

ANSWER: C

The patient's presentation is most suggestive of separation anxiety disorder. This disorder is characterized by developmentally inappropriate and excessive anxiety concerning separation from home or an attachment figure. Patients demonstrate recurrent and excessive distress when faced with such separation. They also demonstrate persistent and excessive worry that a major attachment figure will be lost or harmed. Symptoms must be present for 4 weeks or more, and symptom onset should be before age 18.

REFERENCE

American Psychiatric Association. (2013). *Diagnostic and statistical manual of mental disorders* (5th ed.). Arlington, VA: American Psychiatric Publishing.

19. Which of the following statements about anxiety prevalence is TRUE?

A. Anxiety prevalence is highest among those in the lowest income bracket.
B. Anxiety prevalence is highest among those in the highest income bracket.
C. Anxiety prevalence is highest among the middle class (middle 50% income bracket).
D. Anxiety prevalence does not vary with socioeconomic status.

ANSWER: A

Anxiety prevalence is highest among individuals in the lowest income bracket.

REFERENCE

Merikangas, K. R., & Kalaydjian, A. E. (2009). Anxiety disorders. In B. J. Sadock, V. A. Sadock, P. Ruiz, & H. I. Kaplan (Eds.), *Kaplan and Sadock's comprehensive textbook of psychiatry* (9th ed., p. 1862). Philadelphia, PA: Wolters Kluwer Health/Lippincott Williams and Wilkins.

20. Which of the following statements is TRUE regarding the relationship of alcohol use disorder and anxiety disorders?

A. Sustained abstinence from alcohol among patients with alcohol use disorder results in increased anxiety symptomatology.
B. Patients with alcohol use disorder show lower rates of anxiety disorder than the general population.
C. Children of adults with alcohol use disorder are at no higher risk of developing anxiety disorders than the general population.
D. Rates of alcohol use disorder are higher among individuals with lifelong anxiety disorders than among the general population.

ANSWER: D

Patients with lifelong anxiety disorders have higher rates of alcohol use disorder than the general population. Patients with alcohol use disorder show higher rates of anxiety disorder than the general population, and sustained abstinence from alcohol usually improves anxiety symptoms. Children of adults with alcohol use disorder are at higher risk of developing anxiety disorders. Trait harm avoidance is common in both anxiety disorders and alcohol use disorder.

REFERENCE

Schuckit, M. A., & Hesselbrock, V. (1994). Alcohol dependence and anxiety disorders: What is the relationship? *American Journal of Psychiatry, 151*, 1723–1734.

21. What are the three principal defense mechanisms in phobia?

A. Displacement, projection, and avoidance
B. Projection, avoidance, and intellectualization
C. Humor, sublimation, and displacement
D. Humor, intellectualization, and sublimation

ANSWER: A

Displacement, projection, and avoidance are the three principal defense mechanisms in phobia.

REFERENCE

Sadock, B. J., Sadock, V. A., & Ruiz, P. (2007). *Kaplan and Sadock's synopsis of psychiatry* (10th ed., p. 599). Philadelphia, PA: Lippincott Williams and Wilkins.

22. Specific phobia is observed in what percentage of individuals in the United States?

A. 2%
B. 5%
C. 10%
D. 15%
E. 20%

ANSWER: C

Specific phobia is quite common, seen in approximately 10% of individuals in the United States.

REFERENCE

McClure, E. B., & Pine, D. S. (2009). Clinical features of anxiety disorders. In B. J. Sadock, V. A. Sadock, P. Ruiz, & H. I. Kaplan (Eds.), *Kaplan and Sadock's comprehensive textbook of psychiatry* (9th ed., p. 1849). Philadelphia, PA: Wolters Kluwer Health/Lippincott Williams and Wilkins.

23. Which of the following factors would support a physiological cause of anxiety in medically ill older adults, rather than a psychological cause?

A. The patient has experienced a major life change.
B. The patient has high scores on measures of neuroticism.
C. Anxiety symptoms arise in the absence of psychiatric history or risk factors.
D. There are no new medications or lapses in medication adherence.
E. Anxiety symptoms predate physical illness.

ANSWER: C

The relationship of anxiety and medical illness is complex, as many physical illnesses and medications in late life cause anxiety symptoms on a physiological level, but patients often have a psychological response to the diagnosis of medical illness as well. If anxiety symptoms arise in the absence of psychiatric history or risk factors, a physiological cause should be considered. The other factors would be supportive of psychological origins of anxiety.

REFERENCE

Mohlman, J., Bryant, C., Lenze, E. J., Stanley, M.A., Gum, A., Flint, A....Craske, M.G. (2012). Improving recognition of late life anxiety disorders in *Diagnostic and statistical manual of mental disorders*, fifth edition: Observations and recommendations of the Advisory Committee to the Lifespan Disorders Work Group. *International Journal of Geriatric Psychiatry, 27*, 549–556.

24. Which of the following is TRUE regarding anxiety in neurocognitive disorder?

A. Anxiety tends to worsen with increasing cognitive impairment.
B. Anxiety symptoms may be a prodrome for neurocognitive disorder even 15 years before onset of cognitive decline.
C. New-onset anxiety in mild cognitive impairment may indicate progression toward major neurocognitive disorder.
D. Anxiety is rarely seen in neurocognitive disorder.
E. In major neurocognitive disorder due to Alzheimer's disease, anxiety and depression are observed but are rarely co-morbid with one another.

ANSWER: C

New-onset anxiety in mild cognitive impairment may indicate progression toward major neurocognitive disorder. Agitation, rather than anxiety, is more likely to be present as neurocognitive disorder progresses. Anxiety symptoms more than 10 years before onset of cognitive decline are consistent with a separate anxiety disorder rather than a prodrome. Anxiety is commonly observed in neurocognitive disorder and is often co-morbid with depression in neurocognitive disorder due to Alzheimer's disease.

REFERENCE

Lenze, E. J., Mohlman, J., & Wetherell, J. L. (2015). Anxiety, obsessive-compulsive, and trauma-related disorders. In D. C. Steffens, D. G. Blazer, & M. E. Thakur (Eds.), *The American Psychiatric Publishing textbook of geriatric psychiatry* (5th ed., pp. 358–359). Washington, DC: American Psychiatric Publishing.

25. Social phobia is often difficult to distinguish from agoraphobia, isolative behavior in major depressive disorder, and other diagnoses. Which of the following features would be MOST suggestive of social phobia?

A. Anhedonia
B. Fear in social situations
C. Decreased time spent in social situations
D. Fear of difficult escape
E. Paranoid ideation

ANSWER: B

Patients with a diagnosis of social phobia specifically demonstrate fear or anxiety in social situations. Decreased time spent in social situations is nonspecific. Anhedonia would be characteristic of major depressive disorder. Fear of difficult escape would be seen in agoraphobia. Psychotic symptoms such as paranoid ideation would not be characteristic of social phobia.

REFERENCE

McClure-Tone, E. B., & Pine, D. S. (2009). Clinical features of anxiety disorders. In B. J. Sadock, V. A. Sadock, P. Ruiz, & H. I. Kaplan (Eds.), *Kaplan and Sadock's comprehensive textbook of psychiatry* (9th ed., p. 1849). Philadelphia, PA: Wolters Kluwer Health/Lippincott Williams and Wilkins.

26. What is characteristic of state anxiety, as opposed to trait anxiety?

A. Lifelong pattern of anxiety
B. Hypersensitivity to stimuli
C. Catastrophic thinking
D. Anxiety bound to specific situations
E. Increased psychophysiological reactivity

ANSWER: D

State anxiety includes anxiety bound to specific situations that typically resolves once the stressor has ended. The other options are characteristic of trait anxiety.

REFERENCE

Matorin, A. A., & Ruiz, P. (2009). Clinical manifestations of psychiatric disorders. In B. J. Sadock, V. A. Sadock, P. Ruiz, & H. I. Kaplan (Eds.), *Kaplan and Sadock's comprehensive textbook of psychiatry* (9th ed., p. 1095). Philadelphia, PA: Wolters Kluwer Health/Lippincott Williams and Wilkins.

27. Which of the following is TRUE regarding physiological characteristics of patients with panic disorder?

A. At rest, patients with panic disorder have increased autonomic arousal relative to healthy individuals.
B. Patients with panic disorder have autonomic arousal during panic attacks but return to a normal baseline following the attack.
C. Patients with panic disorder have autonomic arousal during panic attacks and for a period of approximately 60 minutes following the attack, which then resolves.
D. At rest, patients with panic disorder have less autonomic arousal than patients with generalized anxiety disorder.

ANSWER: A

Patients with panic disorder, although they may feel calm between panic attacks, have increased autonomic arousal relative to healthy individuals. They also have more autonomic arousal at rest than do patients with generalized anxiety disorder.

REFERENCE

Grillon, C., & Cornwell, B. R. (2009). Anxiety disorders: Psychophysiological aspects. In B. J. Sadock, V. A. Sadock, P. Ruiz, & H. I. Kaplan (Eds.), *Kaplan and Sadock's comprehensive textbook of psychiatry* (9th ed., pp. 1867–1868). Philadelphia, PA: Wolters Kluwer Health/Lippincott Williams and Wilkins.

28. Which of the following medical conditions can mimic a panic attack?

A. Hypoglycemia
B. Hyperthyroidism
C. Pheochromocytoma
D. Asthma
E. All of the above

ANSWER: E

All of the above medical conditions can mimic a panic attack. Other medical conditions that can resemble a panic attack include hypothyroidism, hyperparathyroidism, seizures, vestibular dysfunction, neoplasms, arrhythmias, and chronic obstructive pulmonary disease.

REFERENCE

McClure-Tone, E. B., & Pine, D. S. (2009). Clinical features of anxiety disorders. In B. J. Sadock, V. A. Sadock, P. Ruiz, & H. I. Kaplan (Eds.), *Kaplan and Sadock's comprehensive textbook of psychiatry* (9th ed., p. 1846). Philadelphia, PA: Wolters Kluwer Health/Lippincott Williams and Wilkins.

29. What is the typical age of onset for panic disorder?

A. Childhood
B. Early adolescence
C. Late adolescence
D. Perimenopausal
E. Late adulthood

ANSWER: C

The typical age of onset for panic disorder is in late adolescence/early adulthood, although onset can occur at any time.

REFERENCE

McClure-Tone, E. B., & Pine, D. S. (2009). Clinical features of anxiety disorders. In B. J. Sadock, V. A. Sadock, P. Ruiz, & H. I. Kaplan (Eds.), *Kaplan and Sadock's comprehensive textbook of psychiatry* (9th ed., p. 1846). Philadelphia, PA: Wolters Kluwer Health/Lippincott Williams and Wilkins.

30. A 9-year-old boy started attending a new school in September. As of December, he had not spoken a single word in class. He used to earn As in all subjects, but his grades have dropped to Bs and Cs because of his apparent refusal to speak. He is a fluent, native English speaker and has no communication difficulties at home or when playing with friends outside of school. This presentation is MOST consistent with which diagnosis?

A. Social anxiety disorder
B. Selective mutism
C. Agoraphobia
D. Generalized anxiety disorder
E. Specific phobia

ANSWER: B

The patient meets criteria for selective mutism: consistent failure to speak in a specific social situation in which there is an expectation for speaking, despite speaking in other situations. The disturbance interferes with educational achievement. Duration of the disturbance is greater than 1 month (not limited to the first month of school). The failure to speak is not attributable to a lack of knowledge of, or comfort with, the spoken language required. The disturbance is not better explained by a communication disorder.

REFERENCE

American Psychiatric Association. (2013). *Diagnostic and statistical manual of mental disorders* (5th ed.). Arlington, VA: American Psychiatric Publishing.

QUESTIONS AND ANSWERS

This chapter has accompanying questions and answers which are available to subscribers as part of the Oxford eLearning platform. To access the questions, follow the link below, or go to http://oxford-elearning.oup.com/books.

http://oxford-elearning.oup.com/books/test/67/10.1093/med/9780190265557.003.0019

20.

SOMATIC SYMPTOM DISORDERS AND FACTITIOUS DISORDERS

Harvinder Singh, Juan Young, Isabella Michna

1. Which of the following disorders is NOT part of the *DSM-5* group of somatic symptom and related disorders?

A. Somatization disorder
B. Factitious disorder
C. Illness anxiety disorder
D. Conversion disorder
E. Somatic symptom disorder

ANSWER: A

Somatization disorder is not part of the *DSM-5* group of somatic symptom and related disorders.

REFERENCE

American Psychiatric Association. (2013). *Diagnostic and statistical manual of mental disorders* (5th ed.). Arlington, VA: American Psychiatric Publishing.

2. Which of the following is the BEST established treatment modality for somatic symptom and related disorders?

A. Antipsychotics
B. Interpersonal psychotherapy (IPT)
C. Antidepressants
D. Benzodiazepines
E. Cognitive behavioral therapy (CBT)

ANSWER: E

CBT is the best established treatment modality for somatic symptom and related disorders.

REFERENCE

Kroenke, K. (2007). Efficacy of treatment for somatoform disorders: A review of randomized controlled trials. *Psychosomatic Medicine, 69*, 881–888.

3. In which of the following conditions are both the mechanism of illness production and the motivation for illness behavior conscious?

A. Somatic symptom disorder
B. Illness anxiety disorder
C. Malingering
D. Factitious disorder
E. Conversion disorder

ANSWER: C

Contrary to the *DSM-IV-TR* somatoform disorders, somatic symptom disorder and illness anxiety disorder focus on the *presence* of distress rather than the *absence* of medical cause. That is, they are not conceptualized as "psychogenic" conditions as was somatization disorder. Nevertheless, somaticizing (translation of psychological distress into somatic complaints) and somatosensory amplification (amplification of somatic symptoms by psychological distress) play a significant role in many, though not all, instances of somatic symptom disorder. In conversion, both the mechanism of illness production (MIP) and the motivation for illness behavior (MIB) are unconscious. In malingering, both MIP and MIB are conscious in that the patient knows what he or she is doing and why (secondary gain). Factitious disorder is characterized by conscious MIP but unconscious MIB.

REFERENCE

Yates, W. R. (2014) Somatic symptom disorders clinical presentation. Retrieved from http://emedicine.medscape.com/article/294908-clinical

4. In which of the following disorders does the individual have the motivation to assume the sick role in the absence of any secondary gain?

A. Malingering
B. Factitious disorder
C. Somatic symptom disorder
D. Illness anxiety disorder
E. Conversion disorder

ANSWER: B

Individuals with factitious disorder have the motivation to assume the sick role despite the absence of any secondary gain.

REFERENCE

Wang, D. L., Powsner, S., & Eisendrath, S. (2009). Factitious disorders. In B. J. Sadock, V. A. Sadock, & P. Ruiz (Eds.), *Kaplan and Sadock's comprehensive textbook of psychiatry* (9th ed., pp. 1949–1964). Philadelphia, PA: Lippincott Williams and Wilkins.

5. Which of the following statements regarding the etiology of somatic symptom disorder is TRUE?

A. Patients unconsciously amplify normal physiological function.
B. Patients misinterpret normal physiological function.
C. Somatic symptom disorder is associated with reduced amygdala volume.
D. Patients often have high autonomic arousal.
E. All of the above.

ANSWER: E

Primary somatic symptom disorders may be associated with a heightened awareness of normal bodily sensations. This heightened awareness may be paired with a cognitive bias to interpret any physical symptom as indicative of medical illness. Autonomic arousal may be high in some patients with somatization. Imaging studies support an association between one or more of the somatic symptom disorders with reduced volume of the brain amygdala and brain connectivity between the amygdala and brain regions controlling executive and motor function.

REFERENCE

van der Kruijs, S. J., Bodde, N. M., Vaessen, M. J., Lazeron, R. H., Vonck, K., Boon, P., Hofman, P. A., Backes, W. H., Aldenkamp, A. P., Jansen, J. F. (2012). Functional connectivity of dissociation in patients with psychogenic non-epileptic seizures. *Journal of Neurology, Neurosurgery and Psychiatry, 83*, 239–247.

6. A 45-year-old man is afraid of having a myocardial infarction since a 50-year-old coworker suffered a myocardial infarction at work 8 months ago. He thinks about having a myocardial infarction several times per day. He checks his blood pressure three times daily and asked his primary care doctor to check routine EKGs every 3 months. He has no symptoms of chest pain or dyspnea on exertion. He denies feeling anxious except for worry about his cardiovascular health. His lipids are normal; however, his low-density lipoprotein level was 5 points higher this year than last, and he was alarmed by this change. His body mass index is normal. There is no family history of coronary artery disease, myocardial infarction, or sudden death. With which diagnosis is this presentation MOST consistent?

A. Adjustment disorder
B. Panic disorder
C. Factitious disorder
D. Conversion disorder
E. Illness anxiety disorder

ANSWER: E

Hypochondriasis is no longer a diagnostic category in *DSM-5*. The patient's presentation is most consistent with illness anxiety disorder. As defined in *DSM-5*, illness anxiety disorder is a preoccupation with having or acquiring a serious illness. Somatic symptoms are *not present or, if present, are only mild in intensity*. If another medical condition is present or there is a high risk for developing a medical condition, the preoccupation is clearly excessive. There is a high level of anxiety about health, and the individual is easily alarmed about personal health status. The individual performs excessive health-related behaviors or exhibits maladaptive avoidance. Illness preoccupation has been present for at least 6 months, but the specific illness that is feared may change over that period.

REFERENCE

American Psychiatric Association. (2013). *Diagnostic and statistical manual of mental disorders* (5th ed.). Arlington, VA: American Psychiatric Publishing.

7. Which of the following is considered a GOOD prognostic factor for conversion disorder (functional neurological symptom disorder)?

A. Long duration of symptoms
B. Female gender
C. Presence of an identifiable stressor
D. Poor premorbid functioning
E. Older age

ANSWER: C

Good prognostic factors for conversion disorder include acute onset of symptoms, short duration of symptoms, healthy premorbid functioning, higher intelligence, absence of coexisting psychopathology, presence of an identifiable stressor, male gender, change in marital status (marriage or divorce), isolated sensory symptoms, very young age, and good premorbid medical health status.

REFERENCE

Allin, M., Streeruwitz, A., & Curtis, V. (2005). Progress in understanding conversion disorder. *Neuropsychiatric Disease and Treatment, 1*, 205–209.

8. Which of the following is considered a POOR prognostic symptom in conversion disorder (functional neurological symptom disorder)?

A. Psychogenic nonepileptic seizure
B. Psychogenic tremor
C. Comorbid medical illness
D. Pending litigation
E. All of the above

ANSWER: E

The following are poor prognostic symptoms in conversion disorder: pseudoseizure (psychogenic nonepileptic seizure), psychogenic tremor, subclinical (undiagnosed) personality pathology, concomitant medical illness, the presence of a stuffed animal brought to the hospital by the patient, poor perception of own well-being, motor symptoms, and pending litigation.

REFERENCE

Allin, M., Streeruwitz, A., & Curtis, V. (2005). Progress in understanding conversion disorder. *Neuropsychiatric Disease and Treatment, 1*, 205–209.

9. Which of the following interventions is recommended for patients with somatic symptom disorder?

A. Acknowledge the patient's symptoms.
B. Schedule regular visits for reassessment.
C. Limit diagnostic testing.
D. Evaluate for and treat diagnosable medical disease.
E. All of the above.

ANSWER: E

All of the above interventions are recommended approaches for treatment of patients with somatic symptom disorder.

REFERENCES

Barsky, A. J., & Borus, J. F. (1999). Functional somatic syndromes. *Annals of Internal Medicine, 130*, 910–921.
Bornschein, S., Forstl, H., & Zilker, T. (2001). Idiopathic environmental intolerances (formerly multiple chemical sensitivity) psychiatric perspectives. *Journal of Internal Medicine, 250*, 309–321.
Yutzy, S. H., & Parish, B. S. (2008). Somatoform disorders. In M. Galanter & H. D. Kleber (Eds.), *The American Psychiatric Publishing textbook of substance abuse treatment* (4th ed., p. 609). Washington, DC: American Psychiatric Publishing.

10. According to *DSM-5*, how many somatic symptoms (distressing or disruptive to daily life) are required for the diagnosis of somatic symptom disorder?

A. One
B. Two
C. Three
D. Four
E. Five

ANSWER: A

The key diagnostic *DSM-5* criteria for somatic symptom disorder include (A) one or more somatic symptoms; (B) excessive thoughts, feelings, or behaviors; and (C) symptom duration typically more than 6 months.

REFERENCE

American Psychiatric Association. (2013). *Diagnostic and statistical manual of mental disorders* (5th ed.). Arlington, VA: American Psychiatric Publishing.

11. A patient with poor adherence to antihypertensive treatment is hospitalized for hypertensive emergency. According to *DSM-5*, this behavior of poor adherence

that influences the course of the patient's medical condition is consistent with which disorder?

A. Illness anxiety disorder
B. Psychological factors affecting other medical conditions
C. Conversion disorder
D. Malingering
E. Factitious disorder

ANSWER: B

According to *DSM-5*, psychological factors affecting other medical conditions are seen when a medical symptom or condition is present and is characterized by psychological or behavioral factors that adversely affect the medical condition in one of the following ways: Factors have influenced the course of the medical condition as shown by a close temporal association between the psychological factors and the development or exacerbation of, or delayed recovery from, the medical condition; factors interfere with the treatment of the medical condition; factors constitute additional well-established health risks for the individual; and factors influence the underlying pathophysiology, precipitating or exacerbating symptoms or necessitating medical attention.

REFERENCE

American Psychiatric Association. (2013). *Diagnostic and statistical manual of mental disorders* (5th ed.). Arlington, VA: American Psychiatric Publishing.

12. Which of the following criteria differentiates malingering from factitious disorder, somatic symptom disorder, illness anxiety disorder, and conversion disorder?

A. The patient provides false information.
B. The patient seeks to be a patient and experience the sick role.
C. Malingering involves the presence of an external incentive.
D. Malingering involves dissociation.
E. None of the above

ANSWER: C

In malingering, there is an external incentive (e.g., avoiding work or obtaining money), whereas factitious disorder has no other incentive than to be a patient and experience the sick role. In malingering and factitious disorder, patients provide false information and behave deceptively, but in somatic symptom disorder, illness anxiety disorder, and conversion disorder, there is no evidence that patients are deceiving clinicians.

REFERENCE

American Psychiatric Association. (2013). *Diagnostic and statistical manual of mental disorders* (5th ed.). Arlington, VA: American Psychiatric Publishing.
Bass, C., & Halligan, P. (2014). Factitious disorders and malingering: Challenges for assessment and management. *Lancet, 383*, 1422–1432.

13. Pseudocyesis is a false belief of __(a)__ that is associated with objective signs and reported symptoms of ___(b)___.

A. a. being pregnant; b. pregnancy
B. a. having a blood disorder; b. leukemia
C. a. near-death experience; b. asystole
D. a. having cancer; b. colorectal cancer
E. a. having a sexually transmitted disease; b. gonorrhea

ANSWER: A

Pseudocyesis is a false belief of being pregnant that is associated with objective signs and reported symptoms of pregnancy. Interestingly, this condition tends to present with the stigmata of pregnancy including expanding abdominal girth *without umbilical eversion*. Polycystic ovarian syndrome should be ruled out in cases of pseudocyesis.

REFERENCE

American Psychiatric Association. (2013). *Diagnostic and statistical manual of mental disorders* (5th ed.). Arlington, VA: American Psychiatric Publishing.

14. A 16-year-old girl is admitted to the epilepsy service for video-EEG monitoring. She has a 2-minute period of unresponsiveness in which she rolls from side to side in the bed. Her eyes are closed during the episode. When the rolling subsides, she opens her eyes and is fully alert and oriented. EEG was largely obscured by muscle artifact. Her presentation is most consistent with which of the following?

A. Generalized tonic–clonic seizure
B. Complex partial seizure
C. Absence seizure
D. Conversion disorder
E. Factitious disorder

ANSWER: D

The patient's presentation is most consistent with psychogenic nonepileptic seizure of conversion disorder (functional neurological symptom disorder). Rolling from side to side is not consistent with a generalized tonic–clonic seizure, complex partial seizure, or absence seizure. There is no tonic period in her movements suggestive of a tonic–clonic seizure. Eyes are also typically open during a generalized tonic–clonic seizure. There is no postictal period in her presentation. Conversion disorder involves neurological symptoms specifically. Factitious disorder is conscious falsification of physical or psychological signs or symptoms to assume the sick role.

REFERENCES

Cragar, D. E., Berry, D. T., Fakhoury, T. A., Cibula, J. E., Schmitt, F. A. (2002). A review of diagnostic techniques in the differential diagnosis of epileptic and nonepileptic seizures. *Neuropsychology Review, 12*, 31–64.
Gulick, T. A., Spinks, I. P., & King, D. W. (1982). Pseudoseizures: Ictal phenomena. *Neurology, 32*, 24.
Gumnit, R. J., & Gates J. R. (1986). Psychogenic seizures. *Epilepsia, 27*(suppl. 2), S124.

15. Which of the following psychiatric diagnoses is NOT associated with conversion disorder?

A. Major depressive disorder
B. Panic disorder
C. Generalized anxiety disorder
D. Substance use disorder
E. Borderline personality disorder

ANSWER: D

There is no significant association of substance use disorder with conversion disorder. Evidence suggests the other diagnoses are significantly associated with conversion disorder.

REFERENCE

Fiszman, A., & Kanner, A. M. (2010). Comorbidities in psychogenic nonepileptic seizures: Depressive, anxiety, and personality disorders. In S. Schacter & W. C. LaFranceJr. (Eds.), *Gates and Rowan's nonepileptic seizures* (3rd ed., p. 225). Cambridge, UK: Cambridge University Press.
Stone, J., Sharpe, M., & Binzer, M. (2004). Motor conversion symptoms and pseudoseizures: A comparison of clinical characteristics. *Psychosomatics, 45*, 492–499.

16. What term refers to the sensation of a foreign body or lump in the throat that is not explained better by a structural lesion, gastroesophageal reflux disease, mucosal abnormality, or esophageal motility disorder?

A. Dysphagia
B. Globus
C. Pseudocyesis
D. Jackhammer esophagus
E. Postcricoid web

ANSWER: B

The term *globus* refers to the sensation of a foreign body or lump in the throat that is not explained better by a structural lesion, gastroesophageal reflux disease, mucosal abnormality, or esophageal motility disorder.

REFERENCE

Aziz, Q., Fass, R., Gyawali, C. P., Miwa, H., Pandolfino, J.E., Zerbib, F. (2016). Functional esophageal disorders. *Gastroenterology*. Feb. epub ahead of print.

17. A 24-year-old woman presents to the emergency room with visual complaints for 4 days. She reports "being blind." She does not appear to be in any distress concerning her symptoms. There is no evidence of blindness on ophthalmologic exam. MRI of the brain is normal. Upon review of the patient's chart, the resident notices that she has been seen by other physicians for myalgia, irritable bowel symptoms, and periodic lower extremity numbness. Further inquiries about her psychiatric history reveal a history of depression and sexual abuse as a child, which the patient reports she has never revealed to anyone else for fear of being stigmatized. Given the history and clinical presentation, which of the following is the MOST likely diagnosis for this individual?

A. Pain disorder
B. Factitious disorder
C. Illness anxiety disorder
D. Conversion disorder
E. Somatic symptom disorder

ANSWER: D

Conversion disorder (functional neurological symptom disorder) presents with signs and symptoms affecting motor and sensory functioning that cannot be explained by a neurological or medical condition. Conversion disorder occurs as a result of stress or emotional crisis. There is an association with comorbid psychiatric conditions, including anxiety, depression, and dissociative disorders. Women are more likely to be diagnosed than men at a 2:1 to 10:1 ratio. Although there may be no organic diagnosis, the symptoms appear real to the patient and can be very distressing.

REFERENCE

Ali, S., Jabeen, S., Pate, R. J., Shahid, M., Chinala, S., Nathani, M., & Shah, R. (2015). Conversion disorder- mind versus body: A review. *Innovations in Clinical Neuroscience*, *12*(5–6), 27–33.

18. Which of the following statements is TRUE regarding factitious disorder?

A. The disorder is more common in males than in females.
B. The most common comorbid psychiatric disorders are anxiety disorders.
C. Patients with the disorder disproportionately work in the healthcare field.
D. Patients typically begin to present at around 40 years of age.
E. Patients with this disorder present with clear secondary gain.

ANSWER: C

This patient is likely presenting with factitious disorder, a disorder that involves the fabrication of physical or psychological symptoms in order to be eligible for admission and undergo medical procedures with no obvious gain. These patients typically wish to assume the "sick role" despite the expenses and difficulties associated with such a role. Studies have reported that approximately half of patients who present with this disorder have an occupation related to healthcare or laboratory work.

REFERENCE

Yates, G. P., & Feldman, M. D. (2016). Factitious disorder: A systematic review of 455 cases in the professional literature. *General Hospital Psychiatry*, *41*, 20–28.

19. Which of the following statements is TRUE regarding somatic symptom disorder?

A. Treatment must always involve pharmacotherapy.
B. Good prognosis is associated with high socioeconomic status and response to treatment of depression and anxiety symptoms.
C. Childhood-onset symptoms usually persist into adulthood.
D. Patients with this disorder must have false beliefs that last at least for 1 year.
E. The presence or absence of ***la belle indifference*** is a reliable feature to differentiate from other disorders.

ANSWER: B

The above presentation suggests that the patient has somatic symptom disorder. This disorder is characterized by 6 months or more of general and nondelusional preoccupation with bodily symptoms that are misinterpreted by the patient as signs of a severe illness. Typically this preoccupation causes enough distress to impair daily functioning. Patients typically have poor insight concerning this disorder. However, patients with a high socioeconomic status and those who respond to treatment of depression and anxiety typically have a good prognosis throughout the course of the disorder.

REFERENCE

Sadock, B. J., & Sadock, V. A. (2014). *Kaplan and Sadock's synopsis of psychiatry: Behavioral sciences/clinical psychiatry* (11th ed.). Philadelphia, PA: Lippincott Williams and Wilkins.

20. A 54-year-old "frequent flyer" with illness anxiety disorder presents to the emergency room with shortness of breath and tachycardia. She has presented to the emergency room 17 times in 6 months with a variety of somatic symptoms, the workup for all of which has been negative. History is notable only for a recent transatlantic flight. What is the next step?

A. Reassure the patient and discharge.
B. Refer to outpatient psychiatry.
C. Order psychiatry consult in emergency room.
D. Admit to inpatient telemetry unit.
E. Proceed with medical workup in emergency room.

ANSWER: E

The patient has symptoms and recent history concerning for pulmonary embolus. Although she has a history of illness anxiety disorder, her medical complaints should be taken seriously and worked up in the emergency room before any referrals are made (although she would benefit from long-term psychiatric services). It would be premature to admit her to any inpatient services before the emergency room workup is completed.

REFERENCE

Wick, J. Y., & Zanni, G. R. (2008). Hypochondria: The worried well. *Consultant Pharmacist*, *23*, 192–194.

QUESTIONS AND ANSWERS

This chapter has accompanying questions and answers which are available to subscribers as part of the Oxford eLearning platform. To access the questions, follow the link below, or go to http://oxford-elearning.oup.com/books.

http://oxford-elearning.oup.com/books/test/67/10.1093/med/9780190265557.003.0020

21.

DISSOCIATIVE DISORDERS

David Matuskey

1. Dissociative identity disorder has been updated to broaden cross-cultural relevance in *DSM*-5 by including which of the following?

A. Speaking in tongues
B. Pathological possession
C. Herbal products
D. Normative spiritual and religious practices

ANSWER: B

The *DSM-5* includes pathological possession. It is a disorder of identity alteration that occurs during an altered state of consciousness. It is attributed to possession by an external spirit, power, deity, or other person.

REFERENCE:

Spiegel, D., et al. (2013). Dissociative disorders in *DSM-5*. *Annual Review of Clinical Psychology, 9*, 299–326. doi:10.1146/annurev-clinpsy-050212-185531. Epub 2013 Feb 1.

2. Which of the following is considered a "positive" dissociative symptom?

A. Derealization
B. Amnesia
C. Aphonia
D. Paralysis

ANSWER: A

Dissociative symptoms can affect all psychological functions and are usually divided into positive and negative symptoms. Positive symptoms include intrusions into awareness and behavior, with accompanying deficits in continuity of subjective experience (e.g., identity fragmentation, depersonalization, derealization). Negative symptoms are the inability to access information or to control mental functions (e.g., amnesia, aphonia, paralysis).

REFERENCE

Spiegel, D., et al. (2013). Dissociative disorders in *DSM-5*. *Annual Review of Clinical Psychology, 9*, 299–326. doi:10.1146/annurev-clinpsy-050212-185531. Epub 2013 Feb 1.

3. Which one of the following diagnoses has a dissociative subtype in *DSM-5*?

A. Major depressive disorder
B. Schizophrenia
C. Post-traumatic stress disorder (PTSD)
D. Obsessive–compulsive disorder (OCD)

ANSWER: C

PTSD has a dissociative subtype, which includes depersonalization and/or derealization.

REFERENCE

American Psychiatric Association. (2013). Trauma- and stressor-related disorders. In *Diagnostic and statistical manual of mental disorders* (5th ed.). t. e. Arlington, VA: American Psychiatric Publishing.

4. Dissociative amnesia is usually differentiated from other amnesias by:

A. An older age at onset of symptoms
B. Lack of precipitating stressors
C. Autobiographical–episodic anterograde amnesia
D. Autobiographical–episodic retrograde amnesia

ANSWER: D

Autobiographical–episodic retrograde amnesia is common in dissociative amnesia and not in neuropsychiatric causes of amnesia (without other deficits). Dissociative amnesia is also characterized by early onset and relationship to stressors. It is less common to have anterograde amnesia.

REFERENCE

Staniloiu, S., & Markowitsch, H. J. (2014). Dissociative amnesia. *Lancet Psychiatry 1*, 226–241.

5. Which of the following neuroimaging modalities generally has NOT found differences in patients with dissociative amnesia relative to controls?

A. Structural MRI
B. Functional MRI
C. PET
D. SPECT

ANSWER: A

Structural MRI does not have clinically significant differences in these patients. Functional MRI, PET, and SPECT have demonstrated metabolic and blood flow differences in memory processing areas.

REFERENCE

Staniloiu, S., & Markowitsch, H. J. (2014). Dissociative amnesia. *Lancet Psychiatry 1*, 226–241.

6. Which one of these is MOST common in the general population?

A. Dissociative identity symptoms
B. Dissociative amnesia symptoms
C. Depersonalization and derealization symptoms
D. Unspecified dissociative symptoms

ANSWER: C

A detached and unreal sense of oneself (depersonalization) or the outside world (derealization) is common, with approximately half of all adults experiencing at least one lifetime transient episode. However, symptomatology that meets full criteria for a disorder of depersonalization and derealization is much less common (approximately 2%).

REFERENCE

American Psychiatric Association. (2013). Dissociative disorders. In *Diagnostic and statistical manual of mental disorders* (5th ed.). Retrieved from http://dsm.psychiatryonline.org/doi/abs/10.1176/appi.books.9780890425596.dsm08

7. Dissociative identity disorder is LEAST associated with which of the following?

A. Increased interpersonal maltreatment
B. Overwhelming early-life events
C. Self-mutilation
D. Low levels of hypnotic capacity

ANSWER: D

Individuals with dissociative identity disorder often have multiple types of interpersonal maltreatment, including overwhelming early-life events such as medical illness. Self-mutilation and suicidal behavior are also common. These individuals usually have greater hypnotic capacity and dissociativity, not lower.

REFERENCE

American Psychiatric Association. (2013). Dissociative disorders. In *Diagnostic and statistical manual of mental disorders* (5th ed.). Retrieved from http://dsm.psychiatryonline.org/doi/abs/10.1176/appi.books.9780890425596.dsm08

8. The type of amnesia MOST common in dissociative amnesia is:

A. Localized amnesia
B. Selective amnesia
C. Generalized amnesia
D. Systematized amnesia

ANSWER: A

The most common form of dissociative amnesia is localized amnesia, a failure to recall events during a specific period of time. Selective amnesia is when the individual can recall some, but not all, of the events during a period of time. Generalized amnesia is a complete loss of memory for one's life history. Systematized amnesia is a loss of a specific category of information.

REFERENCE

American Psychiatric Association. (2013). Dissociative disorders. In *Diagnostic and statistical manual of mental disorders* (5th ed.). Retrieved from http://dsm.psychiatryonline.org/doi/abs/10.1176/appi.books.9780890425596.dsm08

9. Dissociative trance would be categorized in which dissociative disorder?

A. Dissociative amnesia
B. Depersonalization/derealization disorder
C. Other specified dissociative disorder
D. Unspecified dissociative disorder

ANSWER: C

Dissociative trance is characterized by a narrowing or complete loss of awareness of immediate surroundings. This may be accompanied by transient paralysis, loss of consciousness, or stereotyped behaviors of which the individual is unaware and/or feels cannot be controlled. Dissociative trance may be seen as a cultural or religious practice. Other specified dissociative disorder applies to symptoms characteristic of a dissociative disorder that cause clinically significant impairment or problems in social, occupational, or other important areas of functioning but do not meet criteria for any established dissociative disorders.

REFERENCE

American Psychiatric Association. (2013). Dissociative disorders. In *Diagnostic and statistical manual of mental disorders* (5th ed.). Retrieved from http://dsm.psychiatryonline.org/doi/abs/10.1176/appi.books.9780890425596.dsm08

10. Individuals with dissociative identity disorder are LEAST likely to have which comorbidity?

A. Schizophrenia
B. PTSD
C. Conversion disorder
D. Personality disorders
E. Depression

ANSWER: A

Dissociative identity disorder is not associated with schizophrenia but rather with PTSD, depression, personality disorders (especially avoidant and borderline personality disorders), conversion disorder (functional neurological symptom disorder), somatic symptom disorder, eating disorders, substance-related disorders, obsessive–compulsive disorder, and sleep disorders.

REFERENCE

American Psychiatric Association. (2013). Dissociative disorders. In *Diagnostic and statistical manual of mental disorders* (5th ed.). Retrieved from http://dsm.psychiatryonline.org/doi/abs/10.1176/appi.books.9780890425596.dsm08

QUESTIONS AND ANSWERS

This chapter has accompanying questions and answers which are available to subscribers as part of the Oxford eLearning platform. To access the questions, follow the link below, or go to http://oxford-elearning.oup.com/books.

http://oxford-elearning.oup.com/books/test/67/10.1093/med/9780190265557.003.0021

22.

SEXUAL DISORDERS AND GENDER DYSPHORIA

Adefolake Akinsanya

1. Tightening and lifting of the scrotal sac, elevation of the testes, and a 50% increase in the size of the testes during sexual experience is a characteristic of which one of the sexual phases?

A. Desire
B. Excitement
C. Orgasm
D. Resolution
E. Pre-orgasm

ANSWER: B

The excitement phase in males is characterized by tightening and lifting of the scrotal sac, elevation of the testes, and a 50% increase in the size of the testes during sexual experience. There is no change to the scrotum and testes in the orgasmic phase, and they tend to go back to baseline size due to loss of vasocongestion in the resolution phase.

REFERENCE

Sadock, B. J., Sadock, V. A., & Ruiz, P. (2014). Human sexuality and sexual dysfunction. In *Kaplan and Sadock's synopsis of psychiatry* (11th ed., pp. 568–569). Philadelphia, PA: Wolters Kluwer.

2. Experiencing 3 to 15 involuntary contractions of the lower third of the vagina and accompanying strong sustained contractions of the uterus in females during a sexual encounter is a characteristic of what phase?

A. Desire
B. Excitement
C. Orgasm
D. Resolution
E. Pre-orgasm

ANSWER 2: C.

The orgasmic phase in females is characterized by experiencing 3 to 15 involuntary contractions of the lower third of the vagina and accompanying strong sustained contractions of the uterus.

REFERENCE

Sadock, B. J., Sadock, V. A., & Ruiz, P. (2014). Human sexuality and sexual dysfunction. In *Kaplan and Sadock's synopsis of psychiatry* (11th ed., pp. 568–569). Philadelphia, PA: Wolters Kluwer.

3. A 35-year-old female who has been married for 10 years reports pain during sexual intercourse with her husband. She also reports experiencing this same pain last week during a pelvic examination performed by her gynecologist. She describes the pain as feeling as though her vaginal muscles were "cramping." She is concerned because on several occasions this has interfered with sexual intercourse. Which of the following BEST describes the patient's symptoms?

A. Dyspareunia
B. Hypoactive sexual desire
C. Vaginismus
D. Sexual aversion disorder
E. Orgasmic disorder

ANSWER 3: C.

Vaginismus is defined as a painful spasm in the outer third of the vagina that makes intercourse or pelvic examination difficult.

REFERENCE

Sadock, B. J., Sadock, V. A., & Ruiz, P. (2014). Human sexuality and sexual dysfunction. In *Kaplan and Sadock's synopsis of psychiatry* (11th ed., pp. 568–569). Philadelphia, PA: Wolters Kluwer.

4. Which of the following is a sign of sexual addiction?

A. Need for increasing amounts of sexual activity
B. Repeated attempts to limit sexual behavior
C. Persistent high-risk sexual behavior
D. Sexual fantasy as a coping mechanism
E. All of the above

ANSWER 4: E.

All of the above are signs of sexual addiction or compulsive sexual behavior.

REFERENCE

Sadock, B. J., Sadock, V. A., & Ruiz, P. (2009). Normal human sexuality and sexual and gender identity disorders. In *Kaplan and Sadock's comprehensive textbook of psychiatry* (9th ed., p. 2052). Philadelphia, PA: Wolters Kluwer Health/Lippincott Williams and Wilkins.

5. A 26-year-old male is taking fluoxetine for depression. He reports improvement in his mood but also some difficulty during sexual intercourse. Which of the following sexual disorders is the patient MOST likely experiencing?

A. Premature ejaculation
B. Inability to maintain an erection
C. Prolonged erection
D. Delayed orgasm
E. Dyspareunia

ANSWER: D

Fluoxetine and other SSRIs are more likely to be associated with delayed or absent orgasm. As a result, SSRIs are not uncommonly used to treat premature ejaculation.

REFERENCE

Sadock, B. J., Sadock, V. A., & Ruiz, P. (2014). Human sexuality and sexual dysfunction. In *Kaplan and Sadock's synopsis of psychiatry* (11th ed., pp. 568–569). Philadelphia, PA: Wolters Kluwer.

6. Which of the following is the MOST common self-reported sexual dysfunction in women?

A. Sexual desire disorder
B. Sexual arousal disorder
C. Anorgasmia
D. Dyspareunia
E. Vaginismus

ANSWER: A

Sexual desire disorder is the most common self-reported sexual problem in women. Other common self-reported sexual problems include difficulty reaching orgasm and/or maintaining excitement.

REFERENCE

Andreasen, N. C., & Black, D. W. (2011). Sexual dysfunction, paraphilias, and gender identity disorder. In *Introductory textbook of psychiatry* (5th ed., pp. 322–323). Washington, DC: American Psychiatry Publishing.

7. Which of the following is the MOST common self-reported sexual dysfunction in men?

A. Premature ejaculation
B. Difficulty initiating an erection
C. Difficulty maintaining an erection
D. Delayed ejaculation
E. Lack of sexual interest

ANSWER: A

The most common self-reported sexual problem among men is premature ejaculation.

REFERENCE

Andreasen, N. C., & Black, D. W. (2011). Sexual dysfunction, paraphilias, and gender identity disorder. In *Introductory textbook of psychiatry* (5th ed., p. 308). Washington, DC: American Psychiatry Publishing.

8. A 65-year-old happily married postmenopausal female reports difficulty with her sexual life. She states, "Sex is not what it used to be," despite her desire to have sex. Which of the following is she MOST likely to be experiencing?

A. Dyspareunia
B. Anorgasmia
C. Vaginal dryness
D. Sexual arousal disorder
E. Sexual aversion disorder

ANSWER: C

Vaginal dryness due to lack of estrogen after menopause is the most common reason for reduced sexual pleasure in postmenopausal women.

REFERENCE

Sadock, B. J., Sadock, V. A., & Ruiz, P. (2014). Human sexuality and sexual dysfunction. In *Kaplan and Sadock's synopsis of psychiatry* (11th ed., pp. 568–569). Philadelphia, PA: Wolters Kluwer.

9. A 53-year-old man who smokes two packs of cigarettes a day and has a history of untreated hypertension and poorly-controlled diabetes mellitus type 2 reports difficulty maintaining an erection during sexual intercourse with his wife. Which of the following is MOST likely associated with his sexual problem?

A. Untreated hypertension
B. Poorly controlled diabetes
C. Cigarette smoking
D. Sexual arousal disorder
E. Sexual aversion disorder

ANSWER: B

Poorly controlled diabetes affects vascular supply to the penis, with subsequent erectile dysfunction. Although medications used to treat hypertension are associated with erectile dysfunction, untreated hypertension is not associated with erectile dysfunction. Smoking is less likely to cause erectile dysfunction than is untreated diabetes.

REFERENCE

Sadock, B. J., Sadock, V. A., & Ruiz, P. (2014). Human sexuality and sexual dysfunction. In *Kaplan and Sadock's synopsis of psychiatry* (11th ed., pp. 568–569). Philadelphia, PA: Wolters Kluwer.

10. Which of the following is TRUE about sildenafil?

A. Sildenafil is effective in all cases of erectile dysfunction.
B. Sildenafil takes effect about 1 hour after ingestion and can last for up to 4 hours.
C. The mechanism of action of sildenafil includes decreasing the concentration of cGMP.
D. Sildenafil is not contraindicated in persons taking organic nitrates.
E. Common side effects do not include headache and flushing.

ANSWER: B

Sildenafil takes effect within 1 hour and may last for up to 4 hours. It works by increasing the concentration of cGMP, causing vasodilation. Vasodilation of the penis facilitates erection. Use of sildenafil is contraindicated in patients taking organic nitrates because concomitant use of the two drugs can lead to a large, sudden, and sometimes fatal drop in blood pressure. This medication is not effective in all cases of erectile dysfunction. It is ineffective in the absence of sexual stimulation. The most common side effects are headaches, flushing, and dyspepsia.

REFERENCE

Sadock, B. J., Sadock, V. A., & Ruiz, P. (2014). Human sexuality and sexual dysfunction. In *Kaplan and Sadock's synopsis of psychiatry* (11th ed., pp. 568–569). Philadelphia, PA: Wolters Kluwer.

11. A 45-year-old man reports that he is sexually aroused only when his partner humiliates him or beats him to the point of bruising or bleeding. What kind of paraphilia is MOST consistent with this description?

A. Sexual sadism
B. Voyeurism
C. Sexual masochism
D. Fetishism
E. Necrophilia

ANSWER: C

Persons with sexual masochism have a recurrent preoccupation with sexual urges and fantasies involving the act of being personally humiliated, beaten, bound, or otherwise made to suffer. Sexual sadism involves recurrent, intense, sexually arousing fantasies, urges, or behaviors in which the physical suffering of the victim is sexually exciting to the perpetrator. It is often related to rape.

REFERENCE

Sadock, B. J., Sadock, V. A., & Ruiz, P. (2014). Human sexuality and sexual dysfunction. In *Kaplan and Sadock's synopsis of psychiatry* (11th ed., pp. 568–569). Philadelphia, PA: Wolters Kluwer.

12. A 22-year-old man reports that for several years he has been achieving orgasm by rubbing his penis against unaware, fully dressed women on crowded buses. He states that he finds this behavior sexually satisfying and that he has never had an intimate sexual relationship. What kind of paraphilia is MOST consistent with this description?

A. Voyeurism
B. Fetishism
C. Necrophilia
D. Frotteurism
E. Sexual sadism

ANSWER: D

Frotteurism is observed only in men and is characterized by touching or rubbing a nonconsenting person. It often occurs in crowded places. Voyeurism is characterized by secretly watching other people undressing or engaging in sexual activity.

REFERENCE

Sadock, B. J., Sadock, V. A., & Ruiz, P. (2014). Human sexuality and sexual dysfunction. In *Kaplan and Sadock's synopsis of psychiatry* (11th ed., pp. 568–569). Philadelphia, PA: Wolters Kluwer.

13. A 37-year-old male states that for the past 8 months he has had sexual urges and fantasies to dress in female clothing to achieve sexual arousal. He denies being sexually attracted to men and describes his sexual orientation as heterosexual. What kind of paraphilia is MOST consistent with this description?

A. Partialism
B. Transvestism
C. Exhibitionism
D. Voyeurism
E. Frotteurism

ANSWER: B

Transvestism is described in a heterosexual male as fantasies and sexual urges to dress in opposite-gender clothing as a means of arousal.

REFERENCE

Sadock, B. J., Sadock, V. A., & Ruiz, P. (2014). Human sexuality and sexual dysfunction. In *Kaplan and Sadock's synopsis of psychiatry* (11th ed., pp. 568–569). Philadelphia, PA: Wolters Kluwer.

14. Which of the following is defined as the sense of self as being male or female?

A. Gender role
B. Gender identity
C. Sexual identity
D. Sexual orientation
E. Sexual behavior

ANSWER: B

Sexual identity is defined as the pattern of a person's biological sexual characteristics: chromosomes, external genitalia, internal genitalia, hormonal composition, gonads, and secondary sexual characteristics. Gender identity is defined as the sense of self as being male or female. It may or may not agree with physiological sex or gender role. Gender role is the expression of one's gender in society. Sexual orientation is the persisting sexual preference for people of the same sex (homosexual) or people of the opposite sex (heterosexual).

REFERENCE

Sadock, B. J., Sadock, V. A., & Ruiz, P. (2014). Human sexuality and sexual dysfunction. In *Kaplan and Sadock's synopsis of psychiatry* (11th ed., pp. 568–569). Philadelphia, PA: Wolters Kluwer.

15. Which of the following is defined as the pattern of a person's biological sexual characteristics: chromosomes, external genitalia, internal genitalia, hormonal composition, gonads, and secondary sexual characteristics?

A. Gender role
B. Gender identity
C. Sexual identity
D. Sexual orientation
E. Sexual behavior

ANSWER: C

Sexual identity is defined as the pattern of a person's biological sexual characteristics: chromosomes, external genitalia, internal genitalia, hormonal composition, gonads, and secondary sexual characteristics. Gender identity is defined as the sense of self as being male or female. It may or may not agree with physiological sex or gender role. Gender role is the expression of one's gender in society. Sexual orientation is the persisting sexual preference for people of the same sex (homosexual) or people of the opposite sex (heterosexual).

REFERENCE

Sadock, B. J., Sadock, V. A., & Ruiz, P. (2014). Human sexuality and sexual dysfunction. In *Kaplan and Sadock's synopsis of psychiatry* (11th ed., pp. 568–569). Philadelphia, PA: Wolters Kluwer.

16. Which of the following is defined as the expression of one's gender identity in society?

A. Gender role
B. Gender identity
C. Sexual identity
D. Sexual orientation
E. Sexual behavior

ANSWER: A

Gender role is the expression of one's gender in society. Gender identity is defined as the sense of self as being male or female. Sexual identity is defined as the pattern of a person's biological sexual characteristics: chromosomes, external genitalia, internal genitalia, hormonal composition, gonads, and secondary sexual characteristics. It may or may not agree with physiological sex or gender role. Sexual orientation is the persisting sexual preference for people of the same sex (homosexual) or people of the opposite sex (heterosexual).

REFERENCE

Sadock, B. J., Sadock, V. A., & Ruiz, P. (2014). Human sexuality and sexual dysfunction. In *Kaplan and Sadock's synopsis of psychiatry* (11th ed., pp. 568–569). Philadelphia, PA: Wolters Kluwer.

17. Which of the following is defined as the persisting and unchanging preference for people of the same sex (homosexual) or people of the opposite sex (heterosexual)?

A. Gender role
B. Gender identity
C. Sexual identity
D. Sexual orientation
E. Sexual behavior

ANSWER: D

Sexual orientation is the persisting sexual preference for people of the same sex (homosexual) or people of the opposite sex (heterosexual). Gender role is the expression of one's gender in society. Gender identity is defined as the sense of self as being male or female. It may or may not agree with physiological sex or gender role.

Sexual identity is defined as the pattern of a person's biological sexual characteristics: chromosomes, external genitalia, internal genitalia, hormonal composition, gonads, and secondary sexual characteristics.

REFERENCE

Sadock, B. J., Sadock, V. A., & Ruiz, P. (2014). Human sexuality and sexual dysfunction. In *Kaplan and Sadock's synopsis of psychiatry* (11th ed., pp. 568–569). Philadelphia, PA: Wolters Kluwer.

18. Which of the following is TRUE about gender dysphoria?

A. Parents typically report that cross-gender behaviors appear after 3 years of age.
B. Children with gender dysphoria have similar rates of depressive, anxiety, and impulse control disorders as the general population.
C. The most effective therapy is education of parents about acceptance and provision of a supportive environment for the child.
D. Gender dysphoria is about four to five times more common in females than in males.
E. Hormonal and surgical interventions have no effect on depression or quality of life.

ANSWER: B

The term gender dysphoria refers to a marked incongruence between an individual's experienced or expressed gender and the gender assigned at birth. It was previously known as gender identity disorder. Most gender-dysphoric behaviors will become apparent by the age of 3 years, which correlates with the period when children begin to develop a sense of their gender identity. The overall prevalence of male-to-female dysphoria is higher than that of female-to-male, with a sex ratio of four to five gender-assigned boys for each girl. Co-morbid conditions including depression, anxiety, and impulse control disorder are seen in children with gender dysphoria but are not more common than in the general population. Co-morbid mental illness in adults includes substance abuse, self-injurious behavior, suicidality, and completed suicides. The lifetime rate of suicidal thoughts in this population is thought to be about 40%. Effective treatments in children and adolescents include individual, family, and group therapy. Reparative and conversion therapy is not indicated according to practice guidelines of the American Psychiatric Association and the American Academy of Child and Adolescent Psychiatry. Ultimately, hormonal and surgical interventions such as reconstructive surgeries in adulthood might help improve quality of life and reduce depression in these groups of patients.

REFERENCE

Sadock, B. J., Sadock, V. A., & Ruiz, P. (2014). Gender dysphoria. In *Kaplan and Sadock's synopsis of psychiatry* (11th ed., pp. 600–604). Philadelphia, PA: Wolters Kluwer.

19. An 18-year-old female has not reached menarche. Physical exam reveals normal female appearance, Tanner stage 5 breasts, and normal female external genitalia with labial masses. Chromosomal analysis reveals XY karyotype. What is the most likely diagnosis?

A. Turner syndrome
B. Pseudohermaphroditism
C. Androgen insensitivity syndrome
D. Kleinfelter syndrome
E. Adrenogenital syndrome

ANSWER: C

Androgen insensitivity syndrome was formerly called testicular feminization syndrome. Individuals with this syndrome have an XY karyotype, but the tissues are unable to use the testosterone or androgens. The patient appears as a normal female at birth. Sexual characteristics at puberty are usually those of a female. External genitalia appear female with possible labial masses suggestive of cryptorchid testes. Patients typically present to a physician not having reached menarche well into adolescence.

BIBLIOGRAPHY

Sadock, B. J., Sadock, V. A., & Ruiz, P. (2014). Human sexuality and sexual dysfunction. In *Kaplan and Sadock's synopsis of psychiatry* (11th ed., pp. 568–569). Philadelphia, PA: Wolters Kluwer.

20. Patients with gender dysphoria frequently present with traits of which of the following personality disorders?

A. Dependent personality disorder
B. Borderline personality disorder
C. Histrionic personality disorder
D. Schizotypal personality disorder
E. Avoidant personality disorder

ANSWER: B

Depression, substance abuse, and personality disorders are frequently observed among individuals with gender identity disorder. Traits of borderline personality disorder are more commonly seen in these individuals than traits of other personality disorders.

REFERENCE

Andreasen, N. C., & Black, D. W. (2011). Sexual dysfunction, paraphilias, and gender identity disorder. In *Introductory textbook of psychiatry* (5th ed., pp. 322–323). Washington, DC: American Psychiatry Publishing.

QUESTIONS AND ANSWERS

This chapter has accompanying questions and answers which are available to subscribers as part of the Oxford eLearning platform. To access the questions, follow the link below, or go to http://oxford-elearning.oup.com/books.

http://oxford-elearning.oup.com/books/test/67/10.1093/med/9780190265557.003.0022

23.

EATING DISORDERS

Harvinder Singh

1. Which of the following factors is protective against anorexia nervosa?

A. Female sex
B. Infant feeding problems
C. Higher maternal BMI
D. Maternal depression
E. History of undereating

ANSWER: C

Anorexia nervosa is independently predicted by female sex, infant feeding problems, maternal depressive symptoms, and a history of undereating. High self-esteem and higher maternal BMI are protective.

REFERENCE

Nicholls, D. E., & Viner, R. M. (2009). Childhood risk factors for lifetime anorexia nervosa by age 30 years in a national birth cohort. *Journal of the American Academy of Child and Adolescent Psychiatry, 48*, 791–799.

2. A 23-year-old female is involuntarily committed to an inpatient medicine–psychiatry unit for diagnosis of anorexia nervosa, binge eating/purging type. She reports using laxatives frequently to prevent weight gain. With which of the following electrolyte abnormalities is she most likely to present?

A. Hyponatremic–hypochloremic metabolic acidosis
B. Hyponatremic–hyperchloremic metabolic acidosis
C. Hyponatremic–hypochloremic metabolic alkalosis
D. Hyponatremic–hyperchloremic metabolic alkalosis

ANSWER: B

Laxative abuse in anorexia nervosa is associated with hyponatremic–hyperchloremic metabolic acidosis.

REFERENCE

Rosen, D. S., & American Academy of Pediatrics Committee on Adolescence. (2010). Identification and management of eating disorders in children and adolescents. *Pediatrics, 126*, 1240–1253.

3. A 20-year-old female is involuntarily committed to an inpatient medicine–psychiatry unit for diagnosis of anorexia nervosa, binge eating/purging type. She reports inducing vomiting frequently to prevent weight gain. With which of the following electrolyte abnormalities is she most likely to present?

A. Hypokalemic–hypochloremic metabolic acidosis
B. Hypokalemic–hyperchloremic metabolic acidosis
C. Hypokalemic–hypochloremic metabolic alkalosis
D. Hypokalemic–hyperchloremic metabolic alkalosis

ANSWER: C

Anorexia nervosa with frequent self-induced vomiting is associated with hypokalemic-hypochloremic metabolic alkalosis.

REFERENCE

Rosen, D. S., & American Academy of Pediatrics Committee on Adolescence. (2010). Identification and management of eating disorders in children and adolescents. *Pediatrics*, *126*, 1240–1253.

4. Which of the following medications is approved by the FDA for treatment of anorexia nervosa?

A. Fluoxetine
B. Mirtazapine
C. Olanzapine
D. All of the above
E. None of the above

ANSWER: E

There are no FDA-approved medications for anorexia nervosa. Psychopharmacological treatment in anorexia nervosa is generally unhelpful, although fluoxetine may stabilize recovery in patients who have already attained 85% of their expected weight.

REFERENCE

Flament, M. F., Bissada, H., & Spettigue, W. (2012). Evidence-based pharmacotherapy of eating disorders. Int J Neuropsychopharmacol. Mar;15(2):189–207.
Hay, P. J., & Claudino, A. M. (2012). Clinical psychopharmacology of eating disorders: A research update. *International Journal of Neuropsychopharmacology, Mar;15(2):209-22.*

5. Which of the following criteria does NOT apply to a patient with a diagnosis of avoidant/restrictive food intake disorder?

A. The presence of eating disturbance with persistent failure to meet appropriate nutritional needs.
B. This diagnosis is not better explained by lack of available food.
C. This diagnosis is related to the way body weight or shape is experienced by the patient.
D. This diagnosis is not attributable to a concurrent medical condition.

ANSWER: C

Avoidant/restrictive food intake disorder involves an eating/feeding disturbance that is not due to unavailability of food, observation of cultural norms, anorexia nervosa, bulimia nervosa, or a medical condition. Evidence of a disturbance in experience of body shape or weight *excludes* this diagnosis.

REFERENCE

American Psychiatric Association. (2013). *Diagnostic and statistical manual of mental disorders* (5th ed.). Arlington, VA: American Psychiatric Publishing.

6. Which of the following is a risk factor for pica?

A. Family disorganization
B. Pregnancy
C. Epilepsy
D. Intellectual disability
E. All of the above

ANSWER: E

Pica is defined as the persistent ingestion of nonnutritive substances for at least 1 month at an age for which this behavior is developmentally inappropriate. Pica risk factors include parent–child psychopathology, family disorganization, environmental deprivation, pregnancy, epilepsy, brain damage, intellectual disability, and presence of a neurodevelopmental disorder.

REFERENCE

American Psychiatric Association. (2013). *Diagnostic and statistical manual of mental disorders* (5th ed.). Arlington, VA: American Psychiatric Publishing.

7. Which of the following criteria warrants inpatient admission for a patient with anorexia nervosa?

A. Temperature 36.7°C
B. Pulse 60 beats per minute
C. Body weight 85% of expected weight
D. Orthostatic differential of 20 beats per minute

ANSWER: C

Indications for admission for anorexia nervosa in particular include continued weight loss or inability to gain weight despite optimized outpatient care, significant edema, physiological decompensation (including but not limited to life-threatening hyponatremia, hyper- or hypokalemia, cardiac arrhythmia, delirium, or orthostatic differential greater than 30 bpm), temperature less than 36°C, pulse greater than 45 bpm, psychosis, or any other symptoms refractory to outpatient treatment.

REFERENCE

Rio, A., Whelan, K., Goff, L., Reidlinger, D. P., & Smeeton, N. (2013). Occurrence of refeeding syndrome in adults started on artificial nutrition support: Prospective cohort study. *BMJ Open*, *3*(1):e002173.

8. Which of the following medications is approved by the FDA for treatment of bulimia nervosa?

A. Fluoxetine
B. Mirtazapine
C. Olanzapine
D. Bupropion

ANSWER: A

Fluoxetine is FDA approved for treatment of bulimia nervosa. It should be dosed initially 20 mg daily with titration over 1 to 2 weeks to 60 mg daily as tolerated. Some patients may need to begin at a lower dose if side effects are intolerable. A maximum dose of 80 mg daily may be used in some cases.

REFERENCE

Rosen, D. S., & American Academy of Pediatrics Committee on Adolescence. (2010). Identification and management of eating disorders in children and adolescents. *Pediatrics*, *126*, 1240–1253.

9. A patient with a recent diagnosis of anorexia nervosa binge eating/purging type is admitted for medical evaluation. Her weight is below 75% of her expected weight. Which of the following studies should be considered?

A. Serum amylase
B. Serum electrolytes
C. Complete blood count
D. EKG
E. All of the above

ANSWER: E

Recommended medical evaluation of a patient with anorexia nervosa includes complete blood count, urinalysis, and metabolic panel, including phosphorus, TSH, and fasting glucose. Additional considerations based on clinical warrant include serum amylase (for suspected surreptitious vomiting), serum calcium and magnesium with EKG (when the patient is at less than 75% of ideal body weight before starting neuroleptics in particular), dual-energy X-ray absorptiometry (DEXA) scan (when underweight for more than 6 months), and MRI versus head CT plus neuropsychological testing for patients with atypical features (such as hallucinations, delusions, delirium, or persistent cognitive impairment despite weight restoration).

REFERENCE

Yager, J. & Andersen, C. (2005). Clinical practice: Anorexia nervosa. *New England Journal of Medicine*, *353*, 1481–1488.

10. Which of the following treatment approaches has the strongest level of evidence for management of bulimia nervosa?

A. Atypical antipsychotics
B. Tricyclic Antidepressants
C. Benzodiazepines
D. Dialectical–behavioral therapy (DBT)
E. Cognitive–behavioral therapy (CBT)

ANSWER: E

The evidence base for use of CBT as first-line treatment of bulimia nervosa is strong. Although CBT has good acceptability, binge remission rates (cessation of binge eating or purging) at the end of treatments are only 30% to 40%. The listed antidepressants do not have strong evidence supporting their use in bulimia nervosa. Fluoxetine is the main psychotropic medication approved for use in bulimia nervosa by the FDA. There is less evidence of efficacy for other antidepressants.

REFERENCE

Treasure, J., Claudino, A. M., & Zucker, N. (2010). Eating disorders. *Lancet*, *375*, 583–593.

QUESTIONS AND ANSWERS

This chapter has accompanying questions and answers which are available to subscribers as part of the Oxford eLearning platform. To access the questions, follow the link below, or go to http://oxford-elearning.oup.com/books.

http://oxford-elearning.oup.com/books/test/67/10.1093/med/9780190265557.003.0023

24.

IMPULSE CONTROL DISORDERS

Isabella Michna

1. Which of the following statements is TRUE regarding oppositional defiant disorder (ODD)?

A. Severity is indicated by number of settings in which the behavior occurs.
B. The behavior may occur only toward siblings.
C. The diagnosis may not be given to those under 5 years of age.
D. Behaviors are assessed irrespective of the child's gender.
E. The behavior must occur on a daily basis.

ANSWER: A

Mild ODD involves symptoms in one setting. Moderate ODD involves symptoms in at least two settings. Severe ODD involves symptoms in three or more settings. Symptoms must involve at least one other individual who is not a sibling. Children under 5 years of age may qualify for the diagnosis as long as the behavior occurs most days for a period of at least 6 months. For children older than 5 years, the behavior must occur at least once per week for at least 6 months. Behaviors are understood in the context of what is normative for developmental level, gender, and culture.

REFERENCE

American Psychiatric Association. (2013). *Diagnostic and statistical model of mental disorders* (5th ed.). Arlington, VA: American Psychiatric Publishing.

2. Two of the most common co-occurring conditions with oppositional defiant disorder (ODD) are:

A. Attention deficit hyperactivity disorder (ADHD) and conduct disorder
B. Bipolar disorder and intermittent explosive disorder
C. Intellectual disability and social anxiety disorder
D. Language disorder and autism spectrum disorder
E. Borderline personality disorder and intellectual disability

ANSWER: A

ADHD and conduct disorder are the most common co-occurring conditions with ODD.

REFERENCE

Boylan, K., Vaillancourt, T., Boyle, M., & Szatmari, P. (2007). Comorbidity of internalizing disorders in children with oppositional defiant disorder. *European Child and Adolescent Psychiatry, 16*, 484–494.

3. Which of the following is NOT a symptom for the diagnosis of oppositional defiant disorder (ODD) in *DSM-5*?

A. Vindictiveness
B. Angry and irritable mood
C. Argumentative and defiant behavior
D. Truancy

ANSWER: D

The three classes of symptoms outlined in the *DSM-5* criteria for ODD include vindictiveness, angry/irritable mood, and argumentative/defiant behavior.

REFERENCE

American Psychiatric Association. (2013). *Diagnostic and statistical model of mental disorders* (5th ed.). Arlington, VA: American Psychiatric Publishing.

4. The core feature of what disorder exhibits failure to control impulsive and aggressive behavior in response to subjectively experienced provocation that would not typically result in an aggressive outburst?

A. Oppositional defiant disorder
B. Intermittent explosive disorder
C. Conduct disorder
D. Intellectual disability
E. Antisocial personality disorder

ANSWER: B

Although patients with all of the above disorders can demonstrate impulsive or aggressive behaviors, by definition intermittent explosive disorder involves failure to control impulsive and aggressive behavior in response to subjectively experienced provocation that would not typically result in an aggressive outburst.

REFERENCE

American Psychiatric Association. (2013). *Diagnostic and statistical model of mental disorders* (5th ed.). Arlington, VA: American Psychiatric Publishing.

5. A 21-year-old man with a history of oppositional defiant disorder (ODD) presents with impulsive behavioral outbursts two or three times per week that are grossly out of proportion to the stressor. Examples he gives of his behavior include that he punched a hole in the wall of his office and threw a laptop out the window. He also physically threatened a neighbor who was playing loud music but was stopped by a friend before he hit him. He reports that he is unable to control himself and is worried that he may lose his job if this behavior continues. What is his most likely diagnosis?

A. Bipolar disorder
B. ADHD
C. Intermittent explosive disorder
D. Conduct disorder
E. Phencyclidine abuse

ANSWER: C

The patient's presentation is consistent with intermittent explosive disorder, which is characterized by impulsive behavioral outbursts that are out of proportion to the stressor and occur at least twice weekly for 3 months or more. Behavioral outbursts may include damage or destruction of property or physical assault. Outbursts are not premeditated and cause distress or impairment in occupational or interpersonal functioning.

REFERENCE

American Psychiatric Association. (2013). *Diagnostic and statistical model of mental disorders* (5th ed.). Arlington, VA: American Psychiatric Publishing.

6. Childhood-onset obsessive–compulsive disorder (OCD) has a high rate of comorbidity with:

A. Tourette's disorder and ADHD
B. Conduct disorder and intermittent explosive disorder
C. Antisocial personality disorder and ODD
D. Generalized anxiety disorder
E. Disruptive mood dysregulation disorder

ANSWER: A

Childhood-onset OCD is associated with Tourette's disorder and ADHD.

REFERENCE

Matthews, C. A., & Grados, M. A. (2011). Familiality of Tourette syndrome, obsessive–compulsive disorder, and attention-deficit/hyperactivity disorder: Heritability analysis in a large sib-pair sample. *Journal of the American Academy of Child and Adolescent Psychiatry, 50*, 46–54.

7. According to *DSM-5* criteria, four categories of behavior are seen in conduct disorder. Which of the following is NOT one of those categories?

A. Aggression toward people and animals
B. Destruction of property
C. Hyperactivity
D. Deceitfulness or theft
E. Serious violations of rules

ANSWER: C

DSM-5 includes four categories of behavior in conduct disorder: aggression toward people and animals, destruction of property, deceitfulness or theft and serious violation of rules. Hyperactivity is not included in the diagnostic criteria.

REFERENCE

American Psychiatric Association. (2013). *Diagnostic and statistical model of mental disorders* (5th ed.). Arlington, VA: American Psychiatric Publishing.

8. Intermittent explosive disorder exhibits comorbidity with all of the following EXCEPT:

A. Anxiety disorders
B. Psychotic disorders
C. Mood disorders
D. Substance use disorders

ANSWER: B

There is established comorbidity among intermittent explosive disorder and mood, anxiety and substance use disorders.

REFERENCE

Kessler, R. C., Hwang, I., LaBrie, R., Petukhova, M., Sampson, N. A., Winters, K. C. & Shaffer, H. J.. (2006). The prevalence and correlates of *DSM-IV* intermittent explosive disorder in the national comorbidity survey replication. *Archives of General Psychiatry, 63*, 669–678.

9. A 19-year-old woman has been arrested several times for shoplifting. She states she cannot resist the impulse to take things from a store, even though she has enough money to pay for them. Many of the items she takes she has no use for at home, such as men's cologne. She feels an inner sense of relief when she brings the items out of the store. There is no history of aggressive behavior toward others, substance use, or arrests for other reasons. What is the likely diagnosis?

A. Kleptomania
B. Pyromania
C. Conduct disorder
D. Antisocial personality disorder
E. Bipolar disorder type 1

ANSWER: A

Kleptomania involves the impulse to steal objects that may be unneeded and are not obtained for monetary value or out of vengeance or anger. This woman does not meet criteria for antisocial personality disorder or conduct disorder because her behavior appears to be limited to shoplifting. There is no evidence of mood disorder or mania. Pyromania involves purposeful fire setting.

REFERENCE

American Psychiatric Association. (2013). *Diagnostic and statistical model of mental disorders* (5th ed.). Arlington, VA: American Psychiatric Publishing.

10. *DSM-5* outlines "with limited prosocial emotions" as a specifier of conduct disorder. Which of the following characteristics supportive of this diagnosis involves disregard for and lack of concern about the feelings of others?

A. Unconcerned about performance
B. Callousness, lack of empathy
C. Lack of remorse or guilt
D. Shallow or deficient affect

ANSWER: B

Patients who demonstrate callous behavior and lack of empathy show disregard for and lack of concern about the feelings of others. Patients who are unconcerned about performance typically do not worry about problematic performance at school, work, or other activities and do not put forth effort to do well. Patients who show a lack of remorse or guilt do not feel bad when they do something wrong and show a general lack of concern about negative consequences of actions. Patients with shallow or deficient affect do not express feelings or show emotions to others, except in ways that seem shallow, insincere, or superficial.

REFERENCE

American Psychiatric Association. (2013). *Diagnostic and statistical model of mental disorders* (5th ed.). Arlington, VA: American Psychiatric Publishing.

QUESTIONS AND ANSWERS

This chapter has accompanying questions and answers which are available to subscribers as part of the Oxford eLearning platform. To access the questions, follow the link below, or go to http://oxford-elearning.oup.com/books.

http://oxford-elearning.oup.com/books/test/67/10.1093/med/9780190265557.003.0024

25.

ADJUSTMENT DISORDERS

Anil Bachu

1. Which of the following is TRUE about adjustment disorders?

A. They are diagnosed twice as often in women than in men.
B. In children and adolescents, boys are diagnosed as frequently as girls.
C. They are one of the most common psychiatric diagnoses in medically hospitalized patients.
D. Single women are affected more frequently than married women.
E. All of the above.

ANSWER: E

The prevalence of the disorder is from 2% to 8% of the general population. Women are diagnosed with the disorder twice as often as men. Single women are overrepresented in this patient population. In children and adolescents, boys and girls are equally diagnosed. Adjustment disorders are one of the most common psychiatric diagnoses in hospitalized patients for medical and surgical problems. The percentage of individuals in outpatient mental health treatment with a principal diagnosis of an adjustment disorder ranges between 5% and 20%. In a hospital psychiatric consultation setting, adjustment disorder is one of the most common diagnoses, with a prevalence rate of almost 50%.

REFERENCE

American Psychiatric Association. (2013). *Diagnostic and statistical manual of mental disorders* (5th ed., pp. 286–289). Arlington, VA: American Psychiatric Publishing.

Sadock, B. J., & Sadock, V A. (2015). *Kaplan and Sadock's synopsis of psychiatry* (11th ed., pp. 446–450). Philadelphia, PA: Lippincott Williams and Wilkins.

2. A 24-year-old student from Bogotá, Colombia, starts college in the United States. After 1 month, the student's adviser is concerned that she may be depressed. Although the student speaks English well, she does not know anyone in town. Her family is in Bogotá, and she does not anticipate seeing them soon. She has not made many friends. She is not able to concentrate in her classes and is easily irritated. She denies poor sleep, poor appetite, loss of interest in hobbies, feelings of guilt, decreased energy, or suicidal ideation. Which of the following is the MOST likely diagnosis?

A. Major depressive disorder
B. Adjustment disorder
C. Dysthymia
D. Schizotypal personality disorder
E. Schizoid personality disorder

ANSWER: B

According to *DSM-5*, adjustment disorder is the development of emotional or behavioral symptoms in response to an identifiable stressor or stressors occurring within 3 months of the onset of the stressor. It is characterized by marked distress that is out of proportion to the severity or intensity of the stressor, taking into account the external context and the cultural factors that might influence symptom severity and presentation. It is associated with significant impairment in social, occupational, or other important areas of functioning.

REFERENCE

Sadock, B. J., & Sadock, V A. (2015). *Kaplan and Sadock's synopsis of psychiatry* (11th ed., pp. 446–450). Philadelphia, PA: Lippincott Williams and Wilkins.

3. Which of the following is NOT a classification of adjustment disorder in *DSM-5*?

A. With psychotic features
B. With depressed mood
C. With disturbance of conduct
D. With mixed disturbance of emotions and conduct

ANSWER: B

Adjustment disorder with psychotic features is not a category in the *DSM-5*.

REFERENCE

American Psychiatric Association. (2013). *Diagnostic and statistical manual of mental disorders* (5th ed., pp. 286–289). Arlington, VA: American Psychiatric Publishing.

4. A 51-year-old man undergoes a total hip replacement. The surgery was uneventful, and the patient will be discharged to a rehabilitation facility for physical therapy. Nursing staff report that the patient is more anxious and fearful than he was prior to the surgery. The patient acknowledges having trouble sleeping and states he is fearful about leaving the hospital. The mental status exam is otherwise unremarkable. This individual's presentation is MOST consistent with which of the following diagnoses?

A. Generalized anxiety disorder
B. Adjustment disorder with anxiety
C. Acute stress disorder
D. Dependent personality disorder
E. Major depressive disorder

ANSWER: B

Unlike generalized anxiety disorder, adjustment disorder with anxiety requires the presence of a stressor.

REFERENCE

American Psychiatric Association. (2013). *Diagnostic and statistical manual of mental disorders* (5th ed., pp. 286–289). Arlington, VA: American Psychiatric Publishing.

5. A 21-year-old woman returns home from college for her summer break. She appears sad and withdrawn. She does not show any interest in activities with her family, which she used to enjoy. She reports difficulty concentrating at her summer job. Her sleep, appetite, and energy are normal, and she denies suicidal thoughts. She reports a recent stressor, namely, breaking up with her boyfriend 1 week before the end of the semester. What is the MOST likely diagnosis?

A. Major depressive disorder
B. Generalized anxiety disorder
C. Dysthymia
D. Adjustment disorder with depressed mood
E. Adjustment disorder with anxious mood

ANSWER: D

The patient's presentation is most consistent with adjustment disorder with depressed mood. Adjustment disorder is the development of emotional or behavioral symptoms in response to an identifiable stressor that occurs within 3 months of the onset of the stressor and lasts no longer than 6 months after the stressor or its consequences have ceased.

REFERENCE

American Psychiatric Association. (2013). *Diagnostic and statistical manual of mental disorders* (5th ed., pp. 286–289). Arlington, VA: American Psychiatric Publishing.

6. Which of the following would be considered an appropriate first step in the management of adjustment disorder?

A. Cognitive behavioral therapy
B. Group therapy
C. SSRIs
D. Watch and wait
E. Any of the above

ANSWER: E

There is no one specific treatment modality that is considered to be most effective in the management of adjustment disorder. The treatment must be tailored to the patient's history and presenting symptoms. Hence any of the above would be considered an appropriate first step in the management of adjustment disorder.

REFERENCE

Sadock, B. J., Sadock, V. A., & Ruiz, P. (2009). Adjustment disorders. In *Kaplan and Sadock's comprehensive textbook of psychiatry* (9th ed., p. 2194). Philadelphia, PA: Wolters Kluwer Health/Lippincott Williams and Wilkins.

7. Which of the following is an example of behavior that would be observed in adjustment disorder with disturbance of conduct?

A. Reckless driving
B. Vandalism
C. Truancy
D. Aggression
E. All of the above

ANSWER: E

All of these are examples of behaviors seen in adjustment disorder with disturbance of conduct.

REFERENCE

Sadock, B. J., & Sadock, V A. (2015). *Kaplan and Sadock's synopsis of psychiatry* (11th ed., pp. 446–450). Philadelphia, PA: Lippincott Williams and Wilkins.

8. Which of the following disorders has the level of impairment and intensity of symptoms comparable to that of adjustment disorder with depressed mood?

A. Bipolar I disorder
B. Anxiety disorder
C. Major depressive disorder
D. Bipolar II disorder
E. Dysthymic disorder

ANSWER: E

The level of impairment and intensity of symptoms in adjustment disorder with depressed mood are similar to that of dysthymic disorder. Adjustment disorder has minimal intensity of symptoms when compared with major depressive disorder and bipolar disorder.

REFERENCE

Sadock, B. J., & Sadock, V A. (2015). *Kaplan and Sadock's synopsis of psychiatry* (11th ed., pp. 446–450). Philadelphia, PA: Lippincott Williams and Wilkins.

9. Which of the following statements about the psychodynamic origins of adjustment disorder is TRUE?

A. Early childhood trauma may predispose to adjustment disorder later in life.
B. Children who identify with their mother more than their father are at higher risk of developing adjustment disorder.
C. Psychological predisposition to adjustment disorder is independent of the stage of the life cycle.
D. Prior to development of the superego, every child has equal vulnerability to stress.
E. Early childhood trauma increases resilience in adulthood.

ANSWER: A

Children who suffer more early-life trauma tend to develop less mature defense mechanisms. In later life these individuals may have greater difficulty coping with stressors, thus predisposing to adjustment disorder.

REFERENCE

Sadock, B. J., & Sadock, V A. (2015). *Kaplan and Sadock's synopsis of psychiatry* (11th ed., pp. 446–450). Philadelphia, PA: Lippincott Williams and Wilkins.

10. Which of the following stressors could cause adjustment disorder?

A. Single-event stressor
B. Recurrent stressor
C. Continuous stressor
D. Natural disasters
E. All of the above

ANSWER: E

In adjustment disorders, the stressor can be of any type or severity.

REFERENCE

American Psychiatric Association. (2013). *Diagnostic and statistical manual of mental disorders* (5th ed., pp. 286–289). Arlington, VA: American Psychiatric Publishing.

QUESTIONS AND ANSWERS

This chapter has accompanying questions and answers which are available to subscribers as part of the Oxford eLearning platform. To access the questions, follow the link below, or go to http://oxford-elearning.oup.com/books.

http://oxford-elearning.oup.com/books/test/67/10.1093/med/9780190265557.003.0025

26.

PERSONALITY DISORDERS

Waqar Rizvi

1. Which of the following is a mature defense mechanism?

A. Suppression
B. Denial
C. Projection
D. Splitting
E. Projective identification

ANSWER: A

Suppression is a mature defense mechanism that involves the conscious postponement of attention to a conscious impulse of conflict. Other mature defenses include altruism, sublimation, and humor. The other choices above are immature defense mechanisms.

REFERENCE

(2009). *Kaplan and Sadock's comprehensive textbook of psychiatry* (9th ed., pp. 2199–2201). Philadelphia, PA: Lippincott Williams and Wilkins.

2. Which of the following defense mechanisms is characterized by the attribution of one's unrecognized feelings to others?

A. Suppression
B. Denial
C. Projection
D. Splitting
E. Projective identification

ANSWER: C

Projection is characterized by attributing one's unrecognized feelings to others. Individuals externalize their own emotions, impulses, and thoughts that they find to be unacceptable onto others. This defense is common in psychotic disorders and cluster A personality disorders.

REFERENCE

(2003). *Kaplan and Sadock's comprehensive synopsis of psychiatry* (9th ed., p. 802). Philadelphia, PA: Lippincott Williams and Wilkins.

3. Which of the following personality disorders is more prevalent among patients with somatization disorder (*DSM-IV-TR*; somatic symptom disorder in *DSM-5*) than in the general population?

A. Avoidant
B. Borderline
C. Obsessive–compulsive
D. Paranoid
E. All of the above

ANSWER: E

Somatization disorder is commonly co-morbid with many other diagnoses, including major depression, generalized anxiety disorder, psychotic disorders, and personality disorders, including avoidant, paranoid, borderline, and obsessive–compulsive personality disorders.

REFERENCE

(2007). *Kaplan and Sadock's synopsis of psychiatry* (10th ed., pp. 637, 794–802). Philadelphia, PA: Lippincott Williams and Wilkins.

4. Which of the following comorbidities indicates a poorer prognosis in a patient with factitious disorder?

A. Generalized anxiety disorder
B. Antisocial personality disorder
C. Bipolar disorder
D. Major depressive disorder
E. Marijuana abuse disorder

ANSWER: B

In factitious disorder, a co-morbid mood, anxiety, or substance abuse disorder usually indicates a better prognosis. However, co-morbid personality disorders, such as antisocial personality disorder, usually indicate a poorer prognosis.

REFERENCE

(2009). *Kaplan and Sadock's comprehensive textbook of psychiatry* (9th ed., pp. 1957–1959, 2220–2222). Philadelphia, PA: Lippincott Williams and Wilkins.

5. Which of the following personality disorders is most commonly co-morbid with factitious disorder?

A. Paranoid
B. Narcissistic
C. Histrionic
D. Schizotypal
E. Obsessive–compulsive

ANSWER: C

Factitious disorder is often co-morbid with histrionic, borderline, and antisocial personality disorders. The other disorders listed above are not as likely to be co-morbid in patients with factitious disorder.

REFERENCE

(2009). *Kaplan and Sadock's comprehensive textbook of psychiatry* (9th ed., pp. 1957–1961, 2220–2224). Philadelphia, PA: Lippincott Williams and Wilkins.

6. All of the following personality disorders predispose patients to dissociative fugue EXCEPT:

A. Obsessive–compulsive
B. Schizoid
C. Borderline
D. Histrionic

ANSWER: A

Patients with personality disorders, including schizoid, borderline, and histrionic personality disorders, are predisposed to dissociative fugue. Those with obsessive–compulsive personality disorder, however, are not predisposed to dissociative fugue.

REFERENCE

(2007). *Kaplan and Sadock's synopsis of psychiatry* (10th ed., pp. 805–807). Philadelphia, PA: Lippincott Williams and Wilkins.

7. According to the American Psychiatric Association's guidelines for treating patients with borderline personality disorder, which of the following is recommended in the psychotherapeutic treatment process?

A. Therapy is limited to 12 sessions.
B. The therapist must avoid conflict.
C. Roles and responsibilities of the therapist should not be discussed openly.
D. Flexibility is needed because stressful situations occur through the therapeutic process.
E. The therapist should be a passive listener.

ANSWER: D

According to the American Psychiatric Association's guidelines for treating patients with borderline personality disorder, it is recommended that the therapist be flexible because this can encourage rapport with the patient, build trust, and promote adherence with psychotherapy. The other choices are not consistent with the guidelines.

REFERENCE

American Psychiatric Association, Practice Guideline for treating patients with Borderline Personality Disorder; APA guidelines 2015.

8. Which of the following traits is NOT consistent with narcissistic personality disorder?

A. A pervasive pattern of grandiose fantasies or behaviors
B. Interpersonal exploitation of other individuals
C. A need for admiration
D. Oddities or eccentricities in behaviors and communication with others
E. A sense of entitlement

ANSWER: D

Oddities or eccentricities in behaviors and communication with others are characteristic of schizotypal personality disorder. Narcissistic personality disorder is characterized by a pervasive pattern of grandiosity, lack of empathy, need for admiration, sense of entitlement, and the interpersonal exploitation of the rights of others.

REFERENCE

American Psychiatric Association. (2013). *Diagnostic and statistical manual of mental disorders* (5th ed., pp. 669–672). Arlington, VA: American Psychiatric Publishing.

9. Which of the following defense mechanisms is most often associated with individuals with paranoid personality disorder?

A. Projection
B. Splitting
C. Suppression
D. Humor
E. Intellectualization

ANSWER: A

Projection is the defense mechanism most often associated with individuals with paranoid personality disorder. In this defense mechanism, individuals externalize onto others their own emotions, impulses, and thoughts that they find to be unacceptable.

REFERENCE

(2009). *Kaplan and Sadock's comprehensive textbook of psychiatry* (9th ed., pp. 2199–2201). Philadelphia, PA: Lippincott Williams and Wilkins.

10. Which of the following personality disorders is diagnosed more frequently in men than in women?

A. Borderline
B. Dependent
C. Histrionic
D. Antisocial

ANSWER: D

Although antisocial personality disorder can be seen and diagnosed in women, it is much more often seen in and diagnosed in men. The other choices can also be seen and diagnosed in men but are more frequently seen and diagnosed in women.

REFERENCE

(2007). *Kaplan and Sadock's synopsis of psychiatry* (10th ed., pp. 798–799). Philadelphia, PA: Lippincott Williams and Wilkins.

11. According to Otto Kernberg, the borderline level of personality organization involves which of the following?

A. Concrete boundaries between the self and others
B. A lack of anxiety tolerance
C. Consistent sense of self
D. Ego integrity
E. Ideas of reference

ANSWER: B

According to Otto Kernberg, the borderline level of personality organization is characterized by partially blurred boundaries between the self and others, ego weakness (often exemplified by a lack of anxiety tolerance), alternating perceptions of the self and others as either all good or all bad, and primitive defense mechanisms such as projection.

REFERENCE

(2007). *Kaplan and Sadock's synopsis of psychiatry* (10th ed., pp. 799–801). Philadelphia, PA: Lippincott Williams and Wilkins.

12. Which personality disorder is characterized by social inhibition, feelings of inadequacy, and hypersensitivity to negative evaluation?

A. Avoidant
B. Obsessive–compulsive

C. Dependent
D. Schizoid
E. Schizotypal

ANSWER: A

Avoidant personality disorder is characterized by these traits.

REFERENCE

American Psychiatric Association. (2013). *Diagnostic and statistical manual of mental disorders* (5th ed., pp. 672–675). Arlington, VA: American Psychiatric Publishing.

13. Conduct disorder diagnosed prior to age 15 most often evolves into which of the following personality disorders if not appropriately treated?

A. Antisocial
B. Borderline
C. Histrionic
D. Narcissistic
E. Schizoid

ANSWER: A

Conduct disorder most often manifests into antisocial personality disorder when not appropriately treated. These individuals may also have co-morbid narcissistic or other personality disorders, but antisocial personality disorder is most common.

REFERENCE

(2007). *Lewis' child and adolescent psychiatry* (4th ed., pp. 455–460, 474). Philadelphia, PA: Lippincott Williams and Wilkins.

14. Which of the following personality disorders has the strongest association with suicide attempts?

A. Antisocial
B. Borderline
C. Schizotypal
D. Dependent
E. Obsessive–compulsive

ANSWER: B

Borderline personality disorder has the strongest association with suicide attempts.

REFERENCE

(2007). *Kaplan and Sadock's synopsis of psychiatry* (10th ed., pp. 799–801). Philadelphia, PA: Lippincott Williams and Wilkins.

15. Which of the following is recommended for a patient with borderline personality disorder and parasuicidal behaviors?

A. Supportive psychotherapy
B. Interpersonal psychotherapy
C. Psychodynamic psychotherapy
D. Dialectical behavioral therapy
E. Exposure therapy

ANSWER: D

Dialectical behavioral therapy is a form of cognitive behavioral therapy developed by Marsha Linehan, PhD, which has been found to be effective for patients with borderline personality disorder and parasuicidal behaviors.

REFERENCE

(2009). *Kaplan and Sadock's comprehensive textbook of psychiatry* (9th ed., pp. 2222–2223, 2891–2893). Philadelphia, PA: Lippincott Williams and Wilkins.

16. Fragile X syndrome is most often co-morbid with which of the following personality disorders?

A. Antisocial
B. Borderline
C. Schizotypal
D. Dependent
E. Avoidant

ANSWER: C

Fragile X syndrome is co-morbid with a number of psychiatric illnesses, including autism, anxiety disorders, attention deficit hyperactivity disorder, and schizotypal personality disorder.

REFERENCE

(2007). *Kaplan and Sadock's synopsis of psychiatry* (10th ed., pp. 795–797, 1142). Philadelphia, PA: Lippincott Williams and Wilkins.

17. Most personality disorders follow which pattern of evolution as people age into late adulthood?

A. Improving
B. Worsening
C. Enduring
D. Waxing and waning
E. Remitting

ANSWER: C

Studies have shown that, overall, personality disorders tend to be enduring throughout the lives of individuals, well into late adulthood.

REFERENCE

(2007). *Kaplan and Sadock's synopsis of psychiatry* (10th ed., p. 791). Philadelphia, PA: Lippincott Williams and Wilkins.

18. Of the following defense mechanisms, which one is considered the healthiest?

A. Rationalization
B. Sublimation
C. Intellectualization
D. Reaction formation
E. Fantasy

ANSWER: B

Sublimation, suppression, humor, and altruism are mature defense mechanisms.

REFERENCE

(2009). *Kaplan and Sadock's comprehensive textbook of psychiatry* (9th ed., pp. 2199–2201). Philadelphia, PA: Lippincott Williams and Wilkins.

19. Which of the following dimensions assessed on the Temperament and Character Inventory (TCI) is most likely to increase with age?

A. Novelty seeking
B. Harm avoidance
C. Reward dependence
D. Persistence
E. Cooperativeness

ANSWER: E

Among the choices listed, only cooperativeness increases with age in individuals with personality disorders.

REFERENCE

(2009). *Kaplan and Sadock's comprehensive textbook of psychiatry* (9th ed., pp. 2197–2199). Philadelphia, PA: Lippincott Williams and Wilkins.

20. Which of the following personality disorders is most commonly associated with a family history of schizophrenia?

A. Antisocial
B. Borderline
C. Paranoid
D. Schizoid
E. Schizotypal

ANSWER: E

Of all choices listed, the greatest correlation exists between a family history of schizophrenia and schizotypal personality disorder.

REFERENCE

(2007). *Kaplan and Sadock's synopsis of psychiatry* (10th ed., pp. 796–797). Philadelphia, PA: Lippincott Williams and Wilkins.

QUESTIONS AND ANSWERS

This chapter has accompanying questions and answers which are available to subscribers as part of the Oxford eLearning platform. To access the questions, follow the link below, or go to http://oxford-elearning.oup.com/books.

http://oxford-elearning.oup.com/books/test/67/10.1093/med/9780190265557.003.0026

27.

DIAGNOSTIC PROCEDURES

Anil Bachu

1. As part of a comprehensive evaluation, which of the following laboratory tests is MOST appropriate before initiation of treatment with acamprosate?

A. Serum electrolytes
B. Serum albumin
C. Blood urea nitrogen
D. Creatinine clearance
E. Liver function tests

ANSWER: D

Acamprosate is exclusively cleared by the kidneys. Dose adjustment of acamprosate is essential among patients with renal impairment.

REFERENCE

Sadock, B. J., & Sadock V. A. (2009). *Kaplan and Sadock's comprehensive textbook of psychiatry* (9th ed., pp. 3102–3104). Philadelphia, PA: Lippincott Williams and Wilkins.

2. Which of the following blood tests is/are NOT required prior to lithium initiation?

A. TSH
B. Hepatic panel
C. Renal function tests
D. Electrolytes
E. CBC

ANSWER: B

Lithium is renally excreted and may cause renal concentrating defects due to buildup in the cells lining collecting ducts. Because hyponatremia may result in elevated lithium levels, electrolyte levels should be checked prior to treatment with lithium. Lithium may also cause hypothyroidism and leukocytosis and hence TSH and CBC should also be checked prior to treatment with lithium. A hepatic panel should be checked prior to initiation of treatment of medications metabolized in the liver, such as valproic acid.

REFERENCES

Ng, F., Mammen, O. K., Wilting, I., Sachs, G. S., Ferrier, I. N., Cassidy, F., ... & Berk, M. (2009). The International Society for Bipolar Disorder (ISBD) consensus guidelines for the safety monitoring of bipolar disorder treatments. *Bipolar Disorder, 11*(6). doi:10.1111/j 1399 -5618.2009.00737

Sadock, B. J., & Sadock, V. A. (2003). Laboratory tests in psychiatry. In Kaplan & *Sadock's synopsis of psychiatry.* (9th ed., p. 267). Philadelphia, PA: Lippincott Williams and Wilkins.

3. Among patients with narcolepsy, which of the following neuropeptides is DECREASED in the CSF?

A. Melatonin
B. Somatostatin
C. Hypocretin
D. Oxytocin
E. Neurotensin

ANSWER: C

Patients with narcolepsy have low CSF concentrations of hypocretin, a peptide produced in the hypothalamus.

REFERENCE

Dauvilliers, Y., Arnulf, I., & Mignot, E. (2007). Narcolepsy with cataplexy. *Lancet, 369,* 499–511

4. What are the long-term monitoring parameters for patients with bipolar disorder who are treated with valproic acid?

A. Monitor CBC, weight, and liver function test every 3 months for the first year and then annually.
B. Monitor CBC for absolute neutrophil count every 3 months.
C. Monitor TSH, serum calcium, and serum electrolytes every 6 months.
D. Monitor EKG every 3 months.
E. Monitor serum triglycerides and fasting glucose every year.

ANSWER: A

The long-term monitoring parameters for patients taking valproic acid include valproic acid level (during initial therapy and then as clinically indicated), weight, CBC, and liver function tests (every 3 months for the first year and then annually).

REFERENCE

Ng, F., Mammen, O. K., Wilting, I., Sachs, G S., Ferrier, I. N., Cassidy, F., ... & Berk, M. (2009). The International Society for Bipolar Disorder (ISBD) consensus guidelines for the safety monitoring of bipolar disorder treatments. *Bipolar Disorder, 11*(6). doi:10.1111/j 1399-5618.2009.00737

5. Which of the following measures of polysomnography refers to the duration of time from turning off the lights until the onset of Stage 2 (more recently, N2) sleep?

A. Sleep efficiency
B. Sleep latency
C. REM latency
D. Sleep-onset REM period
E. Apnea index

ANSWER: B

Sleep latency refers to the duration of time from turning off the lights until the onset of Stage 2 (or N2) sleep. Sleep efficiency refers to the total sleep time divided by the total time of the sleep record times 100. REM latency is the duration of time from onset of sleep until first REM period. The sleep-onset REM period is the onset of REM sleep within the first 10 minutes of sleep. Apnea index is the number of apneas longer than 10 seconds per hour.

REFERENCE

Sadock, B. J., & Sadock, V. A. (2009). Normal sleep and sleep disorders. In *Kaplan and Sadock's synopsis of psychiatry* (9th ed., p. 2150). Philadelphia, PA: Lippincott Williams and Wilkins. 2150

6. Which of the following medications is MOST likely to cause hyponatremia?

A. Depakote
B. Lithium
C. Lamotrigine
D. Oxcarbazepine
E. Olanzapine

ANSWER: D

Oxcarbazepine may cause hyponatremia, a condition that may lead to delirium, seizures, or coma. Too-rapid correction of hyponatremia can cause osmotic demyelination syndrome (historically central pontine demyelinolysis).

REFERENCE

Van Amelsvoort, T., Bakshi, R., Devaux, C. B., & Schwabe, S. (2006). Hyponatremia associated with carbamazepine and oxcarbazepine therapy: A review. *Epilepsia, 35*. Advance online publication. doi:10.1111/j.1528-1157.1994.tb02930.x

7. At what point in clozapine treatment may the frequency of absolute neutrophil count (ANC) monitoring be reduced to every 4 weeks?

A. 3 months
B. 6 months
C. 12 months
D. 18 months
E. 24 months

ANSWER: C

Obtain at least two baseline ANC levels before initiating clozapine treatment. Patients may transition to less frequent ANC monitoring based on the number of weeks of continuous clozapine therapy and the patient's ANC values. Weekly

ANC monitoring is required for all patients during the first 6 months of treatment. If the ANC remains in the normal range for the first 6 months of therapy (for the general population, ANC greater than or equal to 1,500/μl), monitoring frequency can be reduced to every 2 weeks. If the patient's ANC remains in the normal range for the second 6 months of treatment, ANC monitoring may be reduced to once every 4 weeks.

REFERENCE

Clozapine REMS. (2015). Clozapine and the risk of neutropenia: A guide for healthcare providers. Retrieved from https://www.clozapinerems.com/CpmgClozapineUI/rems/pdf/resources/Clozapine_REMS_HCP_Guide.pdf

8. For patients taking extended-release valproic acid, when should levels be checked relative to the time the medication is administered?

A. Immediately after administration
B. 5 hours after administration
C. 24 hours after administration
D. 18 hours after administration
E. At any time after administration

ANSWER: D

Levels should be checked roughly 18 hours after administration of extended-release valproic acid.

REFERENCE

Reed, R. C., & Dutta, S. (2006). Does it really matter when a blood sample for valproic acid concentration is taken following once-daily administration of divalproex-ER? *Therapeutic Drug Monitoring*, *28*, 413–418.

9. Depersonalization is classified as a disturbance of which of the aspects of the mental status examination?

A. Thought process
B. Thought content
C. Affect
D. Cognition
E. Perception

ANSWER: E

Perceptual disturbances include hallucinations, illusions, depersonalization, and derealization. Depersonalization is a feeling that one is not oneself or that something has changed.

REFERENCE

Sadock, B. J., & Sadock, V. A. (2015). *Kaplan and Sadock's synopsis of psychiatry* (11th ed., pp. 192–283). Philadelphia, PA: Lippincott Williams and Wilkins.

10. When a patient is questioned during a diagnostic interview, her responses are characterized by lack of goal-directedness, with excessive details for each question. Eventually, the patient makes her point. Which of the following describes her thought process?

A. Flight of ideas
B. Clang association
C. Loosening of association
D. Circumstantiality
E. Tangentiality

ANSWER: D

Circumstantiality is a lack of goal-directedness, incorporating tedious and unnecessary details but still arriving at an end point. Tangentiality is a digression from the subject, introducing unrelated thoughts and not arriving at the end point. Loose associations involve jumping from one topic to another with no apparent connection between the topics. In clang associations (from German *klang*, meaning "sound"), word association is based on sound rather than meaning.

REFERENCE

Sadock, B. J., & Sadock, V. A. (2015). *Kaplan and Sadock's synopsis of psychiatry* (11th ed., pp. 192–283). Philadelphia, PA: Lippincott Williams and Wilkins.

11. A 46-year-old male is increasingly worried that his neighbors are monitoring him. He observes them out in the yard often, so he believes that this is "more than just a coincidence." He acknowledges he might be wrong about this, although he thinks it unlikely. This is an example of:

A. Overvalued idea
B. Illusion
C. Thought insertion
D. Ideas of reference
E. Thought perception

ANSWER: A

Overvalued ideas are solitary, abnormal beliefs that are neither delusional nor obsessional, but with which the patient is preoccupied. Overvalued ideas are less strongly held than delusions, as in this example, in which the patient considers he might be wrong.

REFERENCE

McKenna, P. J. (1984). Disorders with overvalued ideas. *British Journal of Psychiatry, 145*, 579–585.

12. A young mother whose son was diagnosed with osteosarcoma reports that she is no longer worried about her son's prognosis. She states she had a dream in which she saw an angel who smiled at her. She believes the dream is a sign that her son is destined to be cured. This is an example of which defense mechanism?

A. Altruism
B. Fantasy
C. Distortion
D. Denial
E. Acceptance

ANSWER: B

Fantasy is an immature defense mechanism that substitutes a less disturbing view of the world in the place of reality to cope with or resolve external conflict. Altruism is a mature defense mechanism described as minimizing internal fears by serving others. Distortion is an immature defense mechanism in which perception of disturbing aspects of external reality is altered in an effort to make them more acceptable. Denial is a pathological defense mechanism to avoid becoming aware of some painful aspect of reality. Acceptance is a mature defense mechanism in which a person assents to the reality of a situation.

REFERENCE

Sadock, B. J., & Sadock, V. A. (2015). *Kaplan and Sadock's synopsis of psychiatry* (11th ed., pp. 192–283). Philadelphia, PA: Lippincott Williams and Wilkins.

13. A 27-year-old female presents for follow-up 2 weeks after her father's death. Since he died, she reports depressed mood and feelings of helplessness. She describes that life is no longer worth living. She is extremely tearful and does not make eye contact. What is the next step in the interview?

A. Leave the room to give her time to compose herself.
B. Offer a tissue and remain silent.
C. Verbally affirm, "It is appropriate to cry."
D. Ask the patient if she has regrets about her relationship with her father.
E. Admit the patient to the psychiatric unit for suicidality.

ANSWER: B

One should always express empathy and then give the control to the patient to build appropriate therapeutic alliance. By offering a tissue to the patient, the physician demonstrates appropriate empathy. Remaining silent initially gives the patient control. Further interview to assess safety would be needed prior to any consideration of admission.

REFERENCE

Sadock, B. J., & Sadock, V. A. (2015). *Kaplan and Sadock's synopsis of psychiatry* (11th ed., pp. 192–283). Philadelphia, PA: Lippincott Williams and Wilkins.

14. In the Montreal Cognitive Assessment, asking the patient to repeat five different words a few minutes after hearing them is an assessment of what?

A. Delayed recall
B. Executive function
C. Attention
D. Registration
E. Abstract thinking

ANSWER: A

Delayed recall is the ability of the patient to repeat the words after a period of time has elapsed. Registration is the ability of the patient to repeat the words immediately after hearing them.

REFERENCE

Julayanont, P., Tangwongchai, S., Hemrungrojn, S., Tunvirachaisakul, C., Phanthumchinda, K., Hongsawat, J., ... & Nasreddine, Z.S. (2015). The Montreal Cognitive Assessment—Basic: A Screening Tool for Mild Cognitive Impairment in Illiterate and Low-Educated Elderly Adults. Journal of the American Geriatrics Society. doi : 10.1111/jgs.13820

15. What kinds of EEG waves are predominant in an awake state?

A. Theta (4–7 Hz)
B. Sharp and spike waves
C. Beta (greater than 13 Hz)
D. Triphasic
E. Alpha (8–12 Hz)

ANSWER: E

Alpha waves predominate in the awake state. The frequencies of electrical activity are divided by frequency and named with Greek letters: delta (less than 4 Hz), theta (4–7 Hz), alpha (8–12 Hz), and beta (greater than 13 Hz).

REFERENCE

Stern, T. A., Fava, M., Wilens, T. E., & Rosenbaum, J. F. (2015). *Massachusetts General Hospital comprehensive clinical psychiatry* (2nd ed., pp. 20–39). Elsevier.

16. Reciting the months of the year backward is a test of which of the following aspects of cognition?

A. Orientation
B. Registration
C. Attention
D. Recall
E. Registration

ANSWER: C

Reciting months of the year backward is a test of attention.

REFERENCE

Sadock, B. J., & Sadock, V. A. (2015). *Kaplan and Sadock's synopsis of psychiatry* (11th ed., pp. 192–283). Philadelphia, PA: Lippincott Williams and Wilkins.

17. Which of the following is a self rated scale?

A. Clinician-Administered PTSD Scale
B. Beck Depression Inventory
C. Hamilton Anxiety Rating Scale
D. Brief Social Phobia Scale
E. Yale–Brown Obsessive–Compulsive Scale

ANSWER: B

The Beck Depression Inventory (BDI) is a self-rated 17-item questionnaire in which patients rate symptoms of depression on a 4-point Likert scale. PTSD can be measured with the Clinician-Administered PTSD Scale (CAPS). The Hamilton Anxiety Rating Scale (HAM-A) is the most commonly used instrument for the evaluation of anxiety symptoms and is a clinician-administered rating scale. The Brief Social Phobia Scale (BSPS) consists of clinician-administered ratings related to social phobia.

The Yale–Brown Obsessive–Compulsive Scale (Y-BOCS) is a clinician-administered semistructured interview designed to measure the severity of obsessive–compulsive symptoms. An optional checklist of 64 specific obsessive and compulsive symptoms precedes the interview.

REFERENCE

Stern, T. A., Fava, M., Wilens, T. E., & Rosenbaum, J. F. (2015). *Massachusetts General Hospital comprehensive clinical psychiatry* (2nd ed., pp. 63–71). Elsevier.

18. Which of the following vitamin deficiencies can present as a hematologic disorder with neuropsychiatric manifestations, including apathy, irritability, cognitive impairment, psychosis, and delirium?

A. Folate
B. Cobalamin
C. Vitamin D
D. Riboflavin
E. Ascorbic acid

ANSWER: B

Cobalamin (vitamin B12) deficiency is characterized by the development of a chronic macrocytic anemia with neurological and psychiatric manifestations that include peripheral neuropathy, apathy, irritability, and depression. Delirium, with associated dementia or psychosis, may also be seen.

REFERENCE

Briani, C., Dalla Torre, C., Citton, V., Manara, R., Pompanin, S., Binotto, G., & Adami, F. (2013). Cobalamin deficiency: Clinical picture and radiological findings. *Nutrients, 5*, 4521–4539.

19. Which of the following assessments is a test of cognition?

A. Mini Mental State Examination
B. Rorschach test
C. Montgomery–Asberg Scale
D. Brief Psychiatric Rating Scale
E. Vineland Adaptive Behavior Scale

ANSWER: A

The Mini Mental State Examination (MMSE) is a 30-point test that assesses cognition in the following ways: orientation, memory, registration, recall, and attention. The Rorschach test is a projective test of personality. The Montgomery–Asberg Scale is an assessment for mood disorders. The Brief Psychiatric Rating Scale is a measure of psychotic symptoms as well as depression and anxiety. The Vineland Adaptive Behavior Scale (VABS-II) is a valid and reliable test to measure a person's adaptive level of functioning, particularly among children with pervasive developmental disorder.

REFERENCES

Aylward, G. (1994). *Practitioner's guide to developmental and psychological testing*. New York, NY: Springer.

Exner, John E. (2002). *The Rorschach: Basic foundations and principles of interpretation* (vol. 1). Hoboken, NJ: Wiley.

Folstein, M., Folstein, S. E., & McHugh, P. R. (1975). "Mini-Mental State": A practical method for grading the cognitive state of patients for the clinician. *Journal of Psychiatric Research*, *12*, 189–198.

Overall, J. E., & Gorham, D. R. (1962). The brief psychiatric rating scale. *Psychological Reports*, *10*, 799–812.

Sadock, B. J., & Sadock, V. A. (2015). *Kaplan and Sadock's synopsis of psychiatry* (11th ed., pp. 192–283). Philadelphia, PA: Lippincott Williams and Wilkins.

Williams, J. B. W., & Kobak, K. A. (2008). Development and reliability of a structured interview guide for the Montgomery–Asberg Depression Rating Scale (SIGMA). *British Journal of Psychiatry*, *192*, 52–58.

20. Which of the following EEG patterns is seen in delirium?

A. Frontal beta activity
B. Right temporal spikes
C. Three-per-second spike and wave patterns
D. Slow waves in alpha and beta wave activity
E. Generalized slow-wave activity consisting of theta and delta waves

ANSWER: E

Generalized slow-wave activity consisting of theta and delta waves is commonly seen in patients with delirium.

REFERENCE

Stern, T. A., Fava, M., Wilens, T. E., & Rosenbaum, J. F. (2015). *Massachusetts General Hospital comprehensive clinical psychiatry* (2nd ed., pp. 173–184). Elsevier.

QUESTIONS AND ANSWERS

This chapter has accompanying questions and answers which are available to subscribers as part of the Oxford eLearning platform. To access the questions, follow the link below, or go to http://oxford-elearning.oup.com/books.

http://oxford-elearning.oup.com/books/test/67/10.1093/med/9780190265557.003.0027

28.

TREATMENT OF PSYCHIATRIC DISORDERS

Harvinder Singh, Miyun Kang, Sarah de Asis, Rajiv Radhakrishnan, Rajesh R. Tampi, Esha Sharma, Geetha Manikkara, Silpa Balachandran, Mahitha Kolli, Suneela Cherlopalle

1. Which of the following statements is FALSE regarding sertraline?

A. Sertraline has the most potent dopamine reuptake inhibition among SSRIs.
B. Alpha-1 receptor antagonism is at least 10-fold greater than that of other SSRIs.
C. Sertraline has greatest potency in blocking serotonin reuptake among SSRIs.
D. Peak plasma levels are lower in young males than in females and older males.
E. Renal impairment does not appreciably influence pharmacokinetics.

ANSWER: C

Among the various SSRIs, sertraline is second only to paroxetine in potency for 5-HT reuptake blockade.

REFERENCES

Hiemke, C., & Härtter, S. (2000). Pharmacokinetics of selective serotonin reuptake inhibitors. *Pharmacology and Therapeutics, 85*, 11–28.
Owens, M. J., Knight, D. L., & Nemeroff, C. B. (2001). Second-generation SSRIs: Human monoamine transporter binding profile of escitalopram and R-fluoxetine. *Biological Psychiatry, 50*, 345–350.

2. Which of the following antidepressants carries the highest risk of weight gain?

A. Fluvoxamine
B. Bupropion
C. Mirtazapine
D. Citalopram
E. Desvenlafaxine

ANSWER: C

The exact mechanism underlying weight gain for mirtazapine is multifactorial. H1 and 5HT2C antagonism by mirtazapine plays a major role. H1activates AMPkinase, which in turn reverses the action of leptin (an appetite-suppressing hormone). Among antidepressants, amitriptyline, mirtazapine, and paroxetine are associated with a greater risk of weight gain.

REFERENCE

Serretti, A., & Mandelli, L.. Antidepressants and body weight: A comprehensive review and meta-analysis. *Journal of Clinical Psychiatry, 71*, 1259–1272.

3. Which of the following is accurate regarding the risk of SSRIs in pregnancy?

A. SSRIs present no appreciable risks in pregnancy.
B. SSRIs should be discontinued by the second trimester to reduce perinatal complications.
C. SNRIs have lower risk than SSRIs in pregnancy
D. Risks and benefits of SSRIs for both mother and baby must be weighed against the potential risks of untreated depression during pregnancy.
E. Only low-dose SSRI should be used in pregnancy.

ANSWER: D

Data on the safety of antidepressants in pregnancy are mixed, but paroxetine in particular appears to have a greater risk of teratogenicity than other SSRIs. It is the only SSRI to have a category D pregnancy status; other SSRIs are category C. SSRIs may increase risk of persistent pulmonary hypertension of the newborn. Untreated depression during pregnancy also increases risk of adverse outcomes for both mother and child, and balancing of risks and benefits of treatment versus no treatment should be conducted on a case-by-case basis. Psychotherapy, electroconvulsive therapy (ECT), repetitive transcranial magnetic stimulation (rTMS), and light therapy pose no known teratogenic risk in pregnancy.

REFERENCE

Patil, A. S., Kuller, J. A., & Rhee, E. H. (2011). Antidepressants in pregnancy: A review of commonly prescribed medications. *Obstetrical and Gynecological Survey, 66*, 777–787.

4. Which of the following medications is FDA approved for treatment of major neurocognitive disorder due to Parkinson's disease?

A. Donepezil
B. Galantamine
C. Rivastigmine
D. Memantine
E. All of the above

ANSWER: C

Rivastigmine is FDA approved for the treatment of dementia secondary to Parkinson's disease.

REFERENCE

Rivastigmine package insert. Retrieved from https://www.pharma.us.novartis.com/product/pi/pdf/exelon.pdf

5. Which medication is approved for the management of major vascular neurocognitive disorder?

A. Donepezil
B. Rivastigmine
C. Memantine
D. Dextromethorphan
E. None of the above

ANSWER: E

Currently, no medication is approved in the United States for the management of vascular neurocognitive disorder. However, randomized clinical evidence supports the use of cholinesterase inhibitors and memantine in vascular neurocognitive disorder.

REFERENCE

Chui, H. C., & Ramirez-Gomez, L. (2016). Vascular cognitive impairment: Diagnosis and treatment. In M. D. Geschwind & C. R. Belkoura (Eds.), *Non-Alzheimer's and atypical dementia* (pp. 43–44). Wiley.

6. Which of the following is an absolute contraindication for ECT?

A. Cerebrovascular accident within the past 3 months
B. Myocardial infarction within the past month
C. Increased intracranial pressure
D. Pregnancy
E. No absolute contraindications.

ANSWER: E

There are no "absolute" medical contraindications to ECT. Whereas each situation described above certainly confers increased risk, ECT remains one of the safest procedures done under sedation in the world. The decision to administer ECT should be made after weighing the risk of severe psychiatric illness against the risks of ECT and sedation. Careful medical evaluation of risk factors should be carried out prior to ECT, with specific attention to modifications of the patient's management and the administration of ECT, which may diminish the level of risk.

REFERENCE

Baghai, T. C., & Möller, H.-J. (2008). Electroconvulsive therapy and its different indications. Dialogues in Clinical Neuroscience, 10(1), 105–117.

7. Which of the following antidepressants has the strongest evidence in support of its safety in breastfeeding women?

A. Fluoxetine
B. Sertraline
C. Citalopram
D. Venlafaxine
E. Desvenlafaxine

ANSWER: B

Sertraline and paroxetine have the most data demonstrating negligible relative infant doses/concentration via breastfeeding.

REFERENCES

Chad, L., Pupco, A., Bozzo, P., & Koren, G. (2013). Update on antidepressant use during breastfeeding. *Canadian Family Physician, 59*(6), 633–634.

Sie, S. D., Wennink, J. M., van Driel, J. J., te Winkel, A. G., Boer, K., Casteelen, G., van Weissenbruch, M. M. (2012). Maternal use of SSRIs, SNRIs and NaSSAs: Practical recommendations during pregnancy and lactation. *Archives of Disease in Childhood Fetal and Neonatal Edition, 97*, F472–F476.

8. Which of the following statements is FALSE regarding antipsychotic medication?

A. Ziprasidone should always be taken with food.
B. Quetiapine has been shown to cause cataracts in beagles.
C. Up to one third of patients on aripiprazole will experience akathisia.
D. Optimal D2 receptor occupancy for reducing extrapyramidal symptoms is 70% 80%.
E. Paliperidone is safer than risperidone in patients with impaired renal clearance capacity.

ANSWER: E

Paliperidone has 80% renal clearance, so it should be avoided in patients with impaired renal function.

REFERENCE

Paliperidone package insert. Revised March 2016. (http://www.invega.com/prescribing-information)

9. Which of the following has been associated with lower risk of upper gastrointestinal bleeding associated with SSRIs?

A. H2-receptor antagonists
B. Sucralfate
C. Cotherapy with aspirin
D. Proton pump inhibitors
E. Bismuth subsalicylate

ANSWER: D

SSRI use may increase the risk of upper gastrointestinal bleeding by about 50%, and concurrent use of Proton pump inhibitors (PPIs) may mitigate this risk. SSRI use with NSAIDs, anticoagulants, and antiplatelet agents increases the risk of gastrointestinal bleeding. Caution should be paid to potential drug–drug interactions via P450 metabolism as many PPIs inhibit P450 isoenzymes (e.g., 2C19) and, therefore, increase SSRI blood levels.

REFERENCES

Andrade, C., Sandarsh, S., Chethan, K. B., Nagesh, K. S. (2010). Serotonin reuptake inhibitor antidepressants and abnormal bleeding: A review for clinicians and a reconsideration of mechanisms. *Journal of Clinical Psychiatry, 71*, 1565–1575.

Gjestad, C., Westin, A. A., & Skogvoll, E. (2015). Effect of proton pump inhibitors on the serum concentrations of the selective serotonin reuptake inhibitors citalopram, escitalopram, and sertraline. *Therapeutic Drug Monitoring, 37*, 90–97.

Targownik, L. E., Bolton, J. M., Metge, C. J., Leung, S., Sareen, J. (2009). Selective serotonin reuptake inhibitors are associated with modest increase in the risk of upper gastrointestinal bleeding. *American Journal of Gastroenterology, 104*, 1475–1482.

10. Which of the following statements is TRUE regarding fluoxetine?

A. It has no active metabolites.
B. Patients with obsessive–compulsive disorder (OCD) typically require lower doses than do patients with depression.
C. Patients with panic disorder should be started on low-dose fluoxetine.
D. There are no known pharmacokinetic drug–drug interactions with fluoxetine.
E. An MAOI may be started safely within 2 weeks of fluoxetine discontinuation.

ANSWER: C

Fluoxetine's active metabolite norfluoxetine has a half-life of 7 to 10 days, which explains why patients should have a 5-week washout after fluoxetine discontinuation before starting an MAOI. Fluoxetine is a potent CYP2D6 inhibitor, and norfluoxetine has moderate inhibitory effects on CYP3A4. As such, there are several known drug interactions via the P450 system. Patients who have panic disorder need a low initial dose of fluoxetine, followed by cautious dose titration. In panic disorder, starting with high doses of SSRIs can precipitate panic attacks. Compared with depression, OCD typically requires higher doses for longer periods of time for response.

REFERENCES

Fluoxetine package insert. Reference ID: 2927282.

Sinclair, L. I., Christmas, D. M., Hood, S. D., Potokar, J. P., Robertson, A., Isaac, A., ..., Davies, S. J. (2009). Antidepressant-induced jitteriness/anxiety syndrome: Systematic review. *British Journal of Psychiatry, 194*, 483–490.

11. Monotherapy with a high-potency, typical antipsychotic is preferred first-line management in which of the following cases?

A. A patient with hallucinations in alcohol withdrawal
B. A patient with phencyclidine (PCP) intoxication
C. A patient with the rigid form of Huntington's disease
D. A patient with stuporous catatonia
E. None of the above

ANSWER: E

High-potency, typical antipsychotics such as haloperidol are best avoided in the above-described conditions. Their use as an adjunct to benzodiazepines for complicated alcohol withdrawal is common practice and generally well tolerated. Low-potency neuroleptics should generally be avoided in delirium due to their anticholinergic effects, which may worsen delirium, and their use in alcohol withdrawal increases the risk of seizures. The use of neuroleptics in PCP intoxication theoretically increases the risk of neuroleptic malignant syndrome. Benzodiazepines are preferred first-line management of agitation in most forms of substance intoxication. Typical neuroleptics may increase the risk of converting catatonia to a malignant form along the lines of neuroleptic malignant syndrome that presents with autonomic instability, elevated creatine kinase, leukocytosis, and so forth. Patients with the rigid form of Huntington's disease are at a higher risk of acute extrapyramidal symptoms with typical antipsychotic medication.

REFERENCE

Kaplan, H. I., Sadock, B. J., Grebb, J. A., & Kaplan, H. I. (1994). *Kaplan and Sadock's synopsis of psychiatry: Behavioral sciences, clinical psychiatry.* Baltimore, MD: Williams and Wilkins.

12. Which of the following medications is contraindicated in the management of typical antipsychotic-induced hypotension?

A. Norepinephrine
B. Epinephrine
C. Metaraminol
D. Fludrocortisone
E. Midodrine

ANSWER: B

Neuroleptic-induced hypotension is mediated by alpha-1 adrenergic blockade. Epinephrine activates alpha and beta adrenergic receptors and when used in the presence of alpha-1 blockade, causes paradoxical reduction of blood pressure due to unopposed relaxation of smooth muscle via beta-2 blockade.

REFERENCE

Gugger, J. J. (2011). Antipsychotic pharmacotherapy and orthostatic hypotension: Identification and management. *CNS Drugs, 25*, 659–671.

13. A drowsy patient in the emergency room is found to have mydriasis, rigidity, restlessness, decreased deep tendon reflexes, tachycardia, and hypotension. Reports from paramedics suggest he overdosed on an unknown quantity of chlorpromazine. Which of the following would be ineffective in the treatment of this patient?

A. Activated charcoal
B. Gastric lavage
C. Emetics
D. IV diazepam
E. Phenytoin

ANSWER: C

The antiemetic action of chlorpromazine would limit the efficacy of emetic medication.

REFERENCE

Kaplan, H. I., Sadock, B. J., Grebb, J. A., & Kaplan, H. I. (1994). *Kaplan and Sadock's synopsis of psychiatry: Behavioral sciences, clinical psychiatry.* Baltimore, MD: Williams and Wilkins.

14. Which of the following is a relative contraindication for the use of typical antipsychotics?

A. Severe cardiac abnormality
B. Uncontrolled epilepsy
C. Tardive dyskinesia
D. Narrow angle of glaucoma
E. All of the above

ANSWER: E

All of the above are contraindications.

REFERENCE

Ovsiew, F. (1993). Contraindications to the use of antipsychotic drugs. *American Journal of Psychiatry, 150*, 1753–1754.

15. Which of the following SSRIs is most effective in the treatment of premature ejaculation?

A. Fluoxetine
B. Clomipramine
C. Paroxetine
D. Sertraline
E. Citalopram

ANSWER: C

Paroxetine has the greatest efficacy in delaying ejaculation.

REFERENCE

Waldinger, M. D., Zwinderman, A. H., Schweitzer, D. H., & Olivier, B. (2004). Relevance of methodological design for the interpretation of efficacy of drug treatment of premature ejaculation: A systematic review and meta-analysis. *International Journal of Impotence Research, 16*, 369–381.

16. Based on studies that systematically screen patients for sexual side effects of SSRIs, what percentage of patients will develop these side effects?

A. Less than 5%
B. 10%
C. 25%
D. More than 50%

ANSWER: D

A recent review of the literature identified that sexual side effects occur in the majority of patients on SSRIs. For instance, sexual side effects were found in 79% of those on citalopram, 70% on fluoxetine, 71% on paroxetine, 80% on sertraline, and 80% on venlafaxine. The purpose of this question is to highlight the striking prevalence of sexual side effects with SSRIs (and SNRIs).

REFERENCE

La Torre, A., Giupponi, G., Duffy, D., Conca, A. (2013). Sexual dysfunction related to psychotropic drugs: A critical review—Part I: Antidepressants. *Pharmcopsychiatry, 46*, 191–199.

17. Which of the following benzodiazepines is the LEAST likely to interact with other medications via P450 metabolism?

A. Alprazolam
B. Lorazepam
C. Diazepam
D. Flurazepam
E. Clonazepam

ANSWER: B

Lorazepam is metabolized by conjugation via glucuronidation (i.e., UGT system, not CYP/P450), which is a form of type II metabolism. Glucuronidation occurs both within the liver and systemically, which is why lorazepam is often preferred over diazepam for alcohol detoxification in patients with severe cirrhosis. Oxazepam and temazepam are metabolized by glucuronidation as well.

REFERENCES

Greenblatt, D. J. (1981). Clinical pharmacokinetics of oxazepam and lorazepam. *Clinical Pharmacokinetics, 6*, 89–105.
Otani, K. (2003). Cytochrome P450 3A4 and benzodiazepines. *Seishin Shinkeigaku Zasshi, 105*, 631–642.

18. Which of the following increases the plasma concentration of lamotrigine?

A. Oral contraceptives
B. Carbamazepine

C. Phenobarbital
D. St. John's wort
E. Valproic acid

ANSWER: E

Valproic acid and sertraline increase lamotrigine levels.

REFERENCE

Lamotrigine package insert. (http://www.accessdata.fda.gov/drugsatfda_docs/label/2009/020241s037s038,020764s030s031lbl.pdf)

19. Which antipsychotic medication is preferred in the management of psychosis in elderly patients with Parkinson's disease?

A. Risperidone
B. Olanzapine
C. Quetiapine
D. Aripiprazole
E. Haloperidol

ANSWER: C

Quetiapine and clozapine are least likely to worsen motor features of Parkinson's disease and/or cause parkinsonian symptoms.

REFERENCE

Steinberg, M., & Lyketsos, C. G. (2012). Atypical antipsychotic use in patients with dementia: Managing safety concerns. *American Journal of Psychiatry, 169*, 900–906.

20. Which of the following statements is TRUE regarding valproic acid?

A. It has no influence on thyroid function tests.
B. It causes chronic kidney disease.
C. Valproic acid–induced hyperammonemia often presents without elevation in alanine and aspartate aminotransferase.
D. It is efficacious for major depressive episodes in bipolar disorder.
E. Its effect on platelets is dose independent.

ANSWER: C

Serum ammonia should always be assayed in patients with delirium who are on valproic acid regardless of whether formal liver function tests (AST, ALT, etc.) are normal. Isolated elevation in ammonia can occur and cause delirium. Valproic acid may falsely alter thyroid function tests, and its effect on platelets is dose dependent. Although effective for mania and maintenance in bipolar disorder, it is not useful for treating major depressive episodes in bipolar disorder. Unlike lithium, it does not cause chronic kidney disease.

REFERENCE

Kaplan, H. I., Sadock, B. J., Grebb, J. A., & Kaplan, H. I. (1994). *Kaplan and Sadock's synopsis of psychiatry: Behavioral sciences, clinical psychiatry.* Baltimore, MD: Williams and Wilkins.

21. Which of the following statements is TRUE regarding lithium?

A. Lithium reduces hippocampal volume.
B. Taking lithium with food alters its absorption.
C. Lithium may be used safely with hemodialysis.
D. Lithium reaches steady state within 24 hours of dose change.
E. Lithium levels greater than 1.0 mEq/L are preferred for mood stabilization.

ANSWER: C

Lithium may actually increase hippocampal and cerebral cortical thickness, and its absorption is not influenced by recent food intake. The half-life of lithium is roughly 24 hours, so steady state requires about 5 days. The lowest lithium trough level that is effective for mood stabilization is preferred; higher levels increase the risk of several medical complications, including chronic kidney disease. Lithium can be used safely with hemodialysis and is typically dosed once after each session of hemodialysis.

REFERENCES

Chiu, C. T., & Chuang, D. M. (2010). Molecular actions and therapeutic potential of lithium in preclinical and clinical studies of CNS disorders. *Pharmacology and Therapeutics, 128*, 281–304.
Chuang, D. M., & Manji, H. K. (2007). In search of the Holy Grail for the treatment of neurodegenerative disorders: Has a simple cation been overlooked? *Biological Psychiatry, 62*, 4–6.

Ikonomov, O. C., & Manji, H. K. (1999). Molecular mechanisms underlying mood stabilization in manic-depressive illness: The phenotype challenge *American Journal of Psychiatry, 156*, 1506–1514.

22. Which of the following would have negligible effect on lithium levels?

A. Dehydration
B. Hydrochlorothiazide
C. Naproxen
D. Sodium depletion
E. Acetaminophen

ANSWER: E

Acetaminophen has no appreciable effect on lithium levels.

REFERENCE

Mary, P. R., & Mohandas, E. (1995). Practical issues in lithium use. *Indian Journal of Psychological Medicine, 18*, 49–60.

23. Which of the following statements in regard to lithium levels is TRUE?

A. Serum levels are increased in cirrhosis.
B. Lithium level corresponds to degree of polyuria.
C. Lithium should be avoided in patients with hypertension.
D. Lithium level equal to or higher than 2.5 mEq/L is a medical emergency only if the patient is symptomatic.
E. Hemodialysis is the most effective way of managing life-threatening lithium toxicity.

ANSWER: B

Lithium is an element that is renally excreted, and liver function has no direct effect on lithium levels. Lithium levels are associated with degree of polyuria, and long-term use may cause irreversible diabetes insipidus. Lithium toxicity is a clinical diagnosis that is confirmed by serum lithium levels. Relatively mild toxicity usually does not occur until serum lithium reaches a level of 1.5 mEq/L (1.5 mmol/L). Levels equal to or greater than 2.5 mEq/L (2.5 mmol/L) constitute a medical emergency, even in patients with limited symptoms.

REFERENCE

Oruch, R., Elderbi, M. A., Khattab, H. A., Pryme, I. F., Lund, A. (2014). Lithium: A review of pharmacology, clinical uses and toxicity. *European Journal of Pharmacology, 740*, 464–473.

24. Which of the following statements about side effects of lithium is TRUE?

A. Clinicians should consult a nephrologist if serum creatinine exceeds 1.6 mg/dl.
B. Lithium should be avoided in patients with suicidality.
C. Hypothyroidism is a contraindication for lithium.
D. It is safe to use lithium with ECT.
E. Cerebellar injury due to lithium is reversible.

ANSWER: A

Lithium can harm renal tubular function. Initially, lithium reduces the ability of the kidneys to concentrate urine, causing dilute polyuria (nephrogenic diabetes insipidus). Over years, this functional deficit can become structural. Biopsy specimens from patients chronically treated with lithium show interstitial fibrosis consistent with chronic interstitial nephritis in more severe cases. Thus, monitoring renal function by serial serum creatinine is an essential part of ongoing lithium therapy. Clinicians should consult a nephrologist and discontinue lithium when the serum creatinine approaches or exceeds 1.6 mg/dl (140 mmol/L). The most important risk factor for renal damage from lithium is repeated episodes of lithium intoxication. Each of the other options is false and highlights key features of lithium: lithium *reduces* suicidality, although because of its potential toxicity, patients with suicidality should be monitored even more closely. Lithium may cause hypothyroidism but this is not a contraindication for use of the medication. Lithium use with ECT enhances post-ECT confusion and so should be avoided. Cerebellar injury due to lithium is typically irreversible (so-called syndrome of irreversible lithium-effectuated neurotoxicity [SILENT]).

REFERENCE

Oruch, R., Elderbi, M. A., Khattab, H. A., Pryme, I. F., Lund, A. (2014). Lithium: A review of pharmacology, clinical uses and toxicity. *European Journal of Pharmacology, 740*, 464–473.

25. Which antipsychotic may reverse neuroleptic-induced hyperprolactinemia?

A. Risperidone
B. Olanzapine
C. Quetiapine
D. Aripiprazole
E. Ziprasidone

ANSWER: D

The addition of aripiprazole rapidly normalizes risperidone-induced hyperprolactinemia.

REFERENCE

Shores, L. E.(2005). Normalization of risperidone-induced hyperprolactinemia with the addition of aripiprazole. *Psychiatry (Edgmont), 2*(3), 42–45.

26. A patient tells you that his spouse found him mowing his yard at 2:00 a.m. a few nights ago. Upon awakening, the patient recalled being unable to sleep earlier that evening, which led him to take several additional "sleeping pills". He says his mind is "blank" for everything else that happened after that. Which of the following medications is most likely to cause this type of amnesia?

A. Hydroxyzine
B. Trazodone
C. Doxepin
D. Zolpidem
E. Suvorexant

ANSWER: D

Numerous cases of anterograde amnesia with bizarre, even dangerous, parasomnias have been reported in the literature. Zolpidem appears to be more likely to cause these than the other "Z-drugs" zaleplon or eszopiclone. Benzodiazepines such as triazolam have been reported to cause anterograde amnesia, but reports are fewer than with zolpidem. Alcohol similarly causes anterograde amnesia in intoxication (known as a blackout or "alcoholic palimpsest"). Anterograde amnesia with barbiturates has led to a condition termed *automatism* whereby a patient forgets having taken a scheduled dose of barbiturate and proceeds to take another, and then another, until he or she either loses consciousness or even experiences fatal respiratory compromise.

REFERENCE

Dolder, C. R., & Nelson, M. H. (2008). Hypnosedative-induced complex behaviors. *CNS Drugs, 22*, 1021–1036.

27. Which of the following statements about bupropion is TRUE?

A. It can be used safely with MAOIs.
B. Weight gain is a common side effect.
C. It has a higher risk of manic overshoot than SSRIs.
D. It may be considered in patients with nonpurging-type anorexia nervosa.
E. Bupropion can cause a false positive urine drug screen for amphetamines.

ANSWER: E

Bupropion can cause a false positive drug screen for amphetamines. It should be avoided with MAOIs for risk of hypertensive crisis, and it often causes weight *loss*. It is widely held to have a *lower* risk of manic overshoot than SSRIs. Its use in anorexia nervosa is effectively contraindicated: It lowers the seizure threshold and may precipitate seizures due to various electrolyte disturbances seen in patients with anorexia nervosa regardless of subtype. Notably, the increased seizure risk is dose dependent and increases markedly over 300 mg total daily dose.

REFERENCES

Casey, E. R., Scott, M. G., Tang, S., Mullins, M. E. (2011). Frequency of false FALSE positive amphetamine screens due to bupropion using the Syva EMIT II immunoassay. *Journal of Medical Toxicology, 7*, 105–108.

Sachs, G. S., Nierenberg, A. A., Calabrese, J. R., Marangell, L. B., Wisniewski, S. R., Gyulai, L., ... Thase, M. E. (2007). Effectiveness of adjunctive antidepressant treatment for bipolar depression. *New England Journal of Medicine, 356*, 1711–1722.

Wellbutrin SR package insert. Retrieved from https://www.gsksource.com/pharma/content/dam/GlaxoSmithKline/US/en/Prescribing_Information/Wellbutrin_SR/pdf/WELLBUTRIN-SR-PI-MG.PDF

28. Which of the following statements about SNRIs is FALSE?

A. Potency order for norepinephrine reuptake inhibition is duloxetine > desvenlafaxine > venlafaxine.
B. SNRIs are more likely to cause gastrointestinal side effects than SSRIs.
C. Emergent discontinuation syndrome is more severe with duloxetine than with venlafaxine.
D. Both venlafaxine and duloxetine are category C for pregnant patients.
E. Desvenlafaxine is an active metabolite of venlafaxine.

ANSWER: C

Duloxetine is a potent 5-HT and norepinephrine reuptake inhibitor, whereas desvenlafaxine is a stronger inhibitor of norepinephrine reuptake than venlafaxine but a less potent inhibitor of norepinephrine reuptake than duloxetine. Gastrointestinal side effects are common with the SNRIs and may have a somewhat greater propensity for causing nausea than do some of the SSRIs. As with the SSRIs, adaptation to this side effect occurs rapidly, in the first 2 to 3 weeks of therapy. The relatively short half-life and low protein binding of venlafaxine, desvenlafaxine, and milnacipran may predispose patients to an increased risk of discontinuation symptoms when the drug is stopped suddenly. Duloxetine's longer half-life and higher protein binding may be associated with a lower frequency of discontinuation symptoms than with venlafaxine. Duloxetine may be safely tapered in most patients by decreasing the total dose by 30 mg per week. Both venlafaxine and duloxetine are category C for pregnant patients. Desvenlafaxine is an active metabolite of venlafaxine.

REFERENCES

Bymaster, F. P., Dreshfield-Ahmad, L. J., Threlkeld, P. G., Shaw, J. L., Thompson, L., Nelson, D. L., ... & Wong, D. T. (2001). Comparative affinity of duloxetine and venlafaxine for serotonin and norepinephrine transporters in vitro and in vivo, human serotonin receptor subtypes, and other neuronal receptors. *Neuropsychopharmacology, 25*, 871–880.

Hosenbocus, S., & Chahal, R. SSRIs and SNRIs: A review of the discontinuation syndrome in children and adolescents. *Journal of the Canadian Academy of Child and Adolescent Psychiatry, 20*, 60–67.

Westanmo, A. D., Gayken, J., & Haight, R. (2005). Duloxetine: A balanced and selective norepinephrine- and serotonin-reuptake inhibitor. *American Journal of Health-System Pharmacy,* 62, 2481–2490.

29. Which of the following statements regarding typical antipsychotics is FALSE?

A. Chlorpromazine can cause benign pigmentation of eyes.
B. Chronic use of chlorpromazine can cause blue-gray skin discoloration.
C. Irreversible retinal pigmentation is associated with thioridazine >1,000 mg/day.
D. Low-potency agents are more likely to cause seizures than high-potency agents.
E. Haloperidol has the greatest anticholinergic effect among typical antipsychotics.

ANSWER: E

Haloperidol has negligible anticholinergic effects.

REFERENCE

Kaplan, H. I., Sadock, B. J., Grebb, J. A., & Kaplan, H. I. (1994). *Kaplan and Sadock's synopsis of psychiatry: Behavioral sciences, clinical psychiatry*. Baltimore, MD: Williams and Wilkins.

30. Pregabalin is FDA approved for which of the following indications?

A. Generalized anxiety disorder
B. Panic disorder
C. Social anxiety disorder
D. Fibromyalgia
E. Bipolar I disordermaintenance treatment

ANSWER: D

Of the above options, pregabalin is FDA approved only for fibromyalgia. It is used off label for panic disorder, generalized anxiety disorder, and social anxiety disorder.

REFERENCE

Stahl, S. M., & Grady, M. M. (2011). *Stahl's essential psychopharmacology: The prescriber's guide* (4th ed.). Cambridge, UK: Cambridge University Press.

31. Transitioning from olanzapine to which other antipsychotic is NOT expected to cause cholinergic rebound?

A. Risperidone
B. Clozapine
C. Aripiprazole

D. Ziprasidone
E. Lurasidone

ANSWER: B

Clozapine and olanzapine have significant anticholinergic activity; therefore, transitioning from one to the other can usually be accomplished with little risk of cholinergic rebound. Risperidone, ziprasidone, lurasidone, and aripiprazole have limited anticholinergic activity. An abrupt transition from olanzapine or clozapine to these agents can cause cholinergic rebound, characterized by excessive salivation, nausea, vomiting, and diarrhea. The risk of cholinergic rebound may be mitigated by initially augmenting a new agent with an anticholinergic medication and subsequently tapered slowly.

REFERENCES

Ganguli, R., Brar, J. S., Mahmoud, R., Berry, S. A., & Pandina, G. J. (2008). Assessment of strategies for switching patients from olanzapine to risperidone: A randomized, open-label, rater-blinded study. *BMC Medicine, 6*, 17.

Henderson, D. C., Nasrallah, R. A., & Goff D. C. (1998). Switching from clozapine to olanzapine in treatment-refractory schizophrenia: Safety, clinical efficacy, and predictors of response. *Journal of Clinical Psychiatry, 59*, 585–588.

32. Which of the following atypical antipsychotics has the lowest risk of extrapyramidal symptoms?

A. Olanzapine
B. Risperidone
C. Clozapine
D. Paliperidone
E. Aripiprazole

ANSWER: C

The risk of extrapyramidal symptoms by class of medication increases from 1 to 5, as follows:

1. Quetiapine and clozapine
2. Aripiprazole, olanzapine, and ziprasidone
3. Paliperidone and risperidone
4. Low-potency conventional neuroleptics
5. High-potency conventional neuroleptics (20%–40%)

REFERENCE

Tandon, R., & Jibson, M. D. (2002). Extrapyramidal side effects of antipsychotic treatment: Scope of problem and impact on outcome. *Annals of Clinical Psychiatry, 14*, 123–129.

33. Which of the following SSRIs is LEAST likely to alter the pharmacokinetics of coadministered medication?

A. Fluoxetine
B. Fluvoxamine
C. Paroxetine
D. Sertraline
E. Citalopram

ANSWER: E

Citalopram and escitalopram are least likely to complicate treatment because of an effect on p450 enzymes.

REFERENCE

Kaplan, H. I., Sadock, B. J., Grebb, J. A., & Kaplan, H. I. (1994). *Kaplan and Sadock's synopsis of psychiatry: Behavioral sciences, clinical psychiatry*. Baltimore, MD: Williams and Wilkins.

34 through 39. Match the following drug interactions with the responsible CYP450 enzyme:

34. Fluvoxamine administered with theophylline raises theophylline plasma concentration.

35. Fluoxetine administered with risperidone worsens parkinsonism.

36. Nefazodone administered with alprazolam raises alprazolam plasma concentration.

37. Fluoxetine administered with triazolam raises triazolam plasma concentration.

38. Carbamazepine autoinduction.

39. Imipramine and cigarette smoking decrease imipramine levels.

A. CYP450 1A2
B. CYP450 2D6
C. CYP450 3A4

ANSWERS:

34. A. Fluvoxamine is an inhibitor of the CYP1 A2 isoenzyme. Theophylline is a substrate of the CYP1 A2 isoenzyme. Hence, fluvoxamine inhibits the metabolism of theophylline, thereby raising its level in the serum.

35. B. Fluoxetine is an inhibitor of the CYP450 2D6 isoenzyme. Risperidone is a substrate of the CYP450 2D6 isoenzyme. Hence, fluoxetine inhibits the metabolism of risperidone, thereby raising its level in the serum. Elevated risperidone level worsens parkinsonism.

36. C. Nefazodone is an inhibitor of the CYP4503 A4 isoenzyme. Alprazolam is a substrate of the CYP4503 A4 isoenzyme. Hence, nefazodone inhibits the metabolism of alprazolam, thereby raising its level in the serum.

37. B. Fluoxetine is an inhibitor of the CYP450 2D6 system. Triazolam is a substrate of the CYP450 2D6 isoenzyme. Hence, fluoxetine inhibits the metabolism of triazolam thereby raising its level in the serum.

38. C. Carbamazepine is both a substrate and an inducer of the CYP450 3A4 isoenzyme. Hence, carbamazepine induces its own metabolism (autoinduction).

39. A. Tobacco is an inducer of the CYP450 1A2 isoenzyme. Imipramine is a substrate of the CYP450 1A2 isoenzyme. Hence, cigarette smoking induces the metabolism of imipramine, thereby decreasing its level in the serum.

REFERENCES

Desai, H. D., Seabolt, J., & Jann, M. W. (2001). Smoking in patients receiving psychotropic medications: A pharmacokinetic perspective. *CNS Drugs, 15*, 469–494.

Fluoxetine package insert. Retrieved from http://www.accessdata.fda.gov/drugsatfda_docs/label/2011/018936s091lbl.pdf

Greene, D. S., Salazar, D. E., Dockens, R. C., Kroboth, P., & Barbhaiya, R. H. (1995). Coadministration of nefazodone and benzodiazepines: III. A pharmacokinetic interaction study with alprazolam. *Journal of Clinical Psychopharmacology, 15*, 399–408.

Michalets, E. L., & Williams, C. R. (2000). Drug interactions with cisapride: Clinical implications. *Clinical Pharmacokinetics, 39*, 49–75.

Ogu, C. C., & Maxa, J. L. (2000). Drug interactions due to cytochrome P450. *Proceedings (Baylor University Medical Center), 13*, 421–423.

Orlando R., Padrini, R., Perazzi, M., De Martin, S., Piccoli, P., & Palatini, P. Liver dysfunction markedly decreases the inhibition of cytochrome P450 1A2-mediated theophylline metabolism by fluvoxamine. *Clinical Pharmacology and Therapeutics, 79*, 489–499.

Pippenger, C. E. (1987). Clinically significant carbamazepine drug interactions: An overview. *Epilepsia, 28*(suppl. 3), S71–S76.

40. Which of the following is FDA approved for suppression of motor and phonic tics in patients with Tourette's syndrome?

A. Risperidone
B. Guanfacine
C. Pimozide
D. Primidone
E. Olanzapine

ANSWER: C

Pimozide is FDA approved for suppression of motor and phonic tics in patients with Tourette's syndrome. Olanzapine, guanfacine, and risperidone are sometimes prescribed off label for this condition. Primidone is not prescribed for Tourette's syndrome.

REFERENCE

Stahl, S. M., & Grady, M. M. (2011). *Stahl's essential psychopharmacology: The prescriber's guide* (4th ed.). Cambridge, UK: Cambridge University Press.

40. Which of the following properties differentiates amphetamine from methylphenidate?

A. Methylphenidate blocks dopamine reuptake; amphetamines also enhance dopamine release.
B. Unlike methylphenidate, amphetamine is a competitive inhibitor at the dopamine transporter.
C. Amphetamine is a competitive inhibitor of vesicular monoamine transporters.
D. Both stereoisomers of methylphenidate are active; only D-amphetamine is active
E. All of the above.

ANSWER: E

All of the above are correct statements.

REFERENCE

Hodgkins, P., Shaw, M., Coghill, D., & Hechtman, L. (2012). Amphetamine and methylphenidate medications for attention-deficit/hyperactivity disorder: Complementary treatment options. *European Child and Adolescent Psychiatry, 21*, 477–492.

41. Which of the following medications is not metabolized by the P450 system?

A. Trazodone
B. Lamotrigine
C. Ziprasidone
D. Clozapine
E. Desvenlafaxine

ANSWER: B

Lamotrigine is metabolized by the uridine 5'-diphosphoglucuronosyl transferase (UGT) system. All others are metabolized through the P450 system.

REFERENCES

Lamotigine package insert. Retrieved from http://www.fda.gov/downloads/AdvisoryCommittees/CommitteesMeetingMaterials/PediatricAdvisoryCommittee/UCM235547.pdf

Prior, T. I., & Baker, G. B. (2003). Interactions between the cytochrome P450 system and the second-generation antipsychotics. *Journal of Psychiatry and Neuroscience, 28*, 99–112.

42. Which of the following is TRUE regarding the efficacy of ECT?

A. Propofol for ECT induction causes less postictal agitation than methohexital.
B. Right unilateral ECT causes fewer cognitive symptoms than bilateral ECT.
C. Stimulus dose is the strongest predictor of ECT treatment outcome.
D. Brief pulse current reduces cognitive effects of ECT.
E. All of the above are true statements.

ANSWER: E

Cognitive impairment is the primary limitation of bitemporal ECT, which is thought to be due to the direct effect on the dominant medial temporal lobe. Current literature suggests that high-dose right unilateral ECT has a comparable efficacy to moderate-dose bitemporal ECT and retains cognitive advantages. Evidence suggests that stimulus dose is the strongest predictor of treatment outcome. Brief pulse has a lower width (0.5–2 ms), which is one of the proposed reasons for its improved cognitive profile. Propofol is the second most commonly used induction agent for ECT. It has higher anticonvulsant properties but lower incidences of postictal agitation compared with methohexital. ECT is the most effective treatment for both unipolar and bipolar depression, with response rates of greater than 80%.

REFERENCES

American Psychiatric Association. (2001). *The practice of electroconvulsive therapy: Recommendations for treatment, training, and privileging: A task force report of the American Psychiatric Association*. Edited by R. Weiner. Washington, DC: American Psychiatric Association.

Sackeim, H. A., Dillingham, E. M., Prudic, J. Cooper, T., McCall, W. V., Rosenquist, P., ... Haskett, R. F. (2009). Effect of concomitant pharmacotherapy on electroconvulsive therapy outcomes: Short-term efficacy and adverse effects. *Archives of General Psychiatry, 66*, 729–737.

43. A 25-year-old man with schizophrenia presents to the emergency room due to florid psychotic decompensation and severe agitation in the context of nonadherence with risperidone. When assertive behavioral interventions are unsuccessful, he is given haloperidol 5 mg intramuscular (IM) followed 30 minutes later by 10 mg IM. Agitation is markedly improved within 20 minutes of the second injection. Shortly thereafter, the patient's voice sounds strangled, and he develops respiratory distress with return of agitation. What should be administered immediately?

A. Haloperidol 10 mg IM
B. Lorazepam 2 mg IM
C. Risperidone 2 mg orally
D. Diphenhydramine 50 mg IM
E. Epinephrine 0.3 mg IM

ANSWER: D

The patient is presenting with features of laryngospasm, a subtype of acute dystonic reaction. Laryngospasm is a medical emergency and is treated with diphenhydramine 50 mg IM/IV (or benztropine 1 mg IM/IV). Very often, haloperidol is combined with lorazepam and diphenhydramine or benztropine for synergistic sedative effect, and, in particular, an anticholinergic medication is added to ward off acute dystonia.

REFERENCES

Criner, G. J., & D'Alonzo, G. E. (2002). *Critical care study guide text and review*. New York, NY: Springer.

Lee, A. S. (1979). Treatment of drug-induced dystonic reactions. *Journal of the American College of Emergency Physicians, 8*, 453–457.

44. Hostile and aggressive behavior may complicate care for patients with schizophrenia. Which of the following antipsychotic medications was shown to have the greatest impact in decreasing hostility in phase 1 of the Clinical Antipsychotic Trials of Intervention Effectiveness (CATIE) trial?

A. Perphenazine
B. Risperidone
C. Olanzapine
D. Quetiapine
E. Ziprasidone

ANSWER: C

Olanzapine was superior in decreasing hostility and aggression over perphenazine and quetiapine at months 1, 3, 6, and 9. It was also significantly superior to ziprasidone at months 1, 3, and 6, and to risperidone at months 3 and 6. The results are consistent with those of a similar post hoc analysis of hostility in first-episode subjects with schizophrenia enrolled in the European First-Episode Schizophrenia Trial (EUFEST), where olanzapine demonstrated advantages over haloperidol, quetiapine, and amisulpride.

REFERENCE

Volavka, J., Czobor, P., Citrome, L., & Van Dorn, R. A. (2014). Effectiveness of antipsychotic drugs against hostility in patients with schizophrenia in the Clinical Antipsychotic Trials of Intervention Effectiveness (CATIE) study. *CNS Spectrums, 19*, 374–381.

45. Which of the following medications for insomnia is safest in older adults?

A. Zolpidem
B. Zaleplon
C. Doxepin
D. Temazepam
E. Ramelteon

ANSWER: E

Ramelteon is the only drug in this list not considered to be potentially inappropriate for use in older adults by the American Geriatrics Society per the Beers criteria. The other medications increase risk of anticholinergic side effects (doxepin) and falls, fractures, and delirium (zolpidem, zaleplon, and temazepam).

REFERENCE

American Geriatrics Society 2015 Beers Criteria Update Expert Panel. (2015). American Geriatrics Society 2015 Updated Beers Criteria for Potentially Inappropriate Medication Use in Older Adults. *Journal of the American Geriatrics Society, 63*, 2227–2246.

46. Which of the following medications is efficacious in treating cataplexy in narcolepsy?

A. Modafinil
B. Methylphenidate
C. Sodium oxybate
D. Ropinirole
E. Melatonin

ANSWER: C

Sodium oxybate is approved by the FDA for both excessive sleepiness and cataplexy in narcolepsy. Modafinil and stimulants are FDA approved for excessive sleepiness in narcolepsy but not for cataplexy. Ropinirole is approved for restless leg syndrome, not narcolepsy.

REFERENCE

Xyrem [sodium oxybate] oral solution US prescribing information. (2014). Palo Alto, CA Jazz Pharmaceuticals, Inc.

47. A 35-year-old female with schizophrenia on risperidone 3 mg at bedtime is diagnosed with breast cancer. Laboratory workup reveals markedly increased prolactin. On evaluation, the patient complains of dysmenorrhea and galactorrhea. Which of the following would be most likely to improve her complaints?

A. Continue risperidone 3 mg PO at bedtime.
B. Taper risperidone and do not rechallenge with antipsychotics.
C. Taper risperidone and switch to paliperidone.
D. Taper risperidone and switch to iloperidone.
E. Taper risperidone and switch to aripiprazole.

ANSWER: E

Special consideration is required when prescribing antipsychotic drugs for patients with an existing diagnosis of breast cancer. In general, first-generation antipsychotics can cause significant elevations in serum prolactin. Antipsychotics that increase prolactin (from 45 to >100 ng/ml) and should be avoided in patients with breast cancer include risperidone, paliperidone, and haloperidol. Antipsychotics that increase prolactin (from 20–50 ng/ml) and should be used with caution in patients with breast cancer include olanzapine, iloperidone, and lurasidone. Antipsychotics that minimally increase prolactin and are preferred in patients with breast cancer include ziprasidone, asenapine, quetiapine, and clozapine. The only antipsychotic that might lower serum prolactin in patients with breast cancer is aripiprazole.

REFERENCE

Rahman, T., Clevenger, C. V., Kaklamani, V., Lauriello, J , Campbell, A., Malwitz, K., & Kirkland, R. S. (2014). Antipsychotic treatment in breast cancer patients. *American Journal of Psychiatry, 171,* 616–621.

48. Which of the following antipsychotics is LEAST likely to exacerbate obsessions and compulsions in patients with OCD co-morbid with schizophrenia?

A. Quetiapine
B. Risperidone
C. Amisulpride
D. Aripiprazole

ANSWER: C

Atypical antipsychotics (dopamine-serotonin antagonists) are more likely to exacerbate obsessive–compulsive symptoms than typical antipsychotics. Atypical antipsychotics block 5HT2A receptors in presynaptic dopamine neurons, which in turn disinhibit dopaminergic activity. This mechanism is postulated to increase obsessive–compulsive symptoms in patients with schizophrenia. Amisulpride has minimal effect on OCD symptoms, as does aripiprazole. Aripiprazole is a 5HT2A and D2 partial antagonist that has been shown to improve obsessive–compulsive symptoms in schizophrenia.

REFERENCES

Hwang, M. Y., & Peter F. Buckley, P. F. (2013). Comorbidities in schizophrenia: Clinical management and conceptual issues. *Psychiatric Annals, 43,* 435–436.

Sayyah, M., Sayyah, M., Boostani, H., Ghaffari, S. M., Hoseini, A.. (2012). Effects of aripiprazole augmentation in treatment-resistant obsessive–compulsive disorder (a double blind clinical trial). *Depression and Anxiety, 29,* 850–854.

49. Which of the following atypical antipsychotics has the shortest half-life?

A. Ziprasidone
B. Iloperidone
C. Asenapine
D. Lurasidone
E. Paliperidone

ANSWER: A

Among the atypical antipsychotics, ziprasidone has the shortest half-life of approximately 7 hours. Ziprasidone must be administered at least twice daily *with food.*

REFERENCE

Preskorn, S. H. (2012). Clinically important differences in the pharmacokinetics of the ten newer "atypical" antipsychotics: Part 1. *Journal of Psychiatric Practice, 18,* 199–204.

50. A 70-year-old man with Parkinson's disease is admitted to the hospital with visual hallucinations. A thorough medical workup has not detected a medical cause for his hallucinations. Which of the following antipsychotics would be most appropriate in treating this patient's symptoms?

A. Ziprasidone
B. Risperidone
C. Quetiapine
D. Cariprazine
E. Iloperidone

ANSWER: C

Atypical antipsychotics quetiapine and clozapine are used to treat psychotic symptoms in individuals with Parkinson's disease that are not amenable to other interventions, including adjustments in the medications used to treat Parkinson's disease.

REFERENCE

Levin, J., Hasan, A., & Höglinger, G. U. (2016). Psychosis in Parkinson disease: Identification, prevention and treatment. *Journal of Neural Transmission (Vienna), 123,* 45–50.

51. A patient with active opioid use disorder is admitted for acute coronary syndrome. Which of the following is recommended for managing opioid withdrawal?

A. Clonidine and avoidance of opioids to prevent drug-seeking behavior
B. Naltrexone for ultrarapid detoxification
C. Tramadol because there is less abuse potential than with opioids
D. Buprenorphine started on the day of admission before withdrawal symptoms begin
E. Methadone plus as-needed morphine

ANSWER: E

Opioid substitution—either methadone or buprenorphine—is first-line management for opioid withdrawal. Buprenorphine should not be administered until a patient is already in withdrawal because it will precipitate withdrawal abruptly. A patient who is using opioids regularly will have increased physiological tolerance and require higher doses for adequate pain relief than opioid-naive patients. Medical admission for opioid detoxification alone is not typically covered by insurance because it is not associated with medical complications (like severe alcohol withdrawal); however, assertive management of opioid withdrawal is critical when withdrawal can complicate medical conditions such as acute coronary syndrome as in this vignette. Ultrarapid detoxification with naltrexone is unsafe and should not be attempted.

REFERENCE

Diaper, A. M., Law, F. D., & Melichar, J. K. (2014). Pharmacological strategies for detoxification. *British Journal of Clinical Pharmacology, 77*, 302–314.

52. Which one of the following drugs is FDA approved for treating bulimia nervosa?

A. Imipramine
B. Bupropion
C. Fluoxetine
D. Venlafaxine
E. Mirtazapine

ANSWER: C

Fluoxetine is indicated for the treatment of bulimia nervosa.

REFERENCE

McElroy, S. L., Guerdjikova, A. I., Mori, N., Keck, P. E. Jr. (2015). Psychopharmacologic treatment of eating disorders: Emerging findings. *Current Psychiatry Reports, 17*(5), 35.

53. Which of the following is useful for treating lithium-induced nephrogenic diabetes insipidus?

A. Imipramine
B. Amiloride
C. Furosemide
D. Fluconazole
E. Cimetidine

ANSWER: B

For nephrogenic diabetes insipidus that does not resolve after the discontinuation of lithium, amiloride may be a beneficial treatment. Amiloride acts via its natriuretic action, causing contraction of extracellular volume and consequent decrease in glomerular filtration while ultimately leading to decreased urine volume. It also reduces the entry of lithium into the distal tubular cells

REFERENCE

Giusti, C. F., Amorim, S. R., Guerra R. A., Portes, E. S.. (2012). Endocrine disturbances related to the use of lithium. *Arquivos Brasileiros de Endocrinologia & Metabologia56*, 153–158.

54. Which of the following can be used safely with an MAOI?

A. Pseudoephedrine
B. Dextromethorphan
C. SSRIs
D. SNRIs
E. Lithium

ANSWER: E

Lithium can be safely used to augment the effects of MAOI antidepressants. Two urgent clinical conditions associated with MAOIs include hypertensive crisis and serotonin syndrome. Hypertensive crises are often caused by dietary tyramine or concurrent use of agents with catecholaminergic activity such as pseudoephedrine.

REFERENCE

Kennedy, S. H., Holt, A., & Baker, G. B. (2009). Monoamine oxidase inhibitors. In B. J. Sadock, V. A. Sadock, & P. Ruiz (Eds.), *Kaplan and Sadock's comprehensive textbook of psychiatry* (9th ed., pp. 3161–3162). Philadelphia, PA: Lippincott Williams and Wilkins.

55. Which of the following agents has NOT been shown to augment the antidepressant effect of SSRIs for a major depressive episode?

A. Lithium
B. Lamotrigine
C. Aripiprazole
D. Mirtazapine
E. Pramipexole

ANSWER: B

The addition of lamotrigine to augment the effects of an SSRI has not shown benefit in the treatment of a major depressive episode.

REFERENCE

Haddad, P. M., Talbot, P. S., Anderson, I. M., McAllister-Williams, R. H. (2015). Managing inadequate antidepressant response in depressive illness. *British Medical Bulletin, 115*, 183–201.

56. Which one of the following drugs is FDA approved for the acute treatment of bipolar depression?

A. Divalproex sodium
B. Lamotrigine
C. Ketamine
D. Quetiapine
E. Paroxetine

ANSWER: D

Among the listed drugs, only quetiapine is FDA approved for the acute treatment of bipolar depression. Olanzapine–fluoxetine combination and lurasidone are also approved in the United States for the acute treatment of bipolar depression.

REFERENCE

McIntyre, R. S., Cha, D. S., Kim, R. D., Mansur, R. B. (2013). A review of FDA-approved treatment options in bipolar depression. *CNS Spectrums, 18*(suppl. 1), 4–20.

57. Which of the following agents is considered first-line management for post-traumatic stress disorder (PTSD)?

A. Sertraline
B. Bupropion
C. Valproic acid
D. Clonazepam
E. Quetiapine

ANSWER: A

The only two medications approved by the FDA for the treatment of PTSD are sertraline and paroxetine. SSRIs are considered first-line agents for PTSD because they have been shown to be effective for all major clusters of PTSD symptoms, including in combat-related PTSD. The data in support of paroxetine and venlafaxine are stronger (as of the time of this publication) than for other SSRIs or SNRIs.

REFERENCES

Jonas, D. E., Cusack, K., Forneris, C. A., Wilkins, T. M., Sonis, J., Middleton, J. C., ... Gaynes, B. N.. (2013). Psychological and pharmacological treatments for adults with posttraumatic stress disorder (PTSD). *Comparative Effectiveness Reviews No. 92.* Agency for Healthcare Research and Quality (US). Report No. 13-EHC011-EF. Retrieved from http://www.ncbi.nlm.nih.gov/pubmedhealth/PMH0055845/

Puetz, T. W., Youngstedt, S. D., & Herring, M. P. (2015) Effects of pharmacotherapy on combat-related PTSD, anxiety, and depression: A systematic review and meta-regression analysis. *PLos ONE, 10*(5), e0126529.

58. Which medication is efficacious for the management of nightmares in PTSD?

A. Trazodone
B. Doxepin
C. Quetiapine
D. Prazosin
E. Clonidine

ANSWER: D

Prazosin is an alpha-1 antagonist initially used for hypertension, and it is efficacious for treating nightmares in PTSD. It is not a hypnotic agent but can improve distressed awakenings related to nightmares. Patients should be warned about potential "first-dose hypotension," in which they develop orthostatic hypotension with the first (or first few) doses within hours of taking the medication or with dose increases. This limits expedient dose titration. Often doses of 8 to 15 mg are needed for full response.

REFERENCE

George, K. C., Kebejian, L., Ruth, L. J., Miller, C. W., Himelhoch, S.. (2016). Meta-analysis of the efficacy and safety of prazosin versus placebo for the treatment of nightmares and sleep disturbances in adults with post-traumatic stress disorder. *Journal of Trauma and Dissociation, 17*(4), 494–510.

59. Which of the following is TRUE regarding naltrexone?

A. It is metabolized by the CYP450 enzyme system.
B. It is safe to be given to patients who are abusing opioid medications.
C. It is available in both oral and injectable forms.
D. Weight gain is a common side effect.
E. Dose adjustment is necessary for patients with mild renal impairment.

ANSWER: C

Naltrexone is available in both oral and injectable forms. It is not metabolized by the CYP450 system, thus reducing risk of drug–drug interactions. Patients must be opioid free for 7 to 10 days before starting treatment. Weight gain is unusual. Dose adjustment is generally not needed for patients with mild renal impairment.

REFERENCE

Stahl, S. M., & Grady, M. M. (2011). *Stahl's essential psychopharmacology: The prescriber's guide* (4th ed.). Cambridge, UK: Cambridge University Press.

60. According to learning theory, which of the following terms best explains the therapeutic aim of exposure therapy for anxiety disorders?

A. Fear extinction
B. Harm avoidance
C. Reward dependence
D. Positive reinforcement
E. Harm reduction

ANSWER: A

Fear extinction (or extinction of the conditional response to trauma cues) best explains the therapeutic aim of exposure therapy. Learning theory gave rise to both classical and operant conditioning. Exposure therapy, in particular, attempts to uncouple exposure to a conditioned stimulus from the fear response by exposing a patient to the conditioned stimulus in a benign environment. Over time, the patient is able to learn that the stimulus itself is benign. Studies of exposure therapy, including, for instance, Prolonged Exposure Therapy and Narrative Exposure Therapy, are nearly uniformly positive, although some have suggested that self-selection bias among patients with PTSD may contribute to these results.

REFERENCE

Cusack, K., Jonas, D. E., Forneris, C. A., Wines, C., Sonis, J., Middleton, J. C., ..., Gaynes, B. N. (2016). Psychological treatments for adults with posttraumatic stress disorder: A systematic review and meta-analysis. *Clinical Psychology Review, 43*, 128–141.

61. What is the role of benzodiazepines in treating PTSD?

A. They are considered first-line treatments.
B. They should be considered but only in conjunction with first-line treatments.
C. They should be used as needed for panic attacks in PTSD.
D. They may be used to enhance outcomes of psychotherapy.
E. They are considered relatively contraindicated.

ANSWER: E

Benzodiazepines are considered relatively contraindicated for the treatment of PTSD. Not only have several randomized clinical studies (both in isolation and in meta-analysis) demonstrated inefficacy of benzodiazepines for PTSD treatment and prevention, but benzodiazepine use has been associated with greater risk of PTSD after a trauma, worse psychotherapy outcomes, and substance use disorders. Benzodiazepines are not recommended as PRNs for panic attacks in any condition. Panic attacks typically last 30 to 60 minutes, but oral benzodiazepines take upwards of an hour to cross the blood–brain barrier for efficacy. Therefore, by the time of benzodiazepine effect, the panic attack has largely if not entirely subsided. Patients are apt to attribute this symptom resolution to the benzodiazepine, thus reinforcing their psychological dependence on the medication due to the post hoc, ergo propter hoc logical fallacy.

REFERENCE

Guina, J., Rossetter, S. R., DeRhodes, B. J., Nahhas, R. W., & Welton, R. S. (2015). Benzodiazepines for PTSD: A systematic review and meta-analysis. *Journal of Psychiatric Practice, 21*, 281–303.

62. After inefficacy with SSRI monotherapy for moderately severe major depression, what is a reasonable next step?

A. Switch to bupropion.
B. Switch to phenelzine.
C. Augment with alprazolam.
D. Augment with risperidone.
E. Use ECT.

ANSWER: A

After poor response with an SSRI, the next reasonable step is either augmentation or switching. Augmentation with bupropion or cognitive behavioral therapy or switching to bupropion, venlafaxine, or cognitive behavioral therapy are the recommended next steps. The American Psychiatric Association guidelines for managing major depression recommend ECT for severe depression or depression with suicidal thoughts or psychotic symptoms.

REFERENCE

American Psychiatric Association. (2010). *Practice guideline for the treatment of patients with major depressive disorder* (3rd ed.). Retrieved from psychiatryonline.org/

63. Vortioxetine, vilazodone, and levomilnacipran are recently FDA approved agents for the treatment of major depressive disorder. Which of the following statements is TRUE of all three medications?

A. Negligible sexual side effects
B. Negligible gastrointestinal side effects
C. Negligible weight gain
D. Negligible effect on sleep

ANSWER: C

No significant weight gain was observed with any of the three medications. Current data are insufficient to make a conclusion regarding sexual functioning. All three medications can cause gastrointestinal side effects. Vilazodone and levomilnacipran can cause insomnia.

REFERENCE

Deardorff, W. J., & Grossberg, G. T. (2014). A review of the clinical efficacy, safety and tolerability of the antidepressants vilazodone, levomilnacipran and vortioxetine. *Expert Opinion on Pharmacotherapy, 15*, 2525–2542.

64. Which of the following classes of agents or modalities of treatment has the strongest data for efficacy in the management of major depressive disorder with atypical features?

A. MAOIs
B. ECT
C. TCAs
D. SSRIs
E. SNRIs

ANSWER: A

MAOIs have greater efficacy than TCAs in treating patients with major depressive disorder with atypical features. Some data support the use of SSRIs, bupropion, and cognitive behavioral therapy. ECT is also an effective treatment. Nevertheless, SSRIs typically remain first-line treatment clinically given their better tolerability.

REFERENCE

American Psychiatric Association. (2010). *Practice guideline for the treatment of patients with major depressive disorder* (3rd ed.). Retrieved from psychiatryonline.org/

65. Repetitive transcranial magnetic stimulation is approved for use in patients with major depressive disorder who have had unsatisfactory response to at least how many antidepressant trials for the current episode of illness?

A. One
B. Two
C. Three
D. Four

ANSWER: A

Repetitive transcranial magnetic stimulation is approved for use in patients with major depressive disorder who have not had a satisfactory response to at least one antidepressant trial.

REFERENCE

American Psychiatric Association. (2010). *Practice guideline for the treatment of patients with major depressive disorder* (3rd ed.). Retrieved from psychiatryonline.org/

66. What is the required minimum washout time between citalopram and a switch to an MAOI?

A. 1 week
B. 2 weeks
C. 5 weeks
D. 8 weeks

ANSWER: B

A 2-week washout period is recommended when transitioning from SSRIs or SNRIs to an MAOI. The one exception is fluoxetine, which requires a washout period of at least 5 weeks prior to starting an MAOI. This is necessary to prevent potentially lethal serotonin syndrome.

REFERENCE

American Psychiatric Association. (2010). *Practice guideline for the treatment of patients with major depressive disorder* (3rd ed.). Retrieved from psychiatryonline.org/

67. Gabapentin is FDA approved for which of the following indications?

A. Restless leg syndrome
B. Anxiety
C. Chronic pain
D. Bipolar disorder
E. Insomnia

ANSWER: A

Among the choices listed, gabapentin (as its prodrug gabapentin enacarbil, trade name Horizant) is FDA approved only for restless leg syndrome. It is frequently prescribed off label for chronic pain but among pain indications is FDA approved only for postherpetic neuralgia.

REFERENCE

Stahl, S. M., & Grady, M. M. (2011). *Stahl's essential psychopharmacology: The prescriber's guide* (4th ed.). Cambridge, UK: Cambridge University Press.

68. Which of the following medications is NOT FDA approved for treatment of acute bipolar mania?

A. Lithium
B. Quetiapine
C. Olanzapine
D. Valproic acid
E. Paliperidone

ANSWER: E

Paliperidone is not FDA approved for the treatment of acute bipolar mania. The other options are all approved.

REFERENCE

Stahl, S. M., & Grady, M. M. (2011). *Stahl's essential psychopharmacology: The prescriber's guide* (4th ed.). Cambridge, UK: Cambridge University Press.

69. Which of the following anticonvulsants is effective for the treatment of behavioral and psychological symptoms of dementia?

A. Carbamazepine
B. Topiramate
C. Lamotrigine
D. Gabapentin
E. None of the above

ANSWER: E

Routine clinical use of carbamazepine or valproic acid in the treatment of behavioral and psychological symptoms of dementia cannot be recommended because the benefits of such treatments are inconsistent. Gabapentin, lamotrigine, and topiramate are also not recommended.

REFERENCE

Konovalov, S., Muralee, S., & Tampi, R. (2008). Anticonvulsants for the treatment of behavioral and psychological symptoms of dementia: A literature review. *International Psychogeriatrics, 20*, 293–308.

70. Which of the following medications is FDA approved for the treatment of delirium?

A. Haloperidol
B. Risperidone
C. Olanzapine
D. Lorazepam
E. None of the above

ANSWER: E

There is no pharmacological intervention approved by the FDA for delirium.

REFERENCE

Campbell, N., Boustani, M. A., Ayub, A., Fox, G. C., Munger, S. L., Ott, C., ..., Singh, R.. (2009). Pharmacological management of delirium in hospitalized adults: A systematic evidence review. *Journal of General Internal Medicine, 24*, 848–853.

71. Which of the following is TRUE regarding management of delirium?

A. Data showed no superiority of risperidone over haloperidol.
B. Data showed superiority of olanzapine over haloperidol.
C. Cholinesterase inhibitors are effective in preventing delirium.
D. Benzodiazepines are effective in treatment of delirium.

ANSWER: A

Data indicate no superiority for atypical antipsychotics over haloperidol in managing delirium.

REFERENCE

Campbell, N., Boustani, M. A., Ayub, A., Fox, G. C., Munger, S. L., Ott, C., ..., Singh, R.. (2009). Pharmacological management of delirium in hospitalized adults: A systematic evidence review. *Journal of General Internal Medicine, 24*, 848–853.

72. The sedating effects of trazodone are attributed to antagonism of all the following receptors EXCEPT:

A. 5-HTA2a
B. D2
C. H1
D. Alpha-1

ANSWER: B

Sedating effects of trazodone are attributed to antagonism of 5-HT21, H1, and alpha-1 adrenergic receptors. They are not related to D2 receptor antagonism.

REFERENCE

McCall, C., & Winkelman, J. W. (2015). The use of hypnotics to treat sleep problems in the elderly. *Psychiatric Annals, 45*, 342–347.

73. Which of the following medications for insomnia has the shortest half-life?

A. Temazepam
B. Triazolam
C. Zolpidem
D. Zaleplon

ANSWER: D

Half-lives of the listed medications are as follows: temazepam: 3.5 to 18.4 hours; triazolam: 1.5 to 5.5 hours; zolpidem: 1.4 to 4.5 hours; zaleplon: 1 hour.

REFERENCE

McCall, C., & Winkelman, J. W. (2015). The use of hypnotics to treat sleep problems in the elderly. *Psychiatric Annals, 45*, 342–347.

74. Polypharmacy is a significant problem for patients with chronic pain. The combination of which of the following pain medications with an SSRI does NOT increase the risk of serotonin syndrome?

A. Tramadol
B. Oxycodone
C. Pregabalin
D. Sumatriptan

ANSWER: C

There is a risk of serotonin syndrome when combining SSRIs or TCAs with tramadol, sumatriptan, oxycodone, orhydrocodone. There is no risk of serotonin syndrome with pregabalin.

REFERENCE

Tobin, M., & Binius, T. (2015). Patients in pain: An approach to evaluation and management. *Psychiatric Annals, 45*, 406–410.

75. Which of the following medications has the largest evidence base for managing aggression in patients with traumatic brain injury?

A. Propranolol
B. Amantadine
C. Carbamazepine
D. Methylphenidate
E. Sertraline

ANSWER: A

Several studies support the use of amantadine, carbamazepine, methylphenidate, and sertraline for management of aggression in individuals with traumatic brain injury. The beta blocker propranolol has the largest evidence base for management of such aggression.

REFERENCE

Aaronson, A., Lloyd, R. B. (2015). Aggression after traumatic brain injury: A review of the current literature. *Psychiatric Annals, 45*, 422–426.

76. Which of the following medications is considered a first-line agent in the management of bipolar disorder in pregnancy?

A. Valproate
B. Lithium
C. Carbamazepine
D. Lamotrigine

ANSWER: B

Lithium is a first-line agent for the management of bipolar disorder in pregnancy despite concerns for increased risk of Ebstein's anomaly. The absolute risk of Ebstein's anomaly is 1 to 2/1,000 in first-trimester exposure as compared with 1/20,000 in the general population.

REFERENCE

Mittal, L., Wichman, C. L., & Byatt, N. (2015). Bipolar disorder in pregnancy and breastfeeding: A practical guide for general psychiatrist. *Psychiatric Annals, 45*, 411–416.

77. Discontinuation of clozapine is recommended in the face of which of the following cardiac issues?

A. QTc prolongation
B. Myocarditis
C. Orthostatic hypotension
D. Sinus tachycardia

ANSWER: B

Myocarditis and cardiomyopathy are both grounds for discontinuation of clozapine.

REFERENCE

Nielsen, J., Correll, C. U., Manu, P., & Kane, J. M. (2013). Termination of clozapine treatment due to medical reasons: When is it warranted and how can it be avoided? *Journal of Clinical Psychiatry, 74*, 603–613.

78. ECT is safe and effective in which trimester of pregnancy?

A. First
B. Second
C. Third
D. All of the above

ANSWER: D

ECT is safe during all trimesters of pregnancy and shows efficacy in all three trimesters.

REFERENCE

Saatcioglu, O., & Tomruk, N. B. (2011). The use of electroconvulsive therapy in pregnancy: A review. *Israel Journal of Psychiatry and Related Sciences, 48*, 6–11.

79. Antipsychotics are frequently used for treatment of behavioral symptoms in dementia and are associated with an increased risk of developing cerebrovascular adverse events (CVAEs). Which of the following statements is TRUE regarding the risk of CVAEs?

A. The risk of CVAEs increases after 3 months of treatment.
B. Cumulative exposure is associated with increased risk.
C. The risk is elevated during the first weeks of treatment.
D. Starting after 1 year, the risk is comparable to that for nonusers.

ANSWER: C

The risk of CVAEs is increased during the first weeks of treatment. The risk decreases over time and is comparable to that for nonusers after 3 months. Cumulative or chronic use is not associated with increased risk.

REFERENCE

Kleijer, B. C., van Marum, R J., Egberts, A. C. G., Jansen, P. A. F., Knol, W., & Heerdink, E. R. Risk of cerebrovascular events in elderly users of antipsychotics. *Journal of Psychopharmacology, 23*, 909–914.

80. Based on the Clinical Antipsychotic Trials of Intervention Effectiveness– Alzheimer's Disease (CATIE-AD), those treated with olanzapine and risperidone had higher rates of the following adverse events than those treated with quetiapine or placebo:

A. Parkinsonism
B. Sedation
C. Cognitive disturbances
D. Increased body weight

ANSWER: A

Parkinsonism or extrapyramidal signs were shown to be more prevalent in those treated with olanzapine and risperidone than in those treated with quetiapine or placebo. Sedation and body weight increased with treatment with antipsychotics. Cognitive disturbances were more common in those treated with olanzapine.

REFERENCE

Schneider, L. S., Tariot, P. N., Dagerman, K. S., Davis, S. M., Hsiao, J. K., Ismail, M. S., ..., Lieberman, J. A.; CATIE-AD Study Group. (2006). Effectiveness of atypical antipsychotic drugs in patients with Alzheimer disease. *New England Journal of Medicine, 355*, 1525–1538.

81. Atomoxetine and stimulant medications are the mainstay of treatment for attention deficit hyperactivity disorder (ADHD). The following medications are nonstimulants that can be used off label as alternative treatments for ADHD:

A. Bupropion, clonidine, imipramine, nortriptyline, modafinil
B. Bupropion, guanfacine, clonidine, imipramine, desipramine
C. Bupropion, clonidine, amitriptyline, nortriptyline, modafinil
D. Bupropion, guanfacine, prazosin, clonidine, modafinil

ANSWER: A

Nonstimulant, non-FDA-approved medications that can be used for the treatment of ADHD include guanfacine, clonidine, bupropion, imipramine, nortriptyline, and modafinil.

REFERENCE

Daughton, J., Liu, H., West, M., Swanson, D., & Kratochvil, C. J. (2010). Practical guide to ADHD pharmacotherapy. *Psychiatric Annals, 40*, 210–217.

82. All of the following benzodiazepines have a parenteral route of administration EXCEPT:

A. Diazepam
B. Chlordiazepoxide
C. Temazepam
D. Lorazepam

ANSWER: C

Diazepam and midazolam can be administered intravenously. Chlordiazepoxide can be administered intramuscularly. Lorazepam can be administered both intravenously and intramuscularly. Temazepam does not have a parenteral route of administration.

REFERENCE

Macaluso, M., Kalia, R., Ali, F., & Khan, A. Y. (2010). The role of benzodiazepine in the treatment of anxiety disorders: A clinical review. *Psychiatric Annals, 40*, 605–610.

83. Which of the following is an evidence-based treatment for PTSD?

A. Cognitive Processing Therapy
B. Prolonged Exposure Therapy
C. Fluoxetine
D. None of the above
E. All of the above

ANSWER: E

Cognitive Processing Therapy and Prolonged Exposure Therapy are evidence-based psychotherapy treatments for PTSD. Cognitive Processing Therapy involves written accounts of the trauma narrative with cognitive restructuring. In Prolonged Exposure Therapy, the trauma narrative is repeated orally during the therapy, and in vivo exposures are utilized to reduce distress and avoid situations impacted by the PTSD. Fluoxetine is an SSRI antidepressant that is used to reduce symptoms of PTSD. Each of these three treatments can help PTSD symptoms related to re-experiencing (such as nightmares), avoidance (such as detachment), and hyperarousal (such as hypervigilance).

REFERENCE

Ursano, R., Bell, C., Eth, S., Friedman, M., Norwood, A., Pfefferbaum, B., ..., Yager, J.; Work Group on ASD and PTSD; Steering Committee on Practice Guidelines. (2004). *Practice guideline for the treatment of patients with acute stress disorder and posttraumatic stress disorder.* Arlington, VA: American Psychiatric Association.

84. Which of the following is the LEAST helpful strategy in the ongoing outpatient treatment of a patient recently hospitalized for a suicide attempt?

A. Suicide prevention contract
B. Regular reassessment of risk
C. Psychoeducation for patient and family
D. Coordination of care with other treatment providers
E. Establishment of rapport between patient and psychiatrist

ANSWER: A

There is limited evidence to support the use of a suicide prevention contract in treatment of a patient with a history of suicide attempt. The other options are all part of a comprehensive treatment approach.

REFERENCE

Jacobs, D. G., Baldessarini, R. J., Conwell, Y., Fawcett, J. A., Horton, L., Meltzer, H., ..., Simon, R. I. (2003). Practice guideline for the assessment and treatment of patients with suicidal behaviors. Retrieved from http://psychiatryonline.org/pb/assets/raw/sitewide/practice_guidelines/guidelines/suicide.pdf

85. A patient taking carbamazepine presents with mouth sores and has bruises over the arms and legs. These are signs of what potentially dangerous side effect?

A. B12 deficiency
B. Eosinophilia
C. Aplastic anemia and agranulocytosis
D. Factor XIII deficiency
E. Vitamin C deficiency

ANSWER: C

Aplastic anemia and agranulocytosis are potential serious side effects, with a five to eight times greater risk among patients who take carbamazepine versus the general population.

REFERENCE

Stahl, S. M., & Grady, M. M. (2011). *Stahl's essential psychopharmacology: The prescriber's guide* (4th ed.). Cambridge, UK: Cambridge University Press.

86. Which of the following medication increases the plasma concentration of carbamazepine?

A. Fluoxetine
B. Phenytoin
C. Phenobarbital
D. Primidone
E. Carbamazepine

ANSWER: A

CYP450 3A4 inhibitors such as fluoxetine, fluvoxamine, and nefazodone can increase the plasma concentration of carbamazepine. The other options are CYP450 3A4 inducers, which can lower the level.

REFERENCE

Stahl, S. M., & Grady, M. M. (2011). *Stahl's essential psychopharmacology: The prescriber's guide* (4th ed.). Cambridge, UK: Cambridge University Press.

87. A typical starting daily dose of prazosin is:

A. 0.1 mg
B. 1 mg
C. 10 mg
D. 100 mg
E. 1,000 mg

ANSWER: B

Prazosin does not typically come in 0.1-mg, 100-mg, or 1,000-mg formulations. Prazosin 10 mg at bedtime can be used for treatment of nightmares in PTSD, but it is not a starting dose because it might abruptly cause hypotension in patients. Prazosin 1 mg at bedtime is a typical daily starting dose.

REFERENCE

Kung S., Espinel, Z., & Lapid, M. I.. (2012). *Treatment of nightmares with prazosin: A systematic review. Mayo Clinic Proceedings, 87,* 890–900.

88. Valproic acid with which of the of PTSD?

A. Irritability
B. Flashbacks
C. Nightmares
D. Avoidance
E. Dissociative amnesia

ANSWER: A

Valproic acid can help with PTSD hyperarousal symptoms, such as irritability, but it is not considered an evidence-based treatment for re-experiencing, avoidance, or memory symptoms.

REFERENCE

Friedman, M. (2006). Posttraumatic stress disorder among military returnees from Afghanistan and Iraq. *American Journal of Psychiatry, 163,* 586–593.

89. Cognitive Processing Therapy typically involves:

A. Audiotaped sessions
B. Detailed written trauma narratives
C. Rating distress during in vivo assignments
D. Sleep diary
E. 20 sessions

ANSWER: B

Unlike Prolonged Exposure Therapy, Cognitive Processing Therapy does not involve audiotaped sessions or rating distress during in vivo assignments. Cognitive Processing Therapy involves writing detailed trauma narratives multiple times during the course of the therapy and does not involve use of a sleep diary (which is used in Cognitive Behavioral Therapy for Insomnia) and is usually 12 sessions long.

REFERENCES

Monson, C., Schnurr, P. P., Resick, P. A., Friedman, M. J., Young-Xu, Y., Stevens, S. P. (2006). Cognitive Processing Therapy for veterans with military-related posttraumatic stress disorder. *Journal of Consulting and Clinical Psychology, 74,* 898–907.

Steenkamp, M., Litz, B. T., Hoge, C. W., Marmar, C. R. (2015). Psychotherapy for military-related PTSD: A review of randomized clinical trials. *JAMA, 314,* 489–500.

90. Prolonged Exposure Therapy involves the use of:

A. Imaginal exposure
B. In vivo exposure
C. Sleep diary
D. Six total sessions
E. A and B

ANSWER: E

Prolonged Exposure Therapy involves the use of both imaginal exposure and in vivo exposure. That is, patients listen to audiotaped sessions involving their verbal narrative of trauma accounts repeatedly during the therapy, as well as doing activities that they usually avoid due to their PTSD. A sleep diary is not part of the Prolonged Exposure Therapy protocol, which generally lasts for about 10 sessions.

REFERENCE

Steenkamp, M., Litz, B. T., Hoge, C. W., Marmar, C. R. (2015). Psychotherapy for military-related PTSD: A review of randomized clinical trials. *JAMA, 314,* 489–500.

91. Which of the following can lower the plasma level of carbamazepine?

A. Phenobarbital
B. Phenytoin
C. Primidone
D. Carbamazepine
E. All of the above

ANSWER: E

All of the above medications can lower plasma levels of carbamazepine, including carbamazepine itself by autoinduction (CYP450 3A4 enzyme).

REFERENCE

Stahl, S. M., & Grady, M. M. (2011). *Stahl's essential psychopharmacology: The prescriber's guide* (4th ed.). Cambridge, UK: Cambridge University Press.

92. A 50-year-old male is in a car accident and is diagnosed with acute stress disorder 1 week later. Which of the following is recommended for his initial treatment plan?

A. Drug testing
B. Providing a safe environment
C. Prazosin
D. Psychological debriefing
E. Cognitive Processing Therapy

ANSWER: B

For acute stress disorder, providing a safe environment with basic needs met is an important part of the treatment plan. Drug testing is not specifically indicated for evaluation or treatment of acute stress disorder. Psychological debriefing might cause worsened outcomes. Prazosin and Cognitive Processing Therapy are treatments that have been use for PTSD, but it is not confirmed that these would be necessary or recommended for acute stress disorder, which may resolve before PTSD develops.

REFERENCE

Ursano, R., Bell, C., Eth, S., Friedman, M., Norwood, A., Pfefferbaum, B., ..., Yager, J.; Work Group on ASD and PTSD; Steering Committee on Practice Guidelines. (2004). *Practice guideline for the treatment of patients with acute stress disorder and posttraumatic stress disorder*. Arlington, VA: American Psychiatric Association.

93. The treatment with the strongest evidence for panic disorder is:

A. Supportive therapy
B. Couples therapy
C. Cognitive behavioral therapy
D. Eye Movement Desensitization and Reprocessing (EMDR)
E. Psychodynamic therapy

ANSWER: C

While there may be case reports for some of the other choices to help panic disorder symptoms, cognitive behavioral therapy (CBT) is considered the treatment of choice for psychotherapy for panic disorder. CBT for panic disorder includes elements of psychoeducation, cognitive restructuring of maladaptive thoughts that can be an obstacle to quick resolution of a panic attack, interoceptive exposures (intentionally creating symptoms that mimic a panic attack), situational exposures (creating a hierarchy of feared or avoided situations), and modifying safety behaviors (such as checking one's pulse) that may be maintaining anxiety about a situation.

REFERENCE

Stein, M., Goin, M. K., Pollack, M. H., Roy-Byrne, P., Sareen, J., Simon, N. M., & Campbell-Sills, L. (2010). *Practice guideline for the treatment of patients with panic disorder*. Arlington, VA: American Psychiatric Association.

94. Which of the following is not indicated for the treatment of panic disorder?

A. Clonazepam
B. Venlafaxine
C. Nortriptyline
D. Gabapentin
E. Sertraline

ANSWER: D

Gabapentin is not specifically indicated for panic disorder. Clonazepam is a benzodiazepine that may reduce panic attack symptoms but should be given short-term given the risks with using benzodiazepines longer-term. Venlafaxine, nortriptyline, and sertraline all may help reduce the frequency of panic attacks.

REFERENCE

Stein, M., Goin, M. K., Pollack, M. H., Roy-Byrne, P., Sareen, J., Simon, N. M., & Campbell-Sills, L. (2010). *Practice guideline for the treatment of patients with panic disorder.* Arlington, VA: American Psychiatric Association.

95. Which psychotherapeutic approach has the largest evidence base for the treatment of suicidal patients?

A. Cognitive behavioral therapy
B. Dialectical behavior therapy
C. Interpersonal therapy
D. Psychoanalysis
E. Group psychotherapy

ANSWER: A

All of the above psychotherapeutic approaches for the treatment of the suicidal patient have shown benefit; however, cognitive behavioral therapy has the largest evidence base.

REFERENCE

Sudak, H. S. (2009). Suicide. In B. J. Sadock, V. A. Sadock, P. Ruiz, & H. I. Kaplan (Eds.), *Kaplan and Sadock's comprehensive textbook of psychiatry* (9th ed., p. 2725). Philadelphia, PA: Wolters Kluwer Health/Lippincott Williams and Wilkins.

96. In treatment of personality disorders, which of the following psychotherapeutic approaches should be avoided?

A. Maintenance of professional objectivity
B. Giving concrete advice on personal and social problems
C. Initial focus on the patient's chief complaint
D. Goal setting
E. Emphasis on healthy lifestyle choices

ANSWER: B

Giving concrete advice on personal and social problems to patients with a variety of personality disorders may elicit resentment, dependence, or noncompliance with treatment. Although specific personality disorders utilize different treatment modalities, there are several general psychotherapeutic principles that can be helpful in treatment of patients with personality disorders. To establish rapport, an initial focus on the patient's chief complaint and an emphasis on healthy lifestyle choices may be helpful, particularly if patients were "forced into treatment" by a friend or family member. Goal setting helps patients to focus the therapy and achieve a sense of accomplishment. Maintenance of professional objectivity is necessary to cope with strong feelings of countertransference.

REFERENCE

Cloninger, C. R., & Svrakic, D. M. (2009). Personality disorders. In B. J. Sadock, V. A. Sadock, P. Ruiz, & H. I. Kaplan (Eds.), *Kaplan and Sadock's comprehensive textbook of psychiatry* (9th ed., pp. 2234–2236). Philadelphia, PA: Wolters Kluwer Health/Lippincott Williams and Wilkins.

97. Which of the following medications prescribed for insomnia is LEAST likely to be habit-forming?

A. Zaleplon
B. Zolpidem
C. Eszopiclone
D. Temazepam
E. Trazodone

ANSWER: E

Trazodone is not habit-forming. Risk of dependence is seen for the other options.

REFERENCE

Stahl, S. M., & Grady, M. M. (2011). *Stahl's essential psychopharmacology: The prescriber's guide* (4th ed.). Cambridge, UK: Cambridge University Press.

98. Which of the following is NOT an acetylcholinesterase inhibitor prescribed for treatment of major neurocognitive disorder due to Alzheimer's disease?

A. Donepezil
B. Rivastigmine
C. Galantamine
D. Memantine

ANSWER: D

Memantine is an NMDA receptor antagonist prescribed for moderate to severe major neurocognitive disorder due to Alzheimer's disease. The other three options are acetylcholinesterase inhibitors.

REFERENCE

Stahl, S. M., & Grady, M. M. (2011). *Stahl's essential psychopharmacology: The prescriber's guide* (4th ed.). Cambridge, UK: Cambridge University Press.

99. Lamotrigine is FDA approved for which of the following indications?

A. Maintenance treatment of bipolar I disorder
B. Acute treatment of bipolar depression
C. Acute treatment of bipolar mania
D. Adjunctive treatment of major depressive disorder
E. Behavioral and psychological symptoms of dementia

ANSWER: A

Although lamotrigine is used off label for bipolar depression, bipolar mania, and major depressive disorder, it is FDA approved only for maintenance treatment of bipolar I disorder. There are no FDA approved medications for the behavioral and psychological symptoms of dementia.

REFERENCE

Stahl, S. M., & Grady, M. M. (2011). *Stahl's essential psychopharmacology: The prescriber's guide* (4th ed.). Cambridge, UK: Cambridge University Press.

100. OCD symptoms may be reduced by all of the following EXCEPT:

A. Fluvoxamine
B. Exposure and Response Prevention Therapy
C. Cognitive restructuring
D. Clonazepam
E. Sertraline

ANSWER: D

Fluvoxamine and sertraline, Exposure and Response Prevention (ERP) Therapy, and cognitive restructuring (i.e., during cognitive behavioral therapy) are all evidence-based methods to treat OCD. Clonazepam is not generally used to treat underlying, core symptoms of OCD.

REFERENCE

Koran, L., Simpson, H. B.. (2013). *Guideline watch: Practice guideline for the treatment of patients with obsessive–compulsive disorder.* Arlington, VA: American Psychiatric Association.

101. Clonidine is FDA approved for treatment of which of the following psychiatric disorders?

A. Tourette's syndrome
B. Opioid withdrawal
C. ADHD
D. PTSD
E. All of the above

ANSWER: C

Although clonidine is commonly used off label for all the above indications, the only psychiatric disorder for which it is FDA approved is ADHD.

REFERENCE

Stahl, S. M., & Grady, M. M. (2011). *Stahl's essential psychopharmacology: The prescriber's guide* (4th ed.). Cambridge, UK: Cambridge University Press.

102. Which of the following medications is NOT FDA approved for the treatment of insomnia?

A. Trazodone
B. Suvorexant
C. Flurazepam
D. Zolpidem
E. Doxepin

ANSWER: A

Although it is commonly used to treat insomnia in individuals with depression, trazodone is not FDA approved for the treatment of insomnia. Suvorexant, flurazepam, zolpidem, and doxepin are all FDA approved for the treatment of insomnia.

REFERENCE

Lee-Iannotti, J. K., & Parish, J. M. (2016). Suvorexant: A promising, novel treatment for insomnia. *Neuropsychiatric Disease and Treatment, 12*, 491–495.

Neubauer, D. N. (2014). New and emerging pharmacotherapeutic approaches for insomnia. *International Review of Psychiatry, 26*, 214–224.

103. Suvorexant exerts its hypnotic effect through which of the following mechanisms?

A. Selective melatonin receptor agonism
B. Selective histamine H1 receptor antagonism
C. Benzodiazepine receptor agonism
D. Orexin receptor antagonism
E. Serotonin antagonism and reuptake inhibition (SARI)

ANSWER: D

Suvorexant exerts its hypnotic effect through orexin (also known as hypocretin) receptor antagonism. Ramelteon is a selective melatonin receptor agonist. Doxepin is a selective histamine H1 receptor antagonist. Benzodiazepine receptor agonism is the mechanism of action for all benzodiazepines and nonbenzodiazepine hypnotics like zolpidem, zaleplon, and eszopiclone. Trazodone is a serotonin antagonist and reuptake inhibitor.

REFERENCES

Fagiolini, A., Comandini, A., Catena Dell'Osso, M., & Kasper, S. (2012). Rediscovering trazodone for the treatment of major depressive disorder. *CNS Drugs, 27*, 1033–1049.

Lee-Iannotti, J. K., & Parish, J. M. (2016). Suvorexant: A promising, novel treatment for insomnia. *Neuropsychiatric Disease and Treatment, 12*, 491–495.

Neubauer, D. N. (2014). New and emerging pharmacotherapeutic approaches for insomnia. *International Review of Psychiatry, 26*, 214–224.

104. Which of the following medications can give a false positive urine drug screen for amphetamines?

A. Valproic acid
B. Acetaminophen
C. Mirtazapine
D. Bupropion
E. Prazosin

ANSWER: D

False positive urine drug screen for amphetamines can occur with the use of bupropion. Other psychotropic medications that can cause false positive urine screens for amphetamines include chlorpromazine and trazodone.

REFERENCE

Brahm, N. C., Yeager, L. L., Fox, M. D., Farmer, K. C., & Palmer, T. A. (2010). Commonly prescribed medications and potential false-positive urine drug screens. *American Journal of Health-System Pharmacy, 67*, 1344–1350.

105. Adding which of the following medications improves antipsychotic-induced sexual dysfunction?

A. Sildenafil
B. Bupropion
C. Mirtazapine
D. Selegiline
E. Benztropine

ANSWER: A

Sexual dysfunction is common among individuals taking antipsychotic medications, with a reported prevalence rate of 45% to 80% among males and 30% to 80% in females. In a randomized controlled trial, the addition of sildenafil was found to reverse sexual dysfunction among males with schizophrenia or delusional disorder when compared with placebo. A randomized controlled study of selegiline versus placebo did not show any benefit for selegiline for antipsychotic-induced sexual dysfunction among men with schizophrenia. There are no controlled studies for the use of bupropion, mirtazapine, or benztropine for the management of antipsychotic-induced sexual dysfunction.

REFERENCES

Berner, M. M., Hagen, M., & Kriston, L. (2007). Management of sexual dysfunction due to antipsychotic drug therapy. *Cochrane Database of Systematic Reviews, 1*, CD003546.

Park, Y. W., Kim, Y., & Lee, J. H. (2012). Antipsychotic-induced sexual dysfunction and its management. *World Journal of Men's Health, 30*, 153–159.

106. A 40-year-old woman who has been treated with haloperidol for delirium in the intensive care unit develops

fever, muscle stiffness, tremor, and altered mental status. Her creatine phosphokinase (CPK) level is also elevated. What is the most likely cause of these symptoms?

A. Serotonin syndrome
B. Toxicity due to haloperidol serum level
C. Neuroleptic malignant syndrome
D. Haloperidol allergy
E. Tardive dyskinesia

ANSWER: C

This individual has developed neuroleptic malignant syndrome (NMS), a severe form of extrapyramidal syndrome that can occur at any time and with any dose of a neuroleptic agent. The risk of NMS is higher with the use of a high-potency antipsychotic agent like haloperidol.

REFERENCE

Seitz, D. P., & Gill, S. S. (2009). Neuroleptic malignant syndrome complicating antipsychotic treatment of delirium or agitation in medical and surgical patients: Case reports and a review of the literature. *Psychosomatics, 50*, 8–15.

107. Which of the following drugs reduces the risk of suicide in patients with bipolar disorder?

A. Valproic acid
B. Haloperidol
C. Lamotrigine
D. Lithium
E. Carbamazepine

ANSWER: D

Lithium may have antisuicidal effects by reducing relapse of mood episodes, decreasing aggression, and possibly reducing impulsivity.

REFERENCE

Cipriani, A., Hawton, K., Stockton, S., & Geddes, J. R. (2013). Lithium in the prevention of suicide in mood disorders: Updated systematic review and meta-analysis. *British Medical Journal, 346*, f3646.

108. Which of the following antipsychotic medications has the highest risk of seizures when used in individuals with schizophrenia and mood disorders?

A. Clozapine
B. Thioridazine
C. Haloperidol
D. Risperidone
E. Aripiprazole

ANSWER: A

A recent study found that the risk of antipsychotic-related seizures was highest for clozapine followed by thioridazine, chlorprothixene, and haloperidol as compared with risperidone and aripiprazole when used in individuals with schizophrenia and mood disorders.

REFERENCE

Wu, C. S., Wang, S. C., Yeh, I. J., & Liu, S. K. (2016). Comparative risk of seizure with use of first- and second-generation antipsychotics in patients with schizophrenia and mood disorders. *Journal of Clinical Psychiatry, 77*, e573–e579.

109. Which one of the following is the MOST common adverse effect associated with the use of trazodone?

A. Priapism
B. Drowsiness
C. Headache
D. Dizziness
E. Dry mouth

ANSWER: B

The most common adverse effect associated with the use of trazodone is drowsiness (somnolence/sedation). This is followed by headache, dizziness, and dry mouth. Priapism is a dramatic but rare adverse effect seen with the use of trazodone. Trazodone should be used with caution in men who have conditions that might predispose them to priapism (e.g., sickle-cell anemia, multiple myeloma) or in men with anatomical deformation of the penis (e.g., cavernosal fibrosis or Peyronie's disease).

REFERENCE

Fagiolini, A, Comandini, A., Catena Dell'Osso, M., & Kasper, S. (2012). Rediscovering trazodone for the treatment of major depressive disorder. *CNS Drugs, 26*, 1033–1049.

110. Which of the following FDA-approved drugs for the treatment of ADHD exerts its therapeutic effects via selective norepinephrine reuptake inhibition?

A. Methylphenidate
B. Atomoxetine
C. Lisdexamfetamine
D. Guanfacine
E. Clonidine

ANSWER: B

Atomoxetine is a selective norepinephrine reuptake inhibitor that is FDA approved for ADHD monotherapy. Guanfacine and clonidine are selective extended-release alpha-2 adrenergic agonists that are approved by the FDA for monotherapy and as adjuncts to stimulants. The stimulants are FDA approved for ADHD monotherapy and are thought to potently increase the extracellular levels of norepinephrine (NE) and dopamine (DA) throughout the brain by blocking NE and DA reuptake. Amphetamines also actively stimulate DA efflux through the DA transporter.

REFERENCES

Chan, E., Fogler, J. M., & Hammerness, P. G. (2016). Treatment of attention-deficit/hyperactivity disorder in adolescents: A systematic review. *JAMA, 315*, 1997–2008.

Spencer, R. C., Devilbiss, D. M., & Berridge, C. W. (2015). The cognition-enhancing effects of psychostimulants involve direct action in the prefrontal cortex. *Biological Psychiatry, 77*, 940–950.

111. Which of the following differentiates the mechanism of action of aripiprazole from other atypical antipsychotics?

A. Partial agonist at 5-HT2A receptors
B. Partial agonist at D2 receptors
C. Partial agonist at 5-HT1A receptors
D. Partial antagonist at 5-HT2A receptors
E. Partial antagonist at 5-HT3 receptors

ANSWER: B

The key feature that differentiates aripiprazole from other atypical antipsychotic medications is that aripiprazole is a partial agonist at the dopamine D_2 receptors.

REFERENCE

Di Sciascio, G., & Riva, M. A. (2015). Aripiprazole: From pharmacological profile to clinical use. *Neuropsychiatric Disease and Treatment, 11*, 2635–2647.

112. Which of the following is the most serious cardiac side effect of clozapine therapy?

A. Bradycardia
B. Hypotension
C. Endocarditis
D. Myocarditis
E. Pericarditis

ANSWER: D

Myocarditis is the most serious cardiac side effect of clozapine therapy. Individuals on clozapine have a 1,000- to 2,000-fold increase in relative risk of myocarditis when compared with the general population. Most cases of myocarditis occur within the first month of treatment. Myocarditis occurs due to acute immunoglobulin E–mediated hypersensitivity (type 1) reaction. Once the diagnosis of myocarditis is made, the clozapine prescription should be stopped immediately. Myocarditis is often considered a relative contraindication to restarting clozapine therapy. Based on common clinical practice and the time course of serious cardiac complications, it is recommended to get a baseline EKG prior to starting clozapine, with follow-up EKG 2 to 4 weeks after initiation and every 6 months thereafter.

REFERENCE

Lundblad, W., Azzam, P. N., Gopalan, P., & Ross, C. A. (2015). Medical management of patients on clozapine: A guide for internists. *Journal of Hospital Medicine, 10*, 537–543.

113. Which of the following is most consistently a dose-related side effect of valproic acid?

A. Liver toxicity
B. Fetal toxicity
C. Weight gain
D. Metabolic side effects
E. Menstrual side effects

ANSWER: C

The dose-dependent side effects of valproate include thrombocytopenia, hair loss, weight gain, and sedation. Chronic exposure to valproate causes liver and pancreatic injury, fetal toxicity, metabolic side effects, and menstrual irregularity.

REFERENCE

Stahl, S. M. (2013). *Stahl's essential psychopharmacology* (4th ed., pp. 373–375). New York, NY: Cambridge University Press.

114. Which of the following is NOT an appropriate reason to proceed with psychiatric treatment without informed consent?

A. The patient is legally deemed incompetent.
B. The patient is admitted to the inpatient unit for a suicide attempt and is refusing medication.
C. There is an acute emergency that poses significant danger to the patient.
D. Therapeutic privilege dictates that the physician can withhold information that would impair the patient's ability to make a competent decision.
E. A competent patient has completed a therapeutic waiver allowing the physician to make choices for them.

ANSWER: B

Even when admitted to an inpatient unit, patients have the right to refuse medications. If the physician believes that the patient's condition warrants treatment, the team may pursue a hearing with a judge for medications against will, but until that point treatment should not proceed without the patient's consent. The other options are circumstances in which treatment may proceed without informed consent from the patient.

REFERENCE

Baron, D. A., Dubin, W. R., & Ning, A. (2009). Other psychiatric emergencies. In B. J. Sadock, V. A. Sadock, P. Ruiz, & H. I. Kaplan (Eds.), *Kaplan and Sadock's comprehensive textbook ofpsychiatry* (9th ed., p. 2744). Philadelphia, PA: Wolters Kluwer Health/Lippincott Williams and Wilkins.

115. A 55-year-old woman presents to your clinic with a 4-month history of depressed mood, low energy, decreased enjoyment in life, and feelings of worthlessness and hopelessness. On review of systems she also reports severe menopausal hot flashes. Which of the following medications is FDA approved for the treatment of both her mood symptoms and hot flashes?

A. Conjugated estrogen
B. Paroxetine
C. Fluoxetine
D. Escitalopram
E. Venlafaxine

ANSWER: B

Paroxetine (Brisdelle, paroxetine mesylate) is FDA approved for the treatment of moderate to severe hot flashes (vasomotor symptoms) associated with menopause. Paroxetine (Pexeva, paroxetine mesylate) is also FDA approved for the treatment of major depressive disorder (MDD), obsessive compulsive disorder (OCD), panic disorder (PD), and generalized anxiety disorder (GAD) in adults. Most SSRIs and SNRIs (fluoxetine being a notable exception) are efficacious for the management of hot flashes. Gabapentin and pregabalin also have evidence in support of their use as nonhormonal treatment of hot flashes.

REFERENCE

FDA approves the first non-hormonal treatment for hot flashes associated with menopause. (2013) Retrieved from ttp://www.fda.gov/NewsEvents/Newsroom/PressAnnouncements/ucm359030.htm
Ruddy, K. J., & Loprinzi, C. L. (2015). Antidepressants decrease hot flashes and improve life quality. *Menopause, 22*, 587–588.

116. Which one of the following is an active metabolite of risperidone?

A. Asenapine
B. Ziprasidone
C. Iloperidone
D. Lurasidone
E. Paliperidone

ANSWER: E

Paliperidone (9-hydroxyrisperidone) is an active metabolite of risperidone.

REFERENCE

Corena-McLeod, M. (2015). Comparative pharmacology of risperidone and paliperidone. Drugs in R&D, *15*, 163–174.

117. Which of the following medications has the lowest weight gain potential when prescribed for the treatment of schizophrenia?

A. Asenapine
B. Iloperidone
C. Paliperidone
D. Lurasidone
E. Risperidone

ANSWER: D

Among the listed drugs, lurasidone has the lowest weight gain potential.

REFERENCE

Musil, R., Obermeier, M., Russ, P., & Hamerle, M. (2015). Weight gain and antipsychotics: A drug safety review. *Expert Opinion on Drug Safety, 14*, 73–96.

118. Vortioxetine is used principally to treat which of the following disorders?

A. Generalized anxiety disorder
B. Major depressive disorder
C. OCD
D. Panic disorder
E. PTSD

ANSWER: B

Vortioxetine is a novel antidepressant with multimodal activity. It is a $5HT_3$, $5HT_7$, and $5HT_{1D}$ receptor antagonist, a $5HT_{1B}$ partial agonist, a $5HT_{1A}$ agonist, and an inhibitor of the serotonin (5-HT) transporter. Vortioxetine has been FDA approved since late 2013 for the treatment of major depressive disorder in adults.

REFERENCE

Baldwin, D. S., Chrones, L., Florea, I., Nielsen, R., Nomikos, G. G., Palo, W., & Reines, E. (2016). The safety and tolerability of vortioxetine: Analysis of data from randomized placebo-controlled trials and open-label extension studies. *Journal of Psychopharmacology, 30*, 242–252.

119. Which of the following is a benefit of ziprasidone relative to most other antipsychotics?

A. Weight gain
B. QTc prolongation
C. Dizziness
D. Nonadherence
E. Sedation

ANSWER: A

A benefit of ziprasidone is lower risk of weight gain relative to most other antipsychotics. Ziprasidone prolongs QTc more than most other antipsychotics. Dizziness is a leading side effect of ziprasidone and other antipsychotics. Nonadherence is a risk with ziprasidone given more complicated dosing instructions than for some other antipsychotics (including twice-daily dosing and the need to take ziprasidone with food). Ziprasidone is moderately sedating, but some patients find it activating when used at a low dose.

REFERENCE

Stahl, S. M., & Grady, M. M. (2011). *Stahl's essential psychopharmacology: The prescriber's guide* (4th ed.). Cambridge, UK: Cambridge University Press.

120. Which of the following is a side effect of anticholinergic medications in the elderly?

A. Delirium
B. Falls
C. Urinary retention
D. Fecal impaction
E. All of the above

ANSWER: E

Anticholinergic medications have extensive side effects in younger adults, but the magnitude and impact of these side effects in older adults can be quite dangerous. In addition to delirium, falls, urinary retention, and fecal impaction, there is increased risk of cognitive impairment, exacerbation of narrow angle glaucoma, tachycardia, angina, and mucosal damage secondary to dry mouth, which may contribute to dental caries and even respiratory infection. These medications should be avoided in the elderly population.

REFERENCE

Gerretsen, P., & Pollock, B. G. (2011). Drugs with anticholinergic properties: A current perspective on use and safety. *Expert Opinion on Drug Safety, 10*, 751–765.

121. Which of the following electrolyte abnormalities is a possible side effect of prolonged treatment with lithium?

A. Hypercalcemia
B. Hypocalcemia
C. Hyponatremia
D. Hypomagnesemia
E. Hyperkalemia

ANSWER: A

Hypercalcemia is a possible adverse effect of long-term lithium use. A recent meta-analysis found that calcium and parathyroid hormone were increased by 10% when compared with normal values in individuals who were treated with lithium versus controls. Hence, calcium levels should be checked at least every 12 months in individuals taking lithium and more frequently if abnormal results are found or the patient has a family history of endocrine abnormalities.

REFERENCE

McKnight, R. F., Adida, M., Budge, K., Stockton, S., Goodwin, G. M., & Geddes, J. R. al. (2012). Lithium toxicity profile: A systematic review and meta-analysis. *Lancet, 379,* 721–728.

122. A 23-year-old woman was admitted to a medical unit for evaluation of cognitive slowing, ataxia, lethargy, drowsiness, nausea, and vomiting developing over 24 hours. She was started on valproic acid for bipolar disorder 4 weeks ago. The dose of the medication was titrated to 2,000 mg a day 1 week ago. On laboratory workup her serum valproic acid level is 87 μg/ml and the ammonia level is 145 μmol/L with normal AST and ALT levels. What is the next best step in the management of this patient's condition?

A. Continue valproic acid at the current dose and closely monitor the patient.
B. Discontinue the valproic acid and closely monitor the patient.
C. Discontinue the valproic acid and start hemodialysis for this patient.
D. Reduce the dosage of valproic acid to 1,000 mg a day and closely monitor the patient.
E. Start peritoneal dialysis on this patient.

ANSWER: B

This patient is presenting with valproate-induced hyperammonemic encephalopathy (VHE). As in this case, elevated ammonia not uncommonly presents with normal liver function tests. This condition is characterized by acute onset of lethargy, impaired consciousness, disorientation, cognitive slowing, and focal neurological deficits. In a case of asymptomatic hyperammonemia, valproic acid can be continued, and the patient can be closely monitored for the development of neurocognitive symptoms. Individuals with mild to moderate symptoms can be treated with a reduction in the dosage of valproic acid. The primary treatment of severe VHE is the withdrawal of valproic acid, which leads to complete recovery in most cases. Hemodialysis is often reserved for cases where the ammonia level is greater than 400 μg/ml or the patient develops significant clinical symptoms. There is some evidence for levocarnitine to treat VHE.

REFERENCE

Chopra, A., Kolla, B. P., Mansukhani, M. P., Netzel, P., & Frye, M. A. (2012). Valproate-induced hyperammonemic encephalopathy: An update on risk factors, clinical correlates and management. *General Hospital Psychiatry, 34,* 290–298.

123. Which of the following medications is NOT considered an appropriate choice for the treatment of depression in individuals with bulimia nervosa?

A. Paroxetine
B. Venlafaxine
C. Bupropion
D. Fluoxetine
E. Vortioxetine

ANSWER: C

Bupropion is not an appropriate medication for the treatment of depression in individuals with bulimia nervosa because its use may cause seizures in these individuals.

REFERENCE

Aigner, M., Treasure, J., Kaye, W., Kasper, S., & WFSBP Task Force On Eating Disorders. (2011). World Federation of Societies of Biological Psychiatry (WFSBP) guidelines for the pharmacological treatment of eating disorders. *World Journal of Biological Psychiatry, 12,* 400–443.

124. Which of the following is a correct statement regarding varenicline?

A. It is a α4β2 nicotinic receptor antagonist.
B. Nausea is the most common adverse effect with its use.
C. It cannot be combined with other smoking cessation medications.
D. It causes clinically important drug–drug interactions when combined with bupropion.
E. It has a half-life of about 4 hours.

ANSWER: B

Varenicline is a partial agonist of the α4β2 nicotinic receptor. The most common adverse event with its use is nausea, which occurs in about 30% of cases. Combining varenicline with other smoking cessation medications can increase the abstinence rates when compared with varenicline alone. Varenicline has no known clinically important drug–drug interactions. It has a half-life of about 24 hours.

REFERENCE

Burke, M. V., Hays, J. T., & Ebbert, J. O. (2016). Varenicline for smoking cessation: A narrative review of efficacy, adverse effects, use in at-risk populations, and adherence. *Patient Preference and Adherence, 10*, 435–441.

125. Which psychotherapeutic approach has the most empirical support for the treatment of borderline personality disorder?

A. Dialectical behavior therapy
B. Cognitive behavioral therapy
C. Interpersonal therapy
D. Problem-solving therapy
E. Supportive therapy

ANSWER: A

Dialectical behavior therapy (DBT) has the most evidence among psychotherapeutic approaches for treatment of borderline personality disorder.

REFERENCE

Rosenthal, M. Z., & Lynch, T. R. (2009). Dialectical behavior therapy. In B. J. Sadock, V. A. Sadock, P. Ruiz, & H. I. Kaplan (Eds.), *Kaplan and Sadock's comprehensive textbook of psychiatry* (9th ed., p. 2884). Philadelphia, PA: Wolters Kluwer Health/Lippincott Williams and Wilkins.

126. An 82-year-old man develops urinary retention, blurry vision, and confusion after taking several extra doses of amitriptyline to help him get to sleep. Blockade of which receptors likely precipitated these symptoms?

A. Dopamine 2 receptors
B. Nicotinic acetylcholine receptors
C. Serotonin 2A receptors
D. Alpha-1 adrenergic receptors
E. Muscarinic acetylcholine receptors

ANSWER: E

Amitriptyline and other tertiary amine TCAs such as imipramine, clomipramine, and doxepin are potent antagonists of muscarinic receptors. The core neurotransmitter aberration in delirium is reduced cholinergic activity at the muscarinic receptors. As in this patient, urinary retention and blurry vision are often symptoms of anticholinergic symptoms. The mnemonic "mad as a hatter (delirium), dry as a bone (anhidrosis), blind as a bat (blurry vision), red as a beet (flushing)" is helpful for remembering the features of the anticholinergic toxidrome.

REFERENCES

Gerretsen, P., & Pollock, B. G. (2011). Drugs with anticholinergic properties: A current perspective on use and safety. *Expert Opinion on Drug Safety, 10*, 751–765.
Mittal, V., Muralee, S., Williamson, D., McEnerney, N., Thomas, J., Cash, M., & Tampi, R. R. (2011). Delirium in the elderly: A comprehensive review. *American Journal of Alzheimer's Disease and Other Dementias, 26*, 97–109.

127. A 72-year-old patient is admitted to the hospital for treatment of pneumonia. Later that evening the patient becomes restless and pulls repeatedly on his IV line. Which of the following interventions should be considered initially?

A. Diphenhydramine 25 mg PO
B. Lorazepam 1 mg PO
C. De-escalation
D. Haloperidol 2 mg IM
E. Soft restraints

ANSWER: C

Behavioral interventions such as de-escalation, correcting sensory deficits, and addressing patients' concerns should be used as first-line treatment approaches for delirium. Haloperidol is commonly used for the treatment of behavioral disturbances of delirium, but its use can result in adverse effects. The use of haloperidol should be reserved for severe agitation that does not respond to dedicated behavioral interventions. Lorazepam and diphenhydramine should not be used because they are likely to worsen delirium. Seclusion and restraint are indicated only as last resorts when all less restrictive interventions have failed.

REFERENCES

Gerretsen, P., & Pollock, B. G. (2011). Drugs with anticholinergic properties: A current perspective on use and safety. *Expert Opinion on Drug Safety, 10,* 751–765.

Mittal, V., Muralee, S., Williamson, D., McEnerney, N., Thomas, J., Cash, M., & Tampi, R. R. (2011). Delirium in the elderly: A comprehensive review. *American Journal of Alzheimer's Disease and Other Dementias, 26,* 97–109.

128. Which of the following medications is MOST likely to contribute to delirium in an elderly patient?

A. Amlodipine
B. Hydrochlorothiazide
C. Propranolol
D. Simvastatin
E. Ranitidine

ANSWER: E

Ranitidine exhibits muscarinic antagonism. The other agents are much less likely to cause delirium.

REFERENCES

Gerretsen, P., & Pollock, B. G. (2011). Drugs with anticholinergic properties: A current perspective on use and safety. *Expert Opinion on Drug Safety, 10,* 751–765.

Mittal, V., Muralee, S., Williamson, D., McEnerney, N., Thomas, J., Cash, M., & Tampi, R. R. (2011). Delirium in the elderly: A comprehensive review. *American Journal of Alzheimer's Disease and Other Dementias, 26,* 97–109.

129. An elderly woman in a nursing facility repeatedly urinates in her bed. When she feels the need to urinate, she rings a bell for assistance to ambulate to the bathroom. Staff members often take 2 to 3 minutes to respond, and the woman becomes incontinent of urine. Which of the following strategies should be implemented first?

A. Scheduled voiding at regular intervals
B. Insertion of permanent urinary catheter
C. Disciplinary action of staff for neglect
D. Initiation of tolterodine 2 mg twice daily
E. Initiation of oxybutynin 5 mg twice daily

ANSWER: A

Behavioral interventions for the management of urinary incontinence should be implemented before initiation of medications. One effective strategy is regularly scheduled voiding. Medications such as tolterodine and oxybutynin are strongly anticholinergic and can cause considerable side effects in the elderly. The staff is taking 2 to 3 minutes to answer the call bell, which does not constitute neglect. A permanent urinary catheter puts the woman at risk of infection.

REFERENCE

Nygaard, I. (2010). Idiopathic urgency urinary incontinence. *New England Journal of Medicine, 363,* 1156–1162.

130. Which of the following statements is TRUE regarding psychotherapy for patients with intellectual disability?

A. Psychotherapy is not indicated because patients cannot engage in treatment.
B. Social skills interventions are useful for adults with intellectual disability, but they generally are not useful for children.
C. Behavioral therapy may be helpful for managing aggressive behaviors.
D. Group therapy should be avoided because it may be overstimulating.
E. Family therapy should be avoided because it may increase stigmatization of the patient.

ANSWER: C

Psychotherapy can be a useful treatment strategy for children and adults with intellectual disability. Evidence exists for use of behavioral, cognitive behavioral, psychodynamic, psychoeducational, and skill-training modalities. Individual, family, and group therapies are all valid approaches.

REFERENCE

King, B. H., Toth, K. E., Hodapp, R. M., & Dykens, E. H. (2009). Intellectual disability. In B. J. Sadock, V. A. Sadock, P. Ruiz, & H. I. Kaplan (Eds.), *Kaplan and Sadock's comprehensive textbook of psychiatry* (9th ed., p. 3467). Philadelphia, PA: Wolters Kluwer Health/ Lippincott Williams and Wilkins.

QUESTIONS AND ANSWERS

This chapter has accompanying questions and answers which are available to subscribers as part of the Oxford eLearning platform. To access the questions, follow the link below, or go to http://oxford-elearning.oup.com/books.

http://oxford-elearning.oup.com/books/test/67/10.1093/med/9780190265557.003.0028

29.

ETHICS

Deepti Challagolla

1. Which of the following is NOT one of the basic principles of ethics?

A. Autonomy
B. Justice
C. Paternalism
D. Nonmaleficence
E. Beneficence

ANSWER: C

Autonomy, justice, beneficence, and nonmaleficence are the four basic ethical principles.

REFERENCE

Sadock, B. J., Sadock, V. A., & Ruiz, P. (Eds.). (2009). *Kaplan and Sadock's comprehensive textbook of psychiatry* (9th ed., p. 4441). Philadelphia, PA: Lippincott Williams and Wilkins.

2. A patient was admitted to a psychiatric unit for suicidal ideation. Before initiating treatment, the treating psychiatrist explains the treatment procedure and obtains the patient's consent to start medication after discussing alternative treatments, risks, and benefits. Which ethical principle did the psychiatrist follow in doing the above?

A. Justice
B. Autonomy
C. Beneficence
D. Paternalism
E. Competence

ANSWER: B

Asking the patient to consent to treatment is an example of respecting a patient's autonomy. The physician must obtain patient's informed consent for tests and treatment. The physician should disclose information that the average person would need to know to make an informed medical decision. This information should include benefits, risks, costs, and alternatives to the proposed treatment. If the patient lacks medical capacity, the physician must obtain informed consent from an appropriate surrogate. Of note, a health care proxy is a document that allows a person to appoint another person (the *agent* of that proxy) to act as a surrogate for medical decisions. Strictly speaking, the word *proxy* should not be used to describe the surrogate for medical decisions.

REFERENCE

Sadock, B. J., Sadock, V. A., & Ruiz, P. (Eds.). (2009). *Kaplan and Sadock's comprehensive textbook of psychiatry* (9th ed., p. 4441). Philadelphia, PA: Lippincott Williams and Wilkins.

3. "First do no harm" refers to which of the basic ethical principles?

A. Beneficence
B. Autonomy
C. Justice
D. Nonmaleficence
E. Fiduciary duty

ANSWER: D

Nonmaleficence is the duty to do no harm. Beneficence is the principle under which physicians help patients and relieve suffering. Autonomy is the principle that a patient has a right to control what happens to his or her own body and make decisions freely and without coercion. Justice is fairness to equal resources/access to care. Fiduciary duty is the principle to work in the patient's best interests.

REFERENCE

Sadock, B. J., Sadock, V. A., & Ruiz, P. (Eds.). (2009). *Kaplan and Sadock's comprehensive textbook of psychiatry* (9th ed., pp. 4441–4443). Philadelphia, PA: Lippincott Williams and Wilkins.

4. A 14-year-old boy is brought by his mother to a neurologist in your group practice. The mother requests that the boy be tested for the *Huntingtin* gene because the boy's father was recently diagnosed with Huntington's disease. What should be the most appropriate response of the neurologist?

A. Do the testing as per the mother's request.
B. Require consent from both parents.
C. Do the testing only if the boy consents.
D. Inform the mother to bring the patient after 18 years.
E. Explain why this test is not appropriate to be performed at this time.

ANSWER: E

Presymptomatic testing for Huntington's disease should be performed only voluntarily at the request of an at-risk patient. It should not be ordered by others, and ordering should not be coerced by others. Such testing should not be ordered in minors who cannot give valid consent. Predictive testing should not be offered to minors or used in cases in which it would determine the carrier state of a relative who did not wish to know. It has also been argued that insurance companies and others with a financial interest should be precluded by law from asking for information on carrier state. Skilled counseling would be essential.

REFERENCE

Craufurd, D. I., & Harris, R. (1986). Ethics of predictive testing for Huntington's chorea: The need for more information. *British Medical Journal (Clinical Research Edition), 293*, 249–251.

5. A patient calls your office 1 hour prior to her actual appointment and informs you that she will not be able to attend that day's session because an emergency came up at work. What would you do in regard to charging the patient for the missed session?

A. Do not charge because she called before her appointment time.
B. Charge for the session if this is a self-pay patient.
C. Charge the patient for not calling well in advance.
D. Cancel all future appointments.
E. The decision to charge depends on advance agreement.

ANSWER: E

Patients need to be informed about a doctor's policies for missed appointments during initial visits. The individual physician determines treatment policies, but patients must know in advance to be able to make an informed decision about whether to accept the doctor's policy or to choose another doctor.

REFERENCE

Kaplan, H. I., Sadock, B. J., Grebb, J. A., & Sadock, V. A. (2007). Ethics in psychiatry. In *Kaplan and Sadock's synopsis of psychiatry: Behavioral sciences, clinical psychiatry* (10th ed., pp. 1383–1391). Baltimore, MD: Williams and Wilkins.

6. What are the ethical guidelines in regard to accepting gifts from patients?

A. Psychiatrists should accept any gift given by a patient to prevent the patient from feeling rejected.
B. Psychiatrists should never accept a gift from a patient.
C. Any gift worth less than $500 can readily be accepted.
D. Accepting a small gift from a patient is acceptable under certain circumstances.
E. None of the above.

ANSWER: D

The details of the case are important in determining whether or not to accept the gift. Exploitation involves using the therapeutic relationship for personal gain, such as hiring a patient or going into business with a patient. A physician should not have any business interactions with a patient aside from payment for treatment.

REFERENCE

Sadock, B. J., Sadock, V. A., & Ruiz, P. (Eds.). (2009). *Kaplan and Sadock's comprehensive textbook of psychiatry* (9th ed., pp. 4444). Philadelphia, PA: Lippincott Williams and Wilkins.

7. A patient can be involuntarily hospitalized under which of the following circumstances?

A. A patient poses imminent danger to him- or herself.
B. A patient poses imminent danger to others.
C. A patient demonstrates inability to meet basic needs.
D. All of the above.

ANSWER: D

Involuntary hospitalization is usually justified by a patient's imminent danger to him or herself or others, or an inability to meet basic needs. To meet these criteria, danger must be likely in the near future and related to a major mental illness.

REFERENCE

American Psychiatric Association. (2015). APA commentary on ethics in practice. Section 3—Practice domains, 3.2 Central ethical and professional practices in psychiatric care, Topic 3.2.6 Involuntary psychiatric treatment. Retrieved from https://www.psychiatry.org/File%20Library/Psychiatrists/Practice/Ethics/APA-Commentary-on-Ethics-in-Practice.pdf

8. Which of the following is NOT required of a psychiatrist to avoid patient abandonment?

A. Give the patient enough time to find a new therapist.
B. Help the patient find a new therapist.
C. Provide a letter of termination.
D. Provide medical records requested by the new therapist.
E. Provide enough medication to last beyond the date of termination.

ANSWER: E

It is unethical for a psychiatrist to terminate a patient without providing a proper referral. It is not unethical to refrain from providing medication beyond the termination date.

REFERENCE

Matrix Medical Communications. (2010). Terminating the treatment relationship. *Psychiatry (Edgmont)*, *7*(1), 40–42. Retrieved from http://www.ncbi.nlm.nih.gov/pmc/articles/PMC2848460/

9. Psychiatrists have an ethical obligation to do all of the following EXCEPT:

A. Report physician impairment
B. Participate in executions
C. Report physician incompetence
D. Report ethical misconduct
E. Report child abuse

ANSWER: B

Psychiatrists should not participate in torture, interrogations, or executions. Psychiatrists have the ethical obligation to report physician impairment, incompetence, and ethical misconduct, as well as to report child (and elder) abuse.

REFERENCE

American Psychiatric Association. (2013). The principles of medical ethics with annotations especially applicable to psychiatry. Section 7, point 5. Retrieved from https://www.psychiatry.org/File%20Library/Psychiatrists/Practice/Ethics/principles-medical-ethics.pdf

10. For how long should a patient's medical records be kept by a psychiatrist?

A. Only as long as the patient is in treatment
B. Until billing is submitted to the patient's insurance company
C. As long as possible
D. Indefinitely
E. Not consistently defined by statutes

ANSWER: E

There is no clear answer. Due to the variety of statutes, regulations, legal principles, and professional obligations affecting psychiatric records, the best risk management advice dictates that records should be kept for as long as possible. The safest and most conservative option is to never destroy patient records (i.e., keep records indefinitely). Perpetual maintenance may seem excessive, but there are many reasons the records may be needed in the future. If records cannot be kept indefinitely, they should be for as long.

REFERENCE

Lambert, K., & Wertheimer, M. (2016, March 2). Retaining patients' psychiatric records. *Psychiatric News*. Retrieved from http://psychnews.psychiatryonline.org/doi/full/10.1176/appi.pn.2016.3a20

11. Which one of the following is considered unethical behavior for a psychiatrist?

A. Transferring the care of a patient after noting romantic feelings toward the patient
B. Avoiding romantic relationships with a patient or ex-patient
C. Treating a new patient with whom the psychiatrist was sexually involved several years ago
D. Seeking supervision for erotic countertransference

ANSWER: C

Sexual activity with current and former patients is unethical. Likewise, any occasion in which the physician interacts with a current or former patient in ways that may preclude an intimate and nonprofessional relationship (as a date, intimate friend, etc.) should be avoided. Sex with patients or former patients is not acceptable under any circumstances. No former sexual partners should be accepted as patients.

REFERENCE

Aravind, V. K., Krishnaram, V. D., & Thasneem, Z. (2012). Boundary crossings and violations in clinical settings. *Indian Journal of Psychological Medicine, 23*, 21–24.

12. A 22-year-old patient recently diagnosed with schizophrenia presents with symptoms of paranoid delusions. He declines medication when he is alone with you but accepts in the presence of his mother, of whom he is paranoid. How should treatment proceed?

A. Do not start the medication because the patient's decision is influenced by the presence of his mother.
B. Start the medication because the patient has provided consent.
C. Await consent from the father.
D. Offer the patient a long-acting injectable medication.
E. Give the medication only when the mother is present.

ANSWER: A

This is a difficult clinical situation, and this question highlights the importance of respecting a patient's autonomy. Autonomy is the principle that a patient has a right to control what happens to his or her own body and make decisions freely and without coercion. Ethically speaking, if a patient cannot provide informed consent for medication, then pursuing surrogate consent from the local probate court (depending on local statute) would be appropriate.

REFERENCES

Matthews, E. (2000). Autonomy and the psychiatric patient. *Journal of Applied Philosophy, 17*, 59–70.
Sjostrand, M., & Helgesson, G. (2008). Coercive treatment and autonomy in psychiatry. *Bioethics, 22*, 113–120.

13. A psychiatrist performing a psychiatric evaluation to determine suitability for employment must inform the patient that:

A. The patient's employer has the right to withhold examination results from the patient.
B. The patient should be truthful.
C. There are limits to the patient's confidentiality.
D. The employer and the psychiatrist determine what information will be released.
E. The patient must comply with the treatment recommendations if treatment is indicated.

ANSWER: C

Patients should be informed of the limits of confidentiality at the beginning of the physician–patient relationship and as events arise that create potential revelations.

REFERENCE

American Psychiatric Association. (2015). APA commentary on ethics in practice. Section 3–Practice domains. 3.2 Central ethical and professional practices in psychiatric care, Topic 3.2.1 Confidentiality. Retrieved from https://www.psychiatry.org/File%20Library/Psychiatrists/Practice/Ethics/APA-Commentary-on-Ethics-in-Practice.pdf

14. Which of the following is an acceptable boundary crossing by a psychiatrist?

A. Meeting a patient over dinner for a session
B. Accepting an expensive wristwatch as a Christmas gift from a patient
C. Visiting a patient with a severe physical illness at home
D. Telling the patient explicit details about the psychiatrist's romantic relationship

ANSWER: C

Boundary violations are transgressions that are immediately harmful, are likely to cause future harm, or are exploitive of the patient. Boundary crossings are deviations from customary behavior, but they do not necessarily harm the patient and may allow for flexibility within the therapy.

REFERENCE

American Psychiatric Association. (2015). APA commentary on ethics in practice. Section 3—Practice domains, 3.2. Central ethical and professional practices in psychiatric care, Topic 3.2.7. Therapeutic boundary-keeping. Retrieved from https://www.psychiatry.org/File%20Library/Psychiatrists/Practice/Ethics/APA-Commentary-on-Ethics-in-Practice.pdf

15. If a patient's spouse emails the psychiatrist with questions regarding the patient's treatment, how should the psychiatrist proceed?

A. Reply to the email and answer the spouse's questions.
B. Call the patient to request verbal permission to communicate with the spouse.
C. Do not reply to the email.
D. Call the spouse to explain that email communication is not permitted.

ANSWER: C

In practices in which email is used as a means of communication, patients should sign a written agreement for communication via email and should be provided with a written policy during the initial visit. Guidelines include that email should not be for emergent or serious issues, and staff will not respond to emails from family members or others.

REFERENCE

Silk, K. R., & Yager, J. (2003). Suggested guidelines for e-mail communication in psychiatric practice. *Journal of Clinical Psychiatry, 64*, 799–806.

16. A psychiatrist refers patients to a drug abuse treatment facility, and she accepts $100 from the facility for each referral. Under which law can she be prosecuted?

A. Anti-Kickback Statute
B. False Claims Act
C. Stark Law
D. HIPAA
E. None of the above

ANSWER: A

The Anti-Kickback Statute prohibits the knowing, willful solicitation, receipt, or remuneration for patient referral or acquisition of goods or services for which payment is made under Medicare/Medicaid. A false claim is a claim submitted for reimbursement that misrepresents the type, price, description, or medical reason that necessitated the expense. The Stark Law prohibits physician self-referral. HIPAA is the Health Insurance Portability and Accountability Act of 1996 that protects health information.

REFERENCE

Yeatts, P. L. (2015). How to comply with the Anti-Kickback Statute. *Journal of the Medical Association of Georgia, 104*(3), 16–17.

17. An example of a false claim is:

A. A service that is billed but never provided
B. A diagnostic code used that does not match the diagnosis of the client
C. Upcoding or billing for a higher level of service than what was provided
D. Billing for unreasonable or unnecessary services
E. All of the above

ANSWER: E

A false claim is a claim submitted for reimbursement that misrepresents the type, price, description, or medical reason that necessitated the expense.

REFERENCE

Sherman, S. E. (1995). The False Claims Act: Litigating scientific misconduct. *Public Health Reports, 110*, 784–789.

18. Which of the following is NOT one of the four basic elements that must be proved by the patient (or a surrogate on behalf of the patient) in order for the plaintiff to prevail in cases of malpractice?

A. Duty of care to the patient
B. Breach of duty
C. Damages caused by breach of duty
D. Deviation from standard of care
E. Injury caused directly by breach of duty

ANSWER: D

The injured patient must show that the physician acted negligently in rendering care and that such negligence resulted in injury. To do so, four legal elements must be proved: a professional duty owed to the patient; breach of such duty; injury caused by the breach; and resulting damages. In terms of the "4 Ds," dereliction of duty directly causes damages. Physicians often deviate from standard of care per patient preference and may do so in a variety of instances where there are countervailing clinical and medical considerations at play.

REFERENCE

Bal, B.S. (2009) An introduction to medical malpractice in the United States. *Clinical Orthopaedics and Related Research, 467*, 339–347.

19. What are the current guidelines to publish scientific papers on patient cases in psychiatry?

A. A treating psychiatrist can publish case reports for scientific advancement.
B. Psychiatrists are prohibited from publishing any case reports of active patients or ex-patients.
C. Case reports can be published only after removing identifying patient information.
D. Scientific papers can be published after receiving verbal approval from patients.
E. A written informed consent is mandatory to publish case reports in psychiatry.

ANSWER: C

Informed consent from the patient is not required to publish case reports, but all identifying information should be hidden to protect the patient's confidentiality.

REFERENCE

Levine, S. B. & Stagno, S. J. (2001). Informed consent for case reports: The ethical dilemma of right to privacy versus pedagogical freedom. *Journal of Psychotherapy Practice and Research, 10*, 193–201.

20. Which of the following is NOT true about informed consent?

A. There are exceptions to informed consent.
B. Information can be withheld by the doctor in special circumstances if it is damaging to the patient.
C. Patients may waive the right to informed consent.
D. All medical situations, even emergencies, require informed consent.
E. Parents should provide informed consent for children.

ANSWER D

The following are the important exceptions to informed consent:

1. Genuine emergencies do not require informed consent. Emergency care occurs in the framework of implied or presumed consent. That is, in emergency situations in which reasonable persons would want the intervention, it is ethical to proceed as if consent exists.
2. Care for children or incompetent patients requires consent from parents or legally recognized surrogates. Assent of incompetent individuals (i.e., acquiescence as opposed to informed consent) is obtained whenever possible.
3. Patients may waive their right to informed consent. This exception, however, presumes competence to do so.
4. The doctrine of therapeutic privilege allows a physician to withhold information if it is truly damaging to the patient, but such exceptions are rare. Withholding information about side-effects of medications in the hope of improving adherence is unacceptable.

REFERENCE

American Psychiatric Association. (2015). APA commentary on ethics in practice. Section 3—Practice domains, 3.2 Central ethical and professional practices in psychiatric care, Topic 3.2.4 Informed consent. Retrieved from https://www.psychiatry.org/File%20Library/Psychiatrists/Practice/Ethics/APA-Commentary-on-Ethics-in-Practice.pdf

QUESTIONS AND ANSWERS

This chapter has accompanying questions and answers which are available to subscribers as part of the Oxford eLearning platform. To access the questions, follow the link below, or go to http://oxford-elearning.oup.com/books.

http://oxford-elearning.oup.com/books/test/67/10.1093/med/9780190265557.003.0029

30.

EPIDEMIOLOGY, BIOSTATISTICS, AND RESEARCH DESIGN

Mark Oldham

1. Which of the following correctly describes the interpretation of a *p* value?

A. The *p* value measures whether an observed result can be attributed to chance.
B. A *p* value of less .01 proves that the alternative hypothesis is false.
C. Higher *p* values indicate greater likelihood that the hypothesis is true.
D. A *p* value of .01 indicates a 1% chance the result is false.
E. Lower *p* values indicate greater practical relevance of results.

ANSWER: A

A *p* value measures whether an observed result can be attributed to chance.

REFERENCE

Nuzzo, R. (2014). Scientific method: Statistical errors. *Nature, 506*, 150–152.

2. An observational cohort study of community-dwelling elders identifies an association between sleeping pills and rate of falls over 12 months. Researchers discover that sleeping pills were prescribed preferentially to those with major neurocognitive disorder. The majority of falls occurred in the same group. Which of the following factors describes the association of sleeping pills with both major neurocognitive disorder and falls?

A. Mediation
B. Correlation
C. Collinearity
D. Confounding
E. Effect modification

ANSWER: D

Confounding occurs when a third variable is associated with both the exposure variable and the outcome of interest. This dual association can distort the "true" relationship between the exposure and outcome in either direction—either strengthening or weakening the statistical association or effect size. One can adjust for confounding using stratification and regression analyses. A mediator variable is a third (often unmeasured) variable that represents the actual mechanism whereby the first variable influences the outcome of interest. Correlation describes an association between two continuous variables. Collinearity (or multicollinearity) is similar to correlation in that two variables are so similar that knowledge of one predicts the other. Effect modification occurs when a third variable alters how the dependent and independent variables are related (e.g., delirium predicts long-term mortality among patients with hip fracture but only among those with baseline dementia).

REFERENCE

Sullivan, L. (2012). *Essentials of biostatistics in public health* (2nd ed., pp. 190–191). Burlington, MA: Jones and Bartlett Learning.

3. Randomization does which of the following?

A. Improves generalizability of results
B. Ensures that each group is equivalent
C. Allows for more sensitive statistical comparisons
D. Enhances the effect size of the studied treatment

E. Attempts to distribute unmeasured variables equally

ANSWER: E

The unique value of randomization is to allocate unmeasured variables as equally as possible. Measured variables can be accounted for using statistical analysis (such as a multivariable regression analysis), but unmeasured variables by definition cannot be controlled. Randomization clarifies the unique effect between the exposure and outcome. Generalizability hinges on sampling, not randomization. Although randomization *attempts* to distribute baseline characteristics equally among groups, randomization can fail. This tends to occur among smaller studies. Effect size is not influenced by randomization.

REFERENCE

Sullivan, L. (2012). *Essentials of biostatistics in public health* (2nd ed., pp. 13–14). Burlington, MA: Jones and Bartlett Learning.

4. A clinician wants to know whether a new medication improves cognitive symptoms in schizophrenia, and only 10% of those eligible for the study are willing to participate. The fact that so few of the eligible subjects agree to participate in this study compromises which of the following in this study?

A. Test-retest reliability
B. Interrater reliability
C. Internal validity
D. External validity
E. Utility

ANSWER: D

External validity describes how well a study generalizes to a broader population, which is compromised if only a small portion of potentially eligible persons agree to participate. Internal validity describes the degree to which each element of a test (such as a self-report scale) accurately represents the construct of interest (i.e., do all the questions accurately depict elements of a major depressive episode?). Reliability speaks to the consistency of a test such as from one test administration to another (test-retest) or between different people administering the test (interrater). Utility is a less-discussed metric but is no less important: it describes the usefulness of a particular test, screening tool, and so forth. A questionnaire that takes 30 minutes to screen for substance abuse would not be useful in a busy primary care clinic.

REFERENCE

Rothwell, P. M. (2005). External validity of randomised controlled trials: "To whom do the results of this trial apply?" *Lancet*, *365*, 82–93.

The following vignette is used for questions 5 through 10:

Ten of 50 patients evaluated at an outpatient clinic were found to have major depression. These patients were also assessed using a new screening questionnaire where a score of 5 or higher was predicted to correspond to major depression. Eight of the patients with major depression were positive on this new screen, whereas 5 of those without depression were also positive.

5. What is the point prevalence of major depression in this sample?

A. 5%
B. 10%
C. 15%
D. 20%
E. 25%

ANSWER: D

The prevalence, defined as the number of cases divided by sample size, is 20% (10/50).

REFERENCE

Sullivan, L. (2012). *Essentials of biostatistics in public health* (2nd ed., p. 26). Burlington, MA: Jones and Bartlett Learning.

6. Does this test have a higher specificity or sensitivity in detecting major depression in this sample?

A. It is more specific (35/40) than sensitive (8/10).
B. It is more specific (35/37) than sensitive (8/13).
C. It is more sensitive (35/40) than specific (8/10).
D. It is more sensitive (35/37) than specific (8/13).
E. Insufficient information is provided to calculate sensitivity and specificity.

ANSWER: A

The test has a sensitivity of 80% (8/10) and specificity of 88% (35/40). Sensitivity is the number of true positives (8) over the total number of those with the condition of

Table 30.1. SPECIFICITY

	MAJOR DEPRESSION	NO MAJOR DEPRESSION	*TOTALS*
Screen positive	8	5	13
Screen negative	2	35	37
Totals	10	40	50

interest (10), which means that the test was 80% sensitive in detecting major depression. Specificity is the number of true negatives (35 = total without depression [40] minus nondepressed patients who screened positive [5]) divided by the number of total without the condition (40) (Table 30.1).

REFERENCE

Sullivan, L. (2012). *Essentials of biostatistics in public health* (2nd ed., pp. 71–72). Burlington, MA: Jones and Bartlett Learning.

7. Based on the test performance in this sample, would this test be more meaningful as a screening instrument or a confirmatory test?

A. Screening instrument
B. Confirmatory test
C. Both
D. Neither

ANSWER: A

Screening or confirmatory instruments are meaningful based on how predictive they are in a particular population. To answer this question, positive and negative predictive values should be considered because, unlike sensitivity and specificity, they incorporate prevalence rates and describe the likelihood of disease. This test has a particularly high negative predictive value (35/37 = 95%), which means that the likelihood of a person having major depression is 5% if negative. Very few depressed patients would be "missed," thus making it good for screening. On the other hand, it has a fairly low positive predictive value (8/13 = 62%). Screening positive on this test means that a patient in this sample has about a two-thirds chance of actually having major depression. This test would yield far too many false positives to be used as a confirmatory test.

REFERENCE

Sullivan, L. (2012). *Essentials of biostatistics in public health* (2nd ed., pp. 71–72). Burlington, MA: Jones and Bartlett Learning.

8. What are the odds that a person screening positive on this test has major depression?

A. 8:5
B. 62%
C. 8:2
D. 80%
E. 8:50

ANSWER: A

Probability (or risk) is reported as a percent and represents the number of a particular outcome divided by the total sample. The probability that a person screening positive on this test has major depression is 5/13 (true positives divided by total positives). However, odds are calculated differently. Odds are calculated as the ratio of number of events to nonevents. This question defines the sample in question as those persons screening positive. Among these, then, events are those with major depression (true positives); nonevents are those without major depression (false positives). Here, the odds are 8 to 5.

REFERENCE

Sullivan, L. (2012). *Essentials of biostatistics in public health* (2nd ed., pp. 28–29). Burlington, MA: Jones and Bartlett Learning.

9. Provided the screening questionnaire yields a continuous value from 0 to 10, which of the following could be used to depict the trade-off between sensitivity and specificity at different cutoff values?

A. Normal distribution
B. Gaussian distribution
C. A nomogram of likelihood ratios
D. Receiver operating characteristic
E. Positive predictive value plotted against negative predictive value

ANSWER: D

The receiver operating characteristic (ROC) is a graphical plot of true positive rate (sensitivity) versus false positive rate (1 − specificity) that is often used to determine discrimination thresholds of screening tests. It is a visual representation of how well a particular test predicts a condition of interest at each cutoff value. An ROC may be depicted as a graph, or the area under the ROC may be reported numerically. An area under the ROC of 50% means that a test has no predictive value (i.e., a positive or negative value remains a 50-50 toss-up) with higher values being more robust tools for predicting the condition of interest. Normal distribution and Gaussian distribution refer to the same probability distribution often depicted as a bell curve, which presumes a random distribution of variables. A nomogram may be used to predict post-test probability. Positive and negative predictive values are not synonymous with sensitivity and specificity.

REFERENCE

Fogel, B. S. (2015). Rating scales and screening tests. In B. S. FogelBS & D. B. Greenberg (Eds.), *Psychiatric care of the medical patient* (3rd ed., pp. 78–79). New York, NY: Oxford University Press.

10. Suppose that this questionnaire has the same sensitivity and specificity in a second sample of patients, and that sample has twice the rate of major depression as the first (in the initial vignette). How does this influence positive and negative predictive values in this second sample?

A. Positive predictive value increases, negative predictive value decreases.
B. Positive predictive value increases, negative predictive value increases.
C. Positive predictive value decreases, negative predictive value decreases.
D. Positive predictive value decreases, negative predictive value increases.
E. Positive and negative predictive values remain the same.

ANSWER: A

Positive and negative predictive values are affected by prevalence, whereas sensitivity and specificity are unique to the test and independent of prevalence. Broadly speaking, with greater prevalence, the likelihood that *any* patient would be positive is greater. As a result, the positive predictive value of a positive test *increases*, whereas the negative predictive value *decreases*. Compare Table 30.1 with Table 30.2. Both screening instruments have 80% sensitivity and 87.5% specificity; however, the prevalence of depression differs in these two samples. The prevalence in the initial sample (in Table 30.1) is 20% (10/50) but 40% (80/200) in the second (Table 30.2). Positive and negative predictive values differ markedly as a result: in the first they are 62% and 95%, respectively, but in the second are 81% and 87%.

Table 30.2. SPECIFICITY

	MAJOR DEPRESSION	NO MAJOR DEPRESSION	*TOTALS*
Screen positive	64	15	79
Screen negative	16	105	121
Totals	80	120	200

REFERENCE

Fogel, B. S. (2015). Rating scales and screening tests. In B. S. FogelBS & D. B. Greenberg (Eds.), *Psychiatric care of the medical patient* (3rd ed., pp. 77–78). New York, NY: Oxford University Press.

The following vignette is used for questions 11 through 13:

One hundred subjects who were eligible for inclusion in a study of repeated transcranial magnetic stimulation (rTMS) for auditory hallucinations were invited to participate. Twenty consented for study enrollment and were randomized equally to rTMS or sham rTMS. Fifty percent of the patients in the rTMS group reported improvement in hallucination intensity versus 20% of those who received sham rTMS.

11. Which of the following statistics would calculate whether the proportion of responders in the rTMS group was statistically superior relative to those who received sham rTMS?

A. Chi-square
B. Pearson's ***r***
C. Paired ***t***-test
D. Hazard ratio
E. Relative risk

ANSWER: A

Chi-square tests can be used to compare the statistical differences in proportions (presented here) between two or more groups. Pearson's *r* calculates correlations between two continuous variables. A *t*-test can determine whether there is a statistical difference between two sets of continuous variables. Hazards are the expected number of events over a given time period, so a hazard ratio compares the hazards of two independent groups. Relative risk is the comparison of one rate with another but does not describe a statistical test of hypothesis testing.

REFERENCE

Sullivan, L. (2012). *Essentials of biostatistics in public health* (2nd ed., pp. 134–135). Burlington, MA: Jones and Bartlett Learning.

12. What bias is most likely to confound these results?

A. Berkson bias
B. Sampling bias
C. Selection bias
D. Response bias
E. Reporting bias

ANSWER: C

Only 20% of those eligible for study inclusion agreed to participate, introducing a type of selection bias (self-selection). This limits the generalizability of this study to the broader population of those with auditory hallucinations. Berkson bias is a form of selection bias among inpatient studies predicated on the factors that lead patients to being hospitalized. Sampling bias refers to how the study subjects were chosen from a larger community. Response bias occurs when only a portion of those sampled respond to a request or element of a study (such as responding to a questionnaire survey). Reporting bias is selective revelation by participants.

REFERENCE

Sullivan, L. (2012). *Essentials of biostatistics in public health* (2nd ed., pp. 12–13). Burlington, MA: Jones and Bartlett Learning.

13. Based on these results, how many subjects would need to be given rTMS before one patient received a "true" response (number needed to treat)?

A. 2
B. 4
C. 5
D. 8
E. 10

ANSWER: B

Number needed to treat is calculated by the inverse of absolute risk reduction (50% minus 20%). The absolute risk reduction is 30%, so the number needed to treat is 3.3. Because people are generally indivisible, the number is rounded up by convention: 4 people needed to treat.

REFERENCE

Centre for Evidence-Based Medicine, Oxford University. (2016). Number needed to treat. Retrieved from http://www.cebm.net/number-needed-to-treat-nnt/

14. What type of study provides information about prevalence of disease in a population at a specific point in time?

A. Cohort
B. Cross-sectional
C. Retrospective
D. Prospective
E. Crossover

ANSWER: B

A cross-sectional study provides information about prevalence of disease in a population at a specific point in time. Cohort studies are longitudinal studies following a group from a well-defined population. Retrospective studies are based on past data, whereas prospective studies observe events as they occur longitudinally. Crossover studies are double-blind studies in which the treatment group becomes the placebo group, and vice versa, such that each group controls for the other.

REFERENCE

(2003). *Kaplan and Sadock's comprehensive synopsis of psychiatry* (9th ed., p. 171). Philadelphia, PA: Lippincott Williams and Wilkins.

15. A researcher wants to determine which factors predict delirium diagnosis (as a dichotomous outcome). What type of regression would be appropriate?

A. Cox regression
B. Single linear regression
C. Multiple linear regression
D. Bayesian regression
E. Logistic regression

ANSWER: E

Logistic regression involves dichotomous outcomes and can incorporate one (single logistic) or several (multiple logistic) independent variables (predictors) for the dependent, dichotomous outcome of interest. Linear regression can also be single or multiple but differs from logistic regression in that the outcome variable is continuous. Cox regression often involves hazard ratios or Meier–Kaplan survival curves and evaluates whether a particular outcome happens more rapidly in one sample relative to another. Bayesian regression is not a formal regression model.

REFERENCE

Sullivan, L. (2012). *Essentials of biostatistics in public health* (2nd ed., pp. 210–211). Burlington, MA: Jones and Bartlett Learning.

16. The number of new cases occurring during a specified period of time, usually 1 year, is called:

A. Prevalence
B. Incidence
C. Distribution
D. Sample
E. Lifetime expectancy

ANSWER: B

Incidence is the number of new cases occurring over a specified time. It is often confused with prevalence, which is the number of existing cases of a disorder. Point prevalence refers to prevalence at a specific point in time, whereas period prevalence refers to prevalence during a specified duration.

REFERENCE

(2003). *Kaplan and Sadock's comprehensive synopsis of psychiatry* (9th ed., pp. 175–177). Philadelphia, PA: Lippincott Williams and Wilkins.

17. A *p* value of .03 means that there is a 3% chance of which of the following?

A. The effect is "real."
B. The result is a false positive.
C. The null hypothesis is true.
D. The alternative hypothesis is true.
E. The results occurred by chance if the null is true.

ANSWER: E

A null hypothesis *assumes* there is no significant relationship between studied groups. In hypothesis testing, a *p* value is the likelihood of obtaining a particular result *presuming the null hypothesis is true.*

REFERENCE

Nuzzo, R. (2014). Scientific method: Statistical errors. *Nature, 506*, 150–152.

18. What study design is most commonly used to evaluate factors associated with very rare outcomes such as teratogenicity of lithium?

A. Randomized trial
B. Prospective cohort study
C. Case control study
D. Case series
E. Case reports

ANSWER: C

Subjects in case control studies are enrolled *based on outcomes*, so this would be the most appropriate study design. In cohort studies, subjects are enrolled based on *exposure*. More recently retrospective cohort studies have been used, but these typically involve the use of national registries in order to obtain sufficient power to detect even a few cases of the outcome of interest. Randomized clinical trials are not feasible because one might have to enroll thousands of subjects to obtain a sufficient number of the outcome of interest. Case series and case reports are descriptive, rather than assessing a hypothesis of cause and effect.

REFERENCE

Gentile, S. (2012). Lithium in pregnancy: The need to treat, the duty to ensure safety. *Expert Opinion on Drug Safety, 11*, 427–437.

19. The proportion of all positive results that are "true positive" is known as:

A. Positive predictive value
B. Negative predictive value
C. Sensitivity
D. Specificity
E. Efficiency

ANSWER: A

The positive predictive value is "true positives" divided by "all positives." The negative predictive value is the proportion of all negative test results that are true negatives. Sensitivity is the true positive rate. Specificity is the true negative rate. Efficiency is the percentage of all results that are true results (positive or negative).

REFERENCE

(2003). *Kaplan and Sadock's comprehensive synopsis of psychiatry* (9th ed., pp. 175–177). Philadelphia, PA: Lippincott Williams and Wilkins.

20. The Hamilton Depression Rating Scale is administered to 100 patients in two separate clinics. Which statistical test would be appropriate to determine whether patients at one of these clinics has higher average scores than the other?

A. Chi-square
B. Fisher's exact test
C. Student's *t*-test
D. Hazard ratio
E. Odds ratio

ANSWER: C

An independent samples *t*-test compares the values of a continuous variable between two groups. Chi-square and Fisher's exact test compare categorical values (including proportions). Hazard ratios describe the ratio of two hazard rates (as calculated in survival analyses), and an odds ratio is the ratio of two odds (as calculated in cohort studies).

REFERENCE

Sullivan, L. (2012). *Essentials of biostatistics in public health* (2nd ed., pp. 138–141). Burlington, MA: Jones and Bartlett Learning.

QUESTIONS AND ANSWERS

This chapter has accompanying questions and answers which are available to subscribers as part of the Oxford eLearning platform. To access the questions, follow the link below, or go to http://oxford-elearning.oup.com/books.

http://oxford-elearning.oup.com/books/test/67/10.1093/med/9780190265557.003.0030

31.

INTERPERSONAL AND COMMUNICATION SKILLS

Deepti Challagolla

1. Which of the following is NOT a strategy to develop patient rapport?

A. Showing empathy
B. Making patients comfortable
C. Showing expertise
D. Making decisions for the patient
E. Being a good listener

ANSWER: D

Several strategies help to develop rapport with patients. The interviewer should be able to put patients at ease; express compassion; evaluate patients' insight and become an ally; show expertise; establish authority as a physician and therapist; and balance the roles of empathic listener, expert, and authority. Doctors should not make decisions for patients or be judgmental.

REFERENCE

(2007). *Kaplan and Sadock's synopsis of psychiatry* (10th ed., pp. 1–2). Philadelphia, PA: Lippincott Williams and Wilkins.

2. During the initial psychiatric evaluation of a new patient, the patient expresses frustration that her last psychiatrist offered only very brief visits and switched medications whenever the patient felt the medications were not helping at the time. The evaluator asks, "Would you like your psychiatrist to listen to and understand you before adjusting medicine?" This is an example of:

A. Clarification
B. Confrontation
C. Interpretation
D. Reframing
E. Redirection

ANSWER: A

Clarification is an attempt to get details from patients about what they have already said.

REFERENCE

(2007). *Kaplan and Sadock's synopsis of psychiatry* (10th ed., pp. 8–9). Philadelphia, PA: Lippincott Williams and Wilkins.

3. Which of the following is an example of an open-ended question?

A. Are you taking the medication?
B. How long have you had difficulty sleeping?
C. How did that happen?
D. You haven't been going to see your doctor, right?
E. Did you sleep OK last night?

ANSWER: C

In general, an interview should begin with broad, open-ended questioning, continue by becoming more specific, and end with detailed direct questioning. Open-ended questions provide genuine answers but have low reliability and precision.

REFERENCE

(2007). *Kaplan and Sadock's synopsis of psychiatry* (10th ed., pp. 8–9). Philadelphia, PA: Lippincott Williams and Wilkins.

4. Nodding one's head and leaning forward in one's chair during an interview are examples of:

A. Reflection
B. Facilitation
C. Confrontation
D. Clarification
E. Interpretation

ANSWER: B

Nodding one's head, leaning forward in the chair, and helping patients continue in the interview by providing both verbal and nonverbal cues that encourage patients to keep talking are examples of facilitation.

REFERENCE

(2007). *Kaplan and Sadock's synopsis of psychiatry* (10th ed., p. 8). Philadelphia, PA: Lippincott Williams and Wilkins.

5. The technique by which a therapist makes a verbal observation about the patient's behavior or thinking, of which the patient may not be aware, is called:

A. Summation
B. Facilitation
C. Interpretation
D. Explanation
E. Reflection

ANSWER: C

This technique is called interpretation and should be used when the therapist has established rapport with the patient. Summation involves summarizing what the patient has said. Facilitation is the use of cues to prompt the patient to continue to talk. Explanation is a technique used to clearly describe the treatment plan. Reflection is an empathic restatement of what the patient has said.

REFERENCE

(2007). *Kaplan and Sadock's synopsis of psychiatry* (10th ed., pp. 8–9). Philadelphia, PA: Lippincott Williams and Wilkins.

6. Which of the following statements best demonstrates the psychotherapeutic principle of interpretation?

A. "Yes, I see what you mean."
B. "Did you say that your aunt had bipolar disorder?"
C. "It's hard for you to depend on me, just as you felt you couldn't depend on your father."
D. "It could be helpful if you could re-establish your routine at home."
E. "It must feel terrible when no one understands your point of view."

ANSWER: C

Interpretation involves the therapist making an observation about the patient's behavior or thinking, of which the patient may not be aware.

REFERENCE

(2007). *Kaplan and Sadock's synopsis of psychiatry* (10th ed., pp. 8–9). Philadelphia, PA: Lippincott Williams and Wilkins.

7. Which of the following best describes countertransference?

A. The activation by the patient of repressed object representations within the therapist
B. An aspect of the patient's self that is acknowledged and consciously projected onto the therapist
C. The therapist's total emotional reaction to the patient, conscious or unconscious
D. A process by which only the therapist contributes to the intersubjective interpretive space between self and therapist
E. The internal reward a therapist gains when a patient improves

ANSWER: C

In psychoanalytic theory, countertransference occurs when the therapist begins to project his or her own unresolved conflicts onto the client. While transference of the client's conflicts onto the therapist is considered a healthy and normal part of psychodynamic therapy, the therapist's job is to remain neutral. At one time, countertransference was widely believed to contaminate the therapeutic relationship. Current thinking is more complex and suggests countertransference can play an important role when those feelings are utilized productively in the therapeutic process.

REFERENCE

(2007). *Kaplan and Sadock's synopsis of psychiatry* (10th ed., pp. 2–3). Philadelphia, PA: Lippincott Williams and Wilkins.

8. A shy 26-year-old woman has never been in a romantic relationship. After 5 months of psychodynamic therapy, she begins to struggle with strong positive feelings toward her male therapist, which she finds hard to accept. This occurs at the same time she is beginning to date someone from work. Her relationship with her colleague is likely an example of:

A. Transference
B. Acting out
C. Countertransference
D. Affection
E. Sublimation

ANSWER: B

Sometimes patients are not aware of their repressed feelings and express them as an action—as this patient is doing with her colleague. The action is repeated in an unconscious manner. For the therapist it is important to try to understand what is being communicated. Transference is generally defined as the set of expectations, beliefs, and emotional responses that a patient brings to the patient–doctor relationship, which are not necessarily based on who the doctor is or how the doctor acts in reality but, rather, on repeated experiences the patient has had with other important authority figures throughout life.

REFERENCE

(2007). *Kaplan and Sadock's synopsis of psychiatry* (10th ed., pp. 1–2). Philadelphia, PA: Lippincott Williams and Wilkins.

9. After several weeks of weekly psychotherapy for recurrent depression and failed relationships, a patient exclaims to the therapist, "You just expect me to trust you when you never reveal a single thing about yourself. I don't know anything about you as a person, not even what kind of training you had, how long you have been practicing, and what kind of success, if any, you have had with patients like me!" How should the therapist respond first?

A. Provide facts about his or her credentials.
B. Explain that self-disclosure is usually not helpful in psychotherapy.
C. Confront the patient's aggressive devaluation of the therapist.
D. Empathize with the patient's fears of trust and feelings of being at a disadvantage.
E. Inquire about the patient's bad experiences with therapy in the past.

ANSWER: D

Empathy is a way of increasing rapport. An empathic psychiatrist may anticipate what is felt before it is spoken and can often help patients articulate what they are feeling. Nonverbal cues, such as body posture and facial expression, are noted. Patients' reactions to the psychiatrist can be understood and clarified. Once the therapist empathizes with the patient, it would not be unreasonable to provide facts about credentials, understanding the patient's need in the context of the therapy.

REFERENCE

(2007). *Kaplan and Sadock's synopsis of psychiatry* (10th ed., pp. 1–2). Philadelphia, PA: Lippincott Williams and Wilkins.

10. According to William Osler, which quality or qualities should a physician possess?

A. Composure
B. Bravery
C. Tenacity
D. Imperturbability
E. All the above

ANSWER: E

William Osler discussed the characteristics and qualities of the physician in his book *Aequanimitas*. They include composure (calmness of mind, bearing, and appearance); bravery (the capacity to face or endure events with courage); tenacity (persistence in attaining a goal or adhering to something valued); and imperturbability (the ability to maintain extreme calm and steadiness).

REFERENCE

(2007). *Kaplan and Sadock's synopsis of psychiatry* (10th ed., pp. 10–11, Table 1-7). Philadelphia, PA: Lippincott Williams and Wilkins.

QUESTIONS AND ANSWERS

This chapter has accompanying questions and answers which are available to subscribers as part of the Oxford eLearning platform. To access the questions, follow the link below, or go to http://oxford-elearning.oup.com/books.

http://oxford-elearning.oup.com/books/test/67/10.1093/med/9780190265557.003.0031

32.

SYSTEMS-BASED PRACTICE ISSUES

Deepti Challagolla

1. Which of the following conditions EXCLUDES patients from receiving hospice care if they receive Medicare Part A benefits?

A. The patient's hospice physician and primary care physician certify that the patient is terminally ill with a life expectancy of 6 months or less.
B. The patient accepts palliative care for comfort instead of care to cure their illness.
C. The patient's hospice physician and primary care physician certify that the patient is terminally ill with a life expectancy of 12 months or less.
D. The patient signs a statement choosing hospice care instead of other Medicare-covered treatments for his or her terminal illness and related conditions.

ANSWER: C

Terminally ill patients who have less than 6 months to live and are eligible for hospital insurance under Medicare Part A and are also eligible for hospice care. The patient must choose to accept palliative care rather than pursuing a cure for his or her illness and sign a statement to that effect.

REFERENCE

Centers for Medicare & Medicaid Services. (2016). Medicare hospice benefits. Retrieved from https://www.medicare.gov/Pubs/pdf/02154.pdf

2. Which of the following is an example of secondary prevention?

A. Deinstitutionalization
B. Depression screening
C. Psychological first aid after acute traumatization
D. Structured day program for patients with schizophrenia
E. Prenatal care to reduce the incidence of intellectual disability in children

ANSWER: B

Secondary prevention is aimed at early disease identification to prevent adverse sequelae. Secondary prevention aims to reduce the impact of a disease or injury that has already occurred. This is done by detecting and treating disease or injury as soon as possible to halt or slow its progress, encouraging personal strategies to prevent re-injury or recurrence, and implementing programs to return people to their original health and level of functioning. Deinstitutionalization and day programs may be a form of tertiary prevention (reducing long-term effects of a chronic disease and enhancing overall quality of life); crisis intervention and prenatal care are primary prevention (preventing psychological conditions such as post-traumatic stress disorder or neurodevelopmental conditions, respectively, before they occur).

REFERENCE

Institute for Work and Health, Toronto. (2016). What researchers mean by...primary, secondary and tertiary prevention. Retrieved from https://www.iwh.on.ca/wrmb/primary-secondary-and-tertiary-prevention.

3. A survey of patients in an addiction treatment program shows that men are four times more likely than women to receive treatment for addiction. Studies have shown that the most prevalent institutional barrier to treatment of addiction in women is:

A. Lack of child care services
B. Treatment staff's reluctance to treat psychopathology in women
C. Women's fear of losing custody of children
D. Lack of addiction screening of women in primary care settings
E. Predominance of male treatment staff

ANSWER: C

Women who have children often fear that admitting a substance use problem will cause them to lose custody of their children. They worry that they will be perceived as irresponsible or neglectful or as "bad mothers" if they admit to substance abuse or dependence.

REFERENCE

Substance Abuse and Mental Health Services Administration. Substance abuse treatment: addressing the specific needs of women. Treatment Improvement Protocol (TIP) Series, No. 51. HHS Publication No. (SMA) 13-4426. Rockville, MD: Substance Abuse and Mental Health Services Administration, 2009.

4. Which is the largest support organization for families of patients with mental illness in the United States?

A. National Alliance on Mental Illness
B. American Psychiatric Association
C. National Institute for Mental Health
D. Joint Commission on Mental Illness and Mental Health
E. American Association for Mental Illness

ANSWER: A

The National Alliance on Mental Illness (NAMI) is the nation's largest grass-roots mental health organization dedicated to building better lives for the millions of Americans affected by mental illness and their families.

REFERENCE

National Alliance on Mental Illness. (2016). *About NAMI*. Retrieved from https://www.nami.org/About-NAMI#sthash.6gRmWYV8.dpuf

5. Which of the following is an example of primary prevention?

A. Twelve-step programs
B. Early identification
C. Psychiatric rehabilitation
D. A mental health education program
E. Reduction of residual effects of mental illness

ANSWER: D

Primary prevention aims to prevent disease or injury before it occurs. This is done by preventing exposures to hazards that cause disease or injury, altering unhealthy or unsafe behaviors that can lead to disease or injury, and increasing resistance to disease or injury should exposure occur.

REFERENCE

Institute for Work and Health, Toronto. (2016). What researchers mean by...primary, secondary and tertiary prevention. Retrieved from https://www.iwh.on.ca/wrmb/primary-secondary-and-tertiary-prevention

6. Which of the following is an example of an advance directive for a patient who is dying?

A. Living trust
B. Durable power of attorney
C. Writ of sanctity
D. Document of accord
E. Family agreement

ANSWER: B

Advance directives are a way to make decisions regarding health care in advance. This document allows people to plan their health care before they become incapacitated or unable to make sound decisions for themselves. Advance directives consist of two documents; a living will and a durable power of attorney for health care (DPOA). The first is a living will, which makes one's wishes known about the type of care that person would want to receive at the end of life. The second document contained in an advance directive is a health care proxy, also known as a durable power of attorney for health care (DPOA). In this document, a person appoints someone to make medical decisions on his or her behalf should the person become incapable of doing so. A living trust is a legal document that is used in all three phases of someone's life: while he or she is alive and well, while he or she is alive but ailing, and after one's death.

REFERENCE

Perez, M. V., Macchi, M. J., & Agranatti, A. F. (2013). Advance directives in the context of end-of-life palliative care. *Current Opinion in Supportive and Palliative Care, 7*, 406–10.

7. What is the purpose of Al-Anon meetings?

A. To help problem gamblers
B. To provide spiritual help for patients with alcohol use disorder
C. To help families and friends of individuals with alcohol use disorder
D. To help a patient with substance use disorder to return to work
E. To provide outpatient rehabilitation for patients with alcohol use disorder

ANSWER: C

Al-Anon helps families and friends of alcoholics, rather than stopping alcoholism in others or assisting with interventions.

REFERENCE

Al-Anon family groups. (2015). Retrieved from http://www.al-anon.alateen.org

8. What is an appropriate recommendation to manage chronic pain for a patient admitted to the hospital who is in a methadone maintenance program?

A. The patient is likely to require higher-than-usual doses of opioids due to tolerance.
B. Staff must refuse to give extra pain medication when requested outside of dosing schedule.
C. Staff should be skilled in recognizing drug-seeking behavior.
D. The patient should be treated with non-opioid medications only.
E. Buprenorphine is preferred while the patient is medically admitted.

ANSWER: A

Many individuals receiving methadone maintenance treatment for opioid use disorder also require treatment for acute or chronic pain, and the presence of pain is known to have a negative impact on patient health and function. However, effective pain management in this population is complicated by many factors, including heightened pain sensitivity, high opioid tolerance, illicit substance use, and variable cross-tolerance to opioid pain medications. Additionally, providers should be attuned to the possibility of opioid-induced hyperalgesia. Treating physicians should prescribe those patients sufficient medication to meet their pain needs, which may be higher than a standard dose due to tolerance.

REFERENCE

Eyler, E. C. (2013). Chronic and acute pain and pain management for patients in methadone maintenance treatment. *American Journal on Addictions, 22*, 75–83.

9. What is mental health parity?

A. Equality for mental health and substance abuse benefits with medical and surgical benefits
B. Equality of physician reimbursement for mental health diagnoses relative to other diagnoses
C. Equal coverage of office visits for psychotherapy and psychopharmacology
D. Free coverage of mental health treatment for incarcerated patients
E. Free coverage of mental health treatment for pregnant patients

ANSWER: A

The Mental Health Parity and Addiction Equity Act of 2008 provides equal benefits for mental health and substance use disorders and for non-mental health disorders by health insurance plans than cover mental health and substance abuse treatments. The Affordable Care Act of 2010 expanded upon this legislation to promote behavioral health prevention and treatment as essential benefits.

REFERENCE

Bartlett, J., & Manderscheid, R. (2016). What does mental health parity really mean for the care of people with serious mental illness? *Psychiatric Clinics of North America, 39*, 331–342.

10. Which of the following is improved with integration of psychiatric services in the primary care setting?

A. Access to psychiatric care
B. Stigma
C. Efficiency of care
D. Patient satisfaction
E. All of the above

ANSWER: E

Integration of mental health care into primary care settings offers a range of benefits.

REFERENCE

Dobbins, M. I., Thomas, S. A., Melton, S. L., & Lee, S.. (2016). Integrated care and the evolution of the multidisciplinary team. *Primary Care*, *43*, 177–190.

11. The recommendation by the US Preventive Services Task Force that all adults be screened for depression where staff-assisted depression care supports are in place to ensure accurate diagnosis, effective treatment, and follow-up represents which of the following types of interventions according to the Institute of Medicine?

A. Universal prevention
B. Selective prevention
C. Indicated prevention
D. Case identification
E. Standard of care

ANSWER: D

The US Institute of Medicine (IOM) has adopted a "protractor" model that stratifies interventions into three phases of prevention, two stages of treatment, and two stages of maintenance. This model has been proposed in contradistinction to the tripartite prevention model (primary, secondary, and tertiary prevention). According to the IOM, screening would represent a form of case identification because the condition is already present and awaits identification.

REFERENCE

Springer, J. F., & Philips, J. (2007). The Institute of Medicine framework and its implications for the advancement of prevention policy, programs and practice. Retrieved from http://ca-sdfsc.org/docs/resources/SDFSC_IOM_Policy.pdf

QUESTIONS AND ANSWERS

This chapter has accompanying questions and answers which are available to subscribers as part of the Oxford eLearning platform. To access the questions, follow the link below, or go to http://oxford-elearning.oup.com/books.

http://oxford-elearning.oup.com/books/test/67/10.1093/med/9780190265557.003.0032

33.

FACTORS AFFECTING PROGNOSIS OR COMPLICATING TREATMENT

Jatinder Chawla, Swapnil Gupta

1. Which of the following features of a depressive episode may be more suggestive of bipolar disorder rather than a recurrent major depressive disorder?

A. Insidious onset of depressive symptoms
B. Postpartum episode
C. Marked anxiety and agitation as opposed to psychomotor retardation
D. Poor acute antidepressant response to lithium

ANSWER: B

Characteristics of a depressive episode occurring as a part of bipolar disorder includes a history of hypomania, onset in the teens, an equal sex ratio, more common postpartum onset, more common acute onset, with higher likelihood of psychomotor retardation as opposed to agitation and anxiety. Further, lithium produces an acute antidepressant effect in bipolar depression that might be absent in unipolar depression.

REFERENCE

Akiskal, H. A. (2002). Classification, diagnosis and boundaries. In M. Maj, H. A. Akiskal, J. J. Lopez-Ibor, & N. Sartorius (Eds.), *Bipolar disorder* (p. 9). Chichester, West Sussex: Wiley.

2. Which of the following is NOT associated with polydipsia in patients with schizophrenia?

A. Neuroleptic use
B. Anticholinergic use
C. Heavy tobacco use
D. Hypertension

ANSWER: D

Polydipsia is compulsive water drinking, usually in excess of 3 liters per day. It can be complicated by water intoxication (i.e., severe hyponatremia, with serum sodium <120 mmol/L), which is potentially fatal, because the associated cerebral edema can result in delirium, seizures, coma, and death. Polydipsia and water intoxication are associated with prolonged hospitalizations, high doses of antipsychotic medications, moderate doses of anticholinergic medications, and heavy smoking.

REFERENCE

American Psychiatric Association. (2004). *Practice guidelines for treatment of patients with schizophrenia* (2nd ed., p. 47). Washington, DC: American Psychiatric Publishing.

3. Mr. J. is an 18-year-old single man who is the son of a wealthy businessman. Although he previously held a 4.0 grade point average, he is placed on academic leave in the context of a psychotic episode. He is admitted to an inpatient facility because of bizarre delusions, disorganized thought process, and declining self-care. He is adherent to antipsychotic medication treatment. He improves clinically, and at the time of discharge, his psychiatrist counsels the family about risk of suicide. Which of the following is NOT a risk factor for suicide in Mr. J.'s case?

A. High socioeconomic status
B. Bizarre delusions
C. Young age of onset
D. Sudden change in environment (admission and discharge)
E. High scholastic achievement

ANSWER: B

Specific risk factors for suicide among persons with schizophrenia are young age, high socioeconomic status, high IQ with a high level of premorbid scholastic achievement, high aspirations and expectations, an early age at onset of illness/first hospitalization, a chronic and deteriorating course with many relapses, and greater insight into the illness. A change in the environment, such as a hospital admission and discharge, may increase the risk of suicidal behavior. Other risk factors include severe depressive and psychotic symptoms, with an increase in the patient's paranoid behavior. Treatment-related factors associated with suicide include inadequate antipsychotic treatment, nonadherence to the medication regimen, and lack of response to medication.

REFERENCE

American Psychiatric Association. (2004). *Practice guidelines for treatment of patients with schizophrenia* (2nd ed., pp. 45–46). Washington, DC: American Psychiatric Publishing.

4. Which of the following is a predictor of nonadherence to pharmacological treatment among patients with mood disorders?

A. Older age
B. Less severe illness
C. Group therapy without individual therapy
D. Co-morbid personality disorder
E. All of the above

ANSWER: D

Predictors of nonadherence to treatment among patients with mood disorders include age younger than 40, co-morbid substance use disorder, co-morbid personality disorder, poor insight, more severe illness, and treatment side effects.

REFERENCE

Pompili, M., Venturini, P., Palermo, M., Stefani, H., Seretti, M.E., Lamis, A....Girardi, P. (2013). Mood disorders medications Predictors of nonadherence—review of the current literature. *Expert Review of Neurotherapeutics, 13*, 809–825.

5. A 50-year-old woman with schizoaffective disorder has been stable for 6 months on olanzapine with no active psychotic or mood symptoms. She presents to the clinic with distressing repetitive thoughts of jumping off a bridge. She reports that she is satisfied with her life, is looking forward to seeing her first grandchild in 2 months, and has no wish to kill herself. However, these thoughts are troubling her very much, and she says, "I cannot get them out of my head." Which of the following is the best strategy to manage this distressing complaint?

A. Switch from olanzapine to clozapine.
B. Hospitalize the patient immediately.
C. Add fluoxetine to the treatment regimen.
D. Add a mood stabilizer to the treatment regimen.
E. Optimize olanzapine dose.

ANSWER: C

This patient is presenting with antipsychotic-induced obsessions. The recommended treatment for treatment-emergent obsessions is the addition of an SSRI such as fluoxetine. Although obsessive–compulsive symptoms typically appear 4 to 8 weeks following initiation of treatment with antipsychotics, they can present as late as 15 months. The antipsychotics most likely to have this side effect are clozapine and olanzapine, followed by risperidone, ziprasidone, and quetiapine. Because clozapine is also likely to cause obsessions, a switch to clozapine is not advisable. Because the thoughts are ego-dystonic and the patient has a strong protective factor of her grandchild, hospitalization is not needed at this time. A mood stabilizer is not indicated in this case.

REFERENCE

Lykouras, L., Alevizos, B., Michalopoulou, P., & Rabavilas, A. (2003). Obsessive–compulsive symptoms induced by atypical antipsychotics: A review of the reported cases. *Progress in Neuro-Psychopharmacology and Biological Psychiatry, 27*, 333–346.

6. Antipsychotic-induced hyperprolactinemia can be managed by switching to which of the following medications?

A. Aripiprazole
B. Chlorpromazine
C. Methylphenidate
D. Fluvoxamine
E. Risperidone

ANSWER: A

A reduction in dose of the offending antipsychotic is the simplest treatment strategy, but its effectiveness is unpredictable, and it carries the risk of precipitating an exacerbation or relapse of psychotic symptoms. Switching the patient to a prolactin-sparing antipsychotic (e.g., aripiprazole, olanzapine, quetiapine, or clozapine) usually proves effective, though there is also a risk of relapse. There are sometimes good reasons to continue treatment with a prolactin-elevating antipsychotic. For example, a long-acting intramuscular depot may be the only way to ensure adequate adherence with antipsychotic treatment, and the risks of relapse may be felt to be too high to justify stopping the depot antipsychotic. In some cases, a dopamine agonist (such as bromocriptine) can be considered.

REFERENCE

Haddad, P. M., & Wieck, A. (2004). Antipsychotic-induced hyperprolactinaemia. *Drugs, 64*, 2291–2314.

7. Which of the following is a predictor of long-term care placement of persons with neurocognitive disorder?

A. Hispanic race
B. Younger age
C. Primary caregiver living in the home
D. Married patient
E. Behavioral and psychological symptoms of dementia

ANSWER: E

Behavioral and psychological symptoms of dementia increase the risk of long-term care placement, as do white race, older age, dementia severity, caregiver burden, and greater functional impairment.

REFERENCE

Cepoiu-Martin, M., Tam-Tham, H., Patten, S., Maxwell, C.J., & Hogan, D.B. (2016). Predictors of long-term care placement in persons with dementia: A systematic review and meta-analysis. *International Journal of Geriatric Psychiatry,* April 4. Epub ahead of print.

8. Which of the following is predictive of poor treatment response to behavioral therapy in panic disorder with agoraphobia?

A. Marital dissatisfaction
B. Catastrophic thoughts
C. Quality of the therapeutic relationship
D. Co-morbid social phobia
E. First episode of panic disorder

ANSWER: B

In a study of patients diagnosed with panic disorder who were receiving a standardized exposure-based behavioral treatment program, severity of agoraphobic complaints, level of depression, motivation for treatment, personality psychopathology, and catastrophic agoraphobic cognitions were related to treatment outcome; whereas the quality of the therapeutic relationship and marital dissatisfaction were not. Catastrophic agoraphobic cognitions were the strongest predictor of poor. Patients frequently distressed by maladaptive cognitions tended to improve less with an exposure-based treatment program.

REFERENCE

Keijsers, G. P., Hoogduin, C. A., & Schaap, C. P. (1994). Prognostic factors in the behavioral treatment of panic disorder with and without agoraphobia. *Behavior Therapy, 25*, 689–708.

9. Poor performance in which of the following neuropsychological domains has been shown to be related to relapses of drinking episodes in alcohol dependence?

A. Cognitive flexibility
B. Social cognition
C. Emotional processing
D. Visuospatial ability
E. Motor speed

ANSWER: A

Neuropsychological studies of substance abuse treatment outcome have generally found that, those who recover show intact functioning on most measures, whereas those who relapse, do poorly on tests of language, abstract reasoning, planning, and cognitive flexibility. These outcomes have been related to involvement of left hemisphere and frontal lobe functions.

REFERENCE

Miller, L. (1991). Predicting relapse and recovery in alcoholism and addiction: Neuropsychology, personality, and cognitive style. *Journal of Substance Abuse Treatment, 8*, 277–291.

10. Which of the following is the best augmenting antipsychotic medication in treatment of obsessive-compulsive disorder (OCD)?

A. Haloperidol
B. Clozapine
C. Quetiapine
D. Olanzapine

ANSWER: A

Antipsychotic augmentation is an effective treatment intervention for OCD among patients who fail to exhibit a treatment response after 12 weeks of maximal therapy with at least one serotonergic agent. Nearly one third of treatment-refractory OCD patients exhibit a treatment response to antipsychotic augmentation. Stratification by specific antipsychotic agent demonstrated strong evidence of efficacy for haloperidol or risperidone augmentation when compared with placebo augmentation.

REFERENCE

Bloch, M. H., Landeros-Weisenberger, A., Kelmendi, B., Coric, V., Bracken, M. B., & Leckman, J. F. (2006). A systematic review: Antipsychotic augmentation with treatment refractory obsessive-compulsive disorder. *Molecular Psychiatry, 11*, 622–632.

11. Which of the following statements is TRUE regarding fertility in women who take antipsychotic medication?

A. Neuroleptics reduce fertility in women with affective psychosis more than in those with nonaffective psychosis.
B. Fertility in women with psychosis is the same as in women without any psychotic disorder.
C. Antipsychotic medications affect fertility in women by reducing libido.
D. Aripiprazole adversely affects fertility more than any other antipsychotic.

ANSWER: A

Treatment with antipsychotics does not appear to influence fertility rates in women with nonaffective psychoses. Women with psychotic disorders have a lower overall general fertility rate than healthy comparison subjects, although fertility was only significantly lower in the women aged 25 and older. This lower fertility rate was less marked in women with affective psychoses.

REFERENCE

Howard, L. M., Kumar, C., Leese, M., & Thornicroft, G. (2002). The general fertility rate in women with psychotic disorders. *American Journal of Psychiatry, 159*, 991–997.

12. A patient treated with clozapine tries to lift his coffee cup, but his arm jerks outward, and the coffee falls to the floor. He feels well otherwise except for isolated incidents of a brief twitch in his arm for the past 2 weeks. His medication was recently increased from 500 mg to 550 mg per day. He mentions the twitches to his doctor, who orders an EEG. The next day, he starts having sudden loss of tone in his left leg, causing him to fall while walking. The most serious consequence of this complication of treatment is:

A. Generalized tonic–clonic seizure
B. Head injury due to fall
C. Meniscal injury
D. Hypokalemia
E. Guillain–Barré syndrome

ANSWER: A

Clozapine-induced myoclonus and "leg-folding" are harbingers of generalized tonic–clonic seizures. The management is an immediate reduction of the dose, if possible, and/or addition of an antiepileptic medication for seizure prophylaxis.

REFERENCE

Sajatovic, M., & Meltzer, H. Y. (1996). Clozapine-induced myoclonus and generalized seizures. *Biological Psychiatry, 39*, 367–370.

13. The highest risk for conversion to schizophrenia seen in which of the following cases?

A. Cocaine-induced psychosis
B. Amphetamine-induced psychosis
C. Alcohol-induced psychosis
D. Cannabis-induced psychosis
E. Nicotine-induced psychosis

ANSWER: D

In a long-term follow-up study, 8-year cumulative risk to receive a schizophrenia spectrum diagnosis was 46% for persons with a diagnosis of cannabis-induced psychosis and 30% for those with an amphetamine-induced psychosis. Although alcohol-induced psychosis was the most common type of substance-induced psychosis, 8-year cumulative risk for subsequent schizophrenia spectrum diagnosis was only 5%. The majority of conversions to a schizophrenia spectrum diagnosis occurred during the first 3 years following the index treatment period, especially for cannabis-induced psychosis.

REFERENCE

Niemi-Pynttäri, J. A., Sund, R., Putkonen, H., Vorma, H., Wahlbeck, K., & Pirkola, S. P. (2013). Substance-induced psychoses converting into schizophrenia: A register-based study of 18,478 Finnish inpatient cases. *Journal of Clinical Psychiatry, 74*, e94–e99.

14. Which of the following is the best predictor of relapse to drinking in patients with alcohol dependence?

A. Difficulty falling asleep
B. Nightmares
C. Sleepwalking
D. Periodic leg movements in sleep
E. Hypersomnolence

ANSWER: A

Difficulty falling asleep is the most replicated, subjective marker of relapse. Consistent with subjective reports, at least two studies found that polysomnography-measured sleep onset latency (i.e., increased time to fall asleep) predicted drinking at at follow-up. One study with actigraphy-measured sleep onset latency also predicted similar outcomes.

REFERENCE

Brower, K. J. (2015). Assessment and treatment of insomnia in adult patients with alcohol use disorders. *Alcohol, 49*, 417–427.

15. All of the following are true about insomnia related to post-traumatic stress disorder (PTSD) EXCEPT:

A. Insomnia in PTSD is related to the long-term prognosis, depressive symptoms, and substance abuse.
B. Cognitive behavioral therapy may be an option to treat PTSD-related insomnia.
C. Quetiapine may be an effective augmenting treatment strategy.
D. Prazosin can be used to treat PTSD-related insomnia.
E. Benzodiazepines are an effective treatment strategy.

ANSWER: E

Evidence suggests that benzodiazepines, TCAs, and MAOIs are not useful for the treatment of PTSD-related sleep disorders. Prazosin, a centrally acting alpha-1 adrenoceptor antagonist, has led to large reductions in nightmares and insomnia in small studies of patients with PTSD. Augmentation of SSRIs with quetiapine, an atypical antipsychotic, may be effective for treatment-resistant nightmares and insomnia, although adverse effects can be significant. Additional medications, including zolpidem, buspirone, gabapentin, and mirtazapine, have been found to improve sleep in patients with PTSD. Large randomized, placebo-controlled trials are needed to confirm these findings. Cognitive behavioral interventions for sleep disruption in patients with PTSD include strategies targeting insomnia and imagery rehearsal therapy for nightmares.

REFERENCE

Maher, M. J., Rego, S. A., & Asnis, G. M. (2006). Sleep disturbances in patients with post-traumatic stress disorder: Epidemiology, impact and approaches to management. *CNS Drugs, 20*, 567–590.

16. Which of the following is most commonly seen as a side effect of disulfiram?

A. Tremor
B. Dysgeusia
C. Tachycardia
D. Constipation
E. Tinnitus

ANSWER: B

Dysgeusia is described as an unpleasant taste in the mouth. Among the above choices, it is most commonly observed as a side effect of disulfiram. In addition, providers should be aware that disulfiram can cause optic neuritis, peripheral neuritis, polyneuritis, peripheral neuropathy, and hepatitis (including both cholestatic and fulminant hepatitis), as well as liver failure resulting in transplant or death.

REFERENCES

Petersen, E. N. (1992). The pharmacology and toxicology of disulfiram and its metabolites. *Acta Psychiatrica Scandinavica, 86*(S369), 7–13.

Disulfiram package insert.

17. One of the strongest risk factors for violence in patients with schizophrenia is:

A. Command auditory hallucinations
B. Alcohol use disorder
C. Poor response to treatment
D. Co-morbid manic symptoms
E. Duration of symptoms

ANSWER: B

Men who abused alcohol and were diagnosed with schizophrenia were 25 times more likely to commit violent crimes than mentally healthy men. The risk of violence for nonalcoholic patients with schizophrenia was 3.6 times, and for other psychoses was 7.7 times. The risk for committing more crimes among alcoholic subjects with schizophrenia was 9.5-fold.

REFERENCE

Räsänen, P., Tähonen, J., Isohanni, M., Rantakallio, P., Lehtonen, J., & Moring, J. (1998). Schizophrenia, alcohol abuse, and violent behavior: A 26-year followup study of an unselected birth cohort. *Schizophrenia Bulletin, 24*, 437–441.

18. Which of the following is NOT a risk factor for completed suicide in patients with borderline personality disorder?

A. Co-morbid psychiatric disorder
B. Another co-morbid cluster B personality disorder
C. High harm avoidance
D. High novelty seeking
E. Co-morbid substance use disorder

ANSWER: C

Patients with borderline personality disorder who commit suicide are more likely to meet the criteria for current and lifetime substance dependence disorders. They have higher levels of current and lifetime psychiatric (historically Axis I, though the pentaxial system was abandoned in *DSM-5*) comorbidity, novelty seeking, impulsivity, hostility, and co-morbid personality disorders, while exhibiting lower levels of harm avoidance. Patients with borderline personality disorder who commit suicide are more likely to have cluster B personality comorbidity.

REFERENCE

McGirr, A., Paris, J., Lesage, A., Renaud, J., & Turecki, G. (2007). Risk factors for suicide completion in borderline personality disorder: A case-control study of cluster B comorbidity and impulsive aggression. *Journal of Clinical Psychiatry, 68*, 721–725.

19. The highest prevalence of co-morbid substance use disorder is found in which of the following conditions?

A. Bipolar disorder
B. Generalized anxiety disorder
C. Antisocial personality disorder
D. Schizophrenia
E. Borderline personality disorder

ANSWER: C

Antisocial personality disorder is the most commonly co-occurring disorder among those with a substance use disorder. Conversely, the National Comorbidity Survey found that almost 80% of all respondents with antisocial personality disorder also had a lifetime substance use disorder. Studies of selected substance misusers show that opioid use disorder has the highest level of co-occurrence with antisocial personality disorder. High prevalence rates of antisocial personality have also been found among users of cocaine, alcohol or solvents.

REFERENCE

Moran, P. (1999). The epidemiology of antisocial personality disorder. *Social Psychiatry and Psychiatric Epidemiology, 34*, 231–242.

20. Which of the following is NOT a predictive factor for psychosocial functioning in schizophrenia?

A. Hallucinations
B. Verbal memory
C. Attention

D. Executive functioning
E. Negative symptoms

ANSWER: A

Verbal memory, processing speed, attention, and severity of negative symptoms are related to subsequent psychosocial outcome. Global psychosocial functioning is predicted by negative symptoms and attention. Verbal memory is a significant predictor of the degree of impairment in recreational activities. Impairment in relationships is predicted by negative symptoms and memory, whereas attention and negative symptoms are predictive of work performance. Verbal memory, processing speed and attention are potential targets for psychosocial interventions to improve outcome.

REFERENCES

Milev, P., Ho, B. C., Arndt, S., & Andreasen, N. C. (2005). Predictive values of neurocognition and negative symptoms on functional outcome in schizophrenia: A longitudinal first-episode study with 7-year follow-up. *American Journal of Psychiatry, 162*, 495–506.

Norman, R. M., Malla, A. K., McLean, T., Voruganti, L. P. N., Cortese, L., McIntosh, E.,... & Rickwood, A. (2000). The relationship of symptoms and level of functioning in schizophrenia to general wellbeing and the Quality of Life Scale. *Acta Psychiatrica Scandinavica, 102*, 303–309.

QUESTIONS AND ANSWERS

This chapter has accompanying questions and answers which are available to subscribers as part of the Oxford eLearning platform. To access the questions, follow the link below, or go to http://oxford-elearning.oup.com/books.

http://oxford-elearning.oup.com/books/test/67/10.1093/med/9780190265557.003.0033

PART IV

CLINICAL VIGNETTES

Edited by Mallika Lavakumar

34.

CLINICAL VIGNETTE

AUTISM SPECTRUM DISORDER

Adefolake Akinsanya

A 22-month-old toddler is brought in at the recommendation of her pediatrician because she orients infrequently when her name is called. She has difficulty in pointing to objects when her mother names them. Furthermore, she is preoccupied with squares, focusing on square objects in her environment.

1. Which of the following diagnoses is suspected?

A. Autism spectrum disorder (ASD)
B. Attention deficit hyperactivity disorder (ADHD)
C. Sterotypic movement disorder
D. Language disorder
E. Specific learning disorder

ANSWER: A

The toddler seems to be demonstrating early signs of autism. The early signs of autism are reduction in eye gaze, shared joint attention, social smiling, orientation to name, and coordination of different modes of communication. Early signs also include delayed babbling and development of gestures. These children may have an unusual tone of voice, demonstrate reduced imitation of actions, and be less likely to engage in imaginative play. Sensory and motor findings include visual fixation on objects, under- or overreaction to sounds, repetitive motor behaviors, and delayed fine and gross motor skills. ADHD is characterized by a pattern of inattention and/or hyperactivity that interferes with function or development. Stereotypic movement disorder refers to repetitive and purposeless motor behavior, early in development, that can often be self-injurious. Language disorder is a disorder of communication, in which the child has persistent difficulties in acquiring and using language across a variety of modalities. Specific learning disorder requires persistence of learning disability in a particular subject (e.g., arithmetic, reading, writing) for 6 months despite provision of additional help. This diagnosis is typically given in school-aged children.

REFERENCE

Anagnostou, E., Zwaigenbaum, L., Szatmari, P., et al. (2014). Autism spectrum disorder: Advances in evidence-based practice. *Canadian Medical Association Journal, 186*, 509–519.

2. By what age can a diagnosis of ASD be made reliably?

A. Autism can reliably be diagnosed at six months
B. Autism can reliably be diagnosed at nine months
C. Autism can reliable be diagnosed at 12 months
D. Autism can reliably be diagnosed by age two
E. Early diagnosis is futile since there are no interventions appropriate for children less than 4 years of age.

ANSWER: D

Many children demonstrate signs of autism as early as 12 months, and the disorder can reliably be diagnosed by 2 years of age. Early diagnosis can provide clarity to families. Early interventions are recommended because they offer optimal benefit for the child and his or her family, particularly because the brain is remarkably plastic in the first 3 years of life. Evidence suggests that integrated developmental and behavioral interventions can improve developmental quotients, functioning, and language skills in children who are 2 years old.

REFERENCE

Dawson, G., Rogers, S., Munson, J., et al. (2010). Randomized, controlled trial of an intervention for toddlers with autism: The Early Start Denver Model. *Pediatrics, 125*, e17–e23.

3. The toddler's parents tell you that their daughter had been doing well until she was 10 months old and that she has been progressively deteriorating over the course of a year. The pediatrician has noted a deceleration in her head circumference, failure to grow, and a loss of previously acquired motor milestones. Prenatal, perinatal, and developmental history prior to 10 months of age did not raise any concerns. What is the likely diagnosis?

A. ASD associated with Rett syndrome
B. Childhood-onset fluency disorder
C. Developmental coordination disorder
D. Specific learning disorder
E. Tourette's syndrome

ANSWER: A

About 10% of cases of autism occur in the context of known genetic conditions such as Rett syndrome, fragile X syndrome, Down syndrome, Angelman syndrome, Prader–Willi syndrome, Williams syndrome, neurofibromatosis type 1, tuberous sclerosis, and phenylketonuria. When this occurs, it should be coded as ASD associated with the relevant neurodevelopmental condition. Rett syndrome is characterized by profound cognitive impairment, poor communication skills, stereotypic hand movements, and pervasive growth failure beginning between ages 6 and 18 months after a period of apparently normal development including acquisition of fine motor skills and language. Childhood-onset fluency disorder is characterized by disturbances in normal fluency and time patterning of speech that manifest as repetition of sounds or syllables, prolongation of sounds, broken words, pauses in speech, word substitutions to avoid problematic words, and repetition of monosyllabic whole words such as I, you, we, and so forth. Developmental coordination disorder is a motor disorder in which the acquisition and execution of motor skills is impaired. A child with a specific learning disorder has persistent difficulties with learning and using academic skills. Domains that are impaired include reading, written expression, and mathematics. Tourette's Syndrome requires both vocal and motor tics for at least a year.

REFERENCE

Percy, A. K. (2011). Rett syndrome: Exploring the autism link. *Archives of Neurology, 68*, 985–989.

4. What is the inheritance pattern for Rett syndrome?

A. Autosomal dominant
B. Autosomal recessive
C. X-linked dominant
D. X-linked recessive
E. Non-Mendelian inheritance

ANSWER: C

Rett syndrome was removed from *DSM-5* because it has a clear genetic basis. It is X-linked dominant. It is caused by mutations in the methyl-CpG binding protein 2 or *MECP2*. This condition is fatal in males by the age of 2.

REFERENCE

National Institute of Neurological Disorders and Stroke, US National Institutes of Health. ( ). Rett syndrome fact sheet. Retrieved from http://www.ninds.nih.gov/disorders/rett/detail_rett.htm

5. Which of the following is TRUE about medication management of ASD?

A. Lorazepam is recommended for insomnia.
B. SSRIs eliminate repetitive behaviors.
C. Melatonin reduces aggression.
D. Valproic acid eliminates repetitive behaviors.
E. Atypical antipsychotics are effective at treating irritability and aggression.

ANSWER: E

Atypical antipsychotics such as risperidone and aripiprazole are efficacious for irritability and aggression. Evidence to date does not support the use of SSRIs for repetitive behaviors or aggression in ASD. Stimulants have been shown to be effective at treating ADHD-like symptoms, and melatonin has a positive effect on initial insomnia (but not aggression).

REFERENCE

Anagnostou, E., Zwaigenbaum, L., Szatmari, P., et al. (2014). Autism spectrum disorder: Advances in evidence-based practice. *Canadian Medical Association Journal, 186*, 509–519.

6. Which of the following is efficacious in ASD?

A. Cognitive behavioral therapy
B. Psychodynamic psychotherapy
C. applied behavior analysis
D. Dialectical behavior therapy
E. Existential psychotherapy

ANSWER: C

Current best practice for preschool-aged children with ASD includes a focus on improving language, cognitive, and adaptive skills using applied behavior analysis (ABA) techniques. ABA involves empirically derived learning to produce changes in behavior that describes antecedents behavior, the behaviors themselves, and their consequences. To date there is no evidence to support the use of cognitive therapy, dialectical behavior therapy, psychodynamic psychotherapy, or existential psychotherapy in the treatment of ASD.

REFERENCE

Reichow, B. (2012). Overview of meta-analysis on early intensive behavioral intervention for young children with autism spectrum disorders. *Journal of Autism and Developmental Disorders, 42*, 512–520.

7. What is the most common psychiatric comorbidity in ASD?

A. ADHD
B. Tourette's syndrome
C. Alcohol use disorder
D. Cocaine use disorder
E. Delusional disorder

ANSWER: A

The most commonly occurring psychiatric comorbidities in ASD are ADHD, anxiety disorders, and depressive disorders.

REFERENCE

Mazzone, L., Ruta, L., & Reale, L. (2012). Psychiatric comorbidities in Asperger syndrome and high functioning autism: Diagnostic challenges. *Annals of General Psychiatry, 11*, 16.

QUESTIONS AND ANSWERS

This chapter has accompanying questions and answers which are available to subscribers as part of the Oxford eLearning platform. To access the questions, follow the link below, or go to http://oxford-elearning.oup.com/books.

http://oxford-elearning.oup.com/books/test/67/10.1093/med/9780190265557.003.0034

35.

CLINICAL VIGNETTE

LEGAL (COMPETENCE TO STAND TRIAL)

Isabella Michna

A 25-year-old man was evaluated by the consultation–liaison psychiatry at the request of the burn surgery service. The man had burned his wife and children using gasoline and subsequently set himself on fire. He was convinced that he and the members of his family were polluted and were going to hell unless their sins were purged with fire. Following medical stabilization, the patient was deemed incompetent to stand trial by a judge.

1. Which of the following is required for a criminal defendant to be competent to stand trial?

A. Absence of psychosis
B. Able to distinguish right from wrong
C. Logical, linear, goal-directed thought process
D. Ninth-grade education level
E. Able to consult with own lawyer and participate in own defense

ANSWER: E

The 1960 Supreme Court Case *Dusky v. United States* outlined the basic standards for determining competence. Competence to stand trial is a legal construct used to identify those criminal defendants who have the requisite mental capacity to understand the nature and objective of the proceedings against them and to participate rationally in preparing their defense. There is no psychiatric disorder, sign, or symptom that automatically implies incompetence.

REFERENCE

Dusky v. United States, 362 U.S. 402, 1960. Retrieved from https://supreme.justia.com/cases/federal/us/362/402/case.html

2. Which of the following ethical principles applies when a psychiatrist determines competence to stand trial?

A. Beneficence
B. Nonmaleficence
C. Autonomy
D. Truth-telling
E. Patient advocacy

ANSWER: D

Conducting a competence-to-stand-trial evaluation may supersede traditional ethical principles of beneficence and nonmaleficence because findings supporting competence to stand trial inevitably enable the court to try, convict, and punish the defendant. For this reason, many psychiatrists do not regard helping the patient as a central task when they are completing competence evaluations. The principles of truth-telling, objectivity, and responsibility to assist in the administration of justice are relevant when determining competence to stand trial.

REFERENCE

Appelbaum, P. S. (1997). A theory of ethics for forensic psychiatry. *Journal of the American Academy of Psychiatry and the Law, 25*, 233–247.

3. Which of the following should a psychiatrist communicate when beginning an evaluation of competence to stand trial?

A. The reason for the evaluation
B. The lack of confidentiality of the interview and findings

C. The right of the evaluee to decline to answer particular questions, with a caveat that noncooperation or refusal may need to be reported
D. The possibility that the psychiatrist will testify regarding the results of the evaluation
E. All of the above

ANSWER: E

When beginning an examination of competence to stand trial, the psychiatrist should attempt to communicate all of the following: the reason for the evaluation, the party who has appointed the psychiatrist, the lack of confidentiality of the interview and findings, the people who will receive the psychiatrist's report, the possibility of the psychiatrist testifying regarding the results of the evaluation, and the right of the evaluee to decline to answer particular questions, with a warning that the psychiatrist may have to report noncooperation or refusal to answer questions to the retaining attorney or to the court.

REFERENCE

Mossman, D., Noffsinger, S. G., Ash, P., Frierson, R. L., Gerbasi, J., Hackett, M., & Zonana, H. V.. (2007). AAPL practice guideline for the forensic psychiatric evaluation of competence to stand trial. *Journal of the American Academy of Psychiatry and the Law, 35*(4 suppl.), S3–S72.

4. When conducting evaluations of competence to stand trial, which of the following statements is true regarding the roles of treating and evaluating psychiatrists?

A. Treating psychiatrists should avoid assessing competence to stand trial on their own patients.
B. A psychiatrist's dual agency does not compromise the therapeutic relationship.
C. A psychiatrist's dual agency does not compromise doctor–patient confidentiality.
D. A psychiatrist's dual agency does not compromise objectivity in the forensic report.
E. Treating psychiatrists are ideally suited to assess competence to stand trial on their own patients.

ANSWER: A

Dual agency occurs when a treating psychiatrist assumes a forensic role with the patient. Because of the medico-legal principles imposed on a psychiatrist when serving in a forensic capacity (namely, that he or she is serving the judicial system rather than the interests of the individual patient), treating psychiatrists should generally avoid conducting forensic evaluations on their own patients. Dual agency can compromise the therapeutic relationship. Determining and reporting competence to stand trial typically involves disclosure to third parties, such as attorneys, and is a violation of confidentiality. Furthermore, given the psychiatrist's preexisting professional relationship and commitment to the patient, his or her objectivity in the forensic process may be compromised. Ideally, independent, nontreating psychiatrists should perform such evaluations.

REFERENCES

Nicholson, R. A., & McNulty, J. L. (1992). Outcome of hospitalization for defendants found incompetent to stand trial. *Behavioral Sciences and the Law, 10*, 371–383.
Strasburger, L. H., Gutheil, T. G., & Brodsky, A. (1997). On wearing two hats: Role conflict in serving as both psychotherapist and expert witness. *American Journal of Psychiatry, 154*, 448–456.

5. Which of the following factors among juvenile offenders undergoing a competence to stand trial assessment predicts likelihood of being found NOT competent to stand trial?

A. Anxiety disorder
B. Over the age of 15
C. Intellectual disability
D. Serious mood disorder
E. Substance use disorder

ANSWER: C

Competence to stand trial assessment of juveniles is a relatively recent phenomenon. Research has found that juvenile offenders under the age of 15, offenders with intellectual disability, or offenders with other neurodevelopmental disorder are more likely to be found incompetent. Youth older than 15 and those with a mood, psychotic, or substance use disorder are less likely to be found incompetent.

REFERENCE

Bath, E., Reba-Harrelson, L., Peace, R., Shen, J., Liu, H.. Correlates of competency to stand trial among youths admitted to a juvenile mental health court. *Journal of the American Academy of Psychiatry and the Law, 43*, 329–339.

6. What is the next step after a criminal defendant is found incompetent to stand trial?

A. The defendant pleads guilty.
B. The defendant is remanded to jail.
C. The defendant released on his or her own recognizance.
D. The defendant pleads not guilty by reason of insanity.
E. The defendant begins the process of having competence restored.

ANSWER: E

Once deemed incompetent to stand trial, the defendant is committed to restoration in either an inpatient or an outpatient setting. Many defendants can be restored to competence in an outpatient setting from a clinical safety and a public safety standpoint, yet a majority of states still require psychiatric hospitalization to evaluate and restore to competence. Dangerousness is a critical factor in determining the location for restoration of competence as are state resources. Note: Competence to stand trial refers to a defendant's ability to participate in his or her own defense, whereas "not guilty by reason of insanity" is predicated on the mental state at the time of the crime.

REFERENCE

Johnson, N. R., & Candilis, P. J. (2015). Outpatient competence restoration: A model and outcomes. *World Journal of Psychiatry, 5*, 228–233.

Miller, R. D. (2003). Hospitalization of criminal defendants for evaluation of competence to stand trial or for restoration of competence: Clinical and legal issues. *Behavioral Sciences and the Law, 21*, 369–391.

7. Once an individual is found incompetent to stand trial and committed to a state psychiatric hospital, treatment begins in order to restore competence. What is the role of compulsory treatment in this setting?

A. Involuntary medication is not allowed.
B. Involuntary medication is allowed if it can restore competence.
C. Involuntary medication is allowed only for dangerousness to self or others.
D. Involuntary medication may be allowed if the defendant disagrees with the charges.
E. Involuntary medication may be given even if the defendant is willing to take medication orally.

ANSWER: B

The case of *Washington v. Harper* was a landmark case that determined that it is constitutional to administer involuntary medications to a defendant who is facing serious criminal charges to render that defendant competent to stand trial, provided that the treatment is medically appropriate, is unlikely to undermine the fairness of the trial, takes into account less coercive alternatives, and is necessary to advance the interests of the trial.

REFERENCE

Washington v. Harper, 494 U.S. 210 (1990). Retrieved from https://supreme.justia.com/cases/federal/us/494/210/

QUESTIONS AND ANSWERS

This chapter has accompanying questions and answers which are available to subscribers as part of the Oxford eLearning platform. To access the questions, follow the link below, or go to http://oxford-elearning.oup.com/books.

http://oxford-elearning.oup.com/books/test/67/10.1093/med/9780190265557.003.0035

36.

CLINICAL VIGNETTE

ETHICS (CAPACITY EVALUATION)

Tobias Wasser

A 73-year-old man with major neurocognitive disorder due to Alzheimer's disease is admitted to the general medicine service for evaluation and management of gastrointestinal bleeding. The patient refuses to undergo upper and lower endoscopy, stating, "No thanks, doc, I've lived a good life." You are consulted by the primary team to assess the patient's capacity to refuse endoscopy.

1. Which of the following are key components of decision-making capacity? (Check all that apply.)

A. Communicate a choice.
B. Understand relevant information.
C. Appreciate the medical consequences of the situation.
D. Offer a rational explanation regarding treatment decision.
E. Agree with the medical provider's recommendation.

ANSWER: A, B, C, D.

Standards for decision-making capacity for consent to treatment vary somewhat across jurisdictions. Generally they embody the abilities to communicate a choice, to understand the relevant information, to appreciate the medical consequences of the situation, and to reason about treatment choices. The mnemonic "CRAM" is a common means of recalling these four elements (*c*ommunicate decision, *r*elevant information understood, *a*ppreciate risks/benefits and alternatives, and *m*anipulate information in a rational, reality-based fashion).

REFERENCE

Appelbaum, P. S. (2007). Clinical practice: Assessment of patients' competence to consent to treatment. *New England Journal of Medicine, 357,* 1834–1840.

2. Who is capable of assessing a patient's decision-making capacity for medical decisions?

A. Only a psychiatrist
B. Only a psychiatrist with clinical expertise in this area
C. Any physician
D. A psychologist
E. A registered nurse or a physician

ANSWER: C

Not only may any treating physician assess a patient's decision-making capacity, but a physician should assess capacity to make medical decisions whenever providing care. Physicians are obligated to ensure that patients provide informed consent when making medical decisions such as consenting to a procedure or taking medication. A treating nonpsychiatric physician has the advantage of greater familiarity with the patient and with available treatment options. Psychiatric consultation may be helpful in complex cases.

REFERENCE

Ganzini, L., Volicer, L., Nelson, W., Derse, A. (2003). Pitfalls in assessment of decision-making capacity. *Psychosomatics, 44,* 237–243.

3. A diagnosis of which of the following conditions indicates that a patient inevitably lacks decision-making capacity?

A. Stroke
B. Dementia
C. Depression
D. Schizophrenia
E. None of the above

ANSWER: E

Any diagnosis that compromises mentation can lead to impairment in decision-making capacity. Neurocognitive disorders such as delirium or dementia (major neurocognitive disorder in *DSM-5*) commonly impair decision-making capacity, but most diagnoses encompass a range of severity. Therefore, no diagnosis automatically means that decision-making capacity is impaired.

REFERENCE

Rosenstein, D. L., & Miller, F. G. (2011). Ethical issues. In J. L. Levenson (Ed.), *Textbook of psychosomatic medicine: Psychiatric care of the medically ill* (2nd ed., pp. 33–44). Washington, DC: American Psychiatric Publishing.

4. Which of the following pieces of information relevant to the patient's treatment decision must be provided to the patient before a conclusion regarding decision-making capacity can be made? (Check all that apply.)

A. The wishes of the patient's family
B. The nature of the patient's condition
C. The nature and purpose of the proposed treatment
D. The risks and benefits of the proposed treatment
E. The risks and benefits of alternative treatments, including the option of forgoing treatment

ANSWER: B, C, D, E.

The first step in assessing for decision-making capacity is to ensure that the information relevant to making an informed decision has been communicated to the patient. Typically, such disclosure includes the nature of the patient's condition, the nature and purpose of the proposed treatment, and the risks and benefits of the proposed treatment and of alternative treatments, including the option of no treatment. Because such disclosure cannot be presumed, either the evaluator should ask a physician responsible for the patient's care to disclose the relevant information again in the evaluator's presence or the evaluator should undertake the disclosure.

REFERENCE

Appelbaum, P. S. (2007). Clinical practice: Assessment of patients' competence to consent to treatment. *New England Journal of Medicine, 357*, 1834–1840.

5. Which cognitive screening test has been found to best correlate with clinical judgment of incapacity for medical decision-making?

A. Young Mania Rating Scale
B. Beck Depression Inventory
C. Brief Psychiatric Rating Scale
D. Mini-Mental State Examination
E. Minnesota Multiphasic Personality Inventory

ANSWER: D

The Mini-Mental State Examination (MMSE) correlates with clinical judgments of incapacity, and it may have some use in identifying patients at the high and low ends of the range of capacity, especially among elderly persons with cognitive impairment. MMSE scores of less than 19 are highly likely to be associated with impaired decision-making capacity.

REFERENCE

Appelbaum, P. S. (2007). Clinical practice: Assessment of patients' competence to consent to treatment. *New England Journal of Medicine, 357*, 1834–1840.

6. If the patient above is deemed to lack decision-making capacity, which guiding principle must be called upon to determine the appropriate course of action?

A. Autonomy
B. Paternalism
C. Beneficence
D. Best interests
E. Substituted judgment

ANSWER: E

When a patient lacks the capacity to make a decision, a substitute decision-maker must be sought. For patients with advance directives, either the treatment choice or the appointment of a surrogate decision-maker should take effect. In the absence of an advance directive, the patient's family should be contacted. Many states have statutes indicating the order in which family members may be approached. In general, the order is first the spouse, then the adult children, parents, and siblings, followed by other relatives. Paternalism refers to the physician serving as a parent, making decisions for that patient even at the expense of autonomy. The legal doctrine of parens patriae (for "parent of the nation") provides justification for appointment of a conservator or guardian (depending on jurisdiction) to protect citizens who are otherwise unable to protect or provide adequately for themselves. Conservators/guardians are statutorily charged to adhere to the "best interests" principle, rather than a "substituted judgment." Beneficence refers to the principle of acting to benefit the patient. Autonomy refers to the patient's right to make decisions pertaining to his or her healthcare.

REFERENCE

Beauchamp, T. L., & Childress, J. L. (2012). Moral principles. In T. L. Beauchamp & J. L. Childress (Eds.), *Principles of biomedical ethics* (7th ed.). New York, NY: Oxford University Press.

7. Which of the following statements is TRUE regarding consultations for decision-making capacity?

A. They constitute about half of psychiatric consultation requests in general hospitals.
B. They commonly find that a patient retains decision-making capacity.
C. Decision-making capacity is more often than not obvious to both consultee and consultant.
D. Capacity consultations are often a euphemism for managing a frustrating patient care situation.
E. Capacity consultation requests are sometimes an appeal for help by the primary team in addressing a moral or ethical question.

ANSWER: B, C. D, E.

Capacity evaluation requests account for a growing proportion of requests for consultations made to psychiatric consultation–liaison services, though they do not account for half of consult requests. In about a third of cases it is clear that even though the explicit consultation question is about decision-making capacity, there is a "hidden" consultation question. Often this "hidden" question is ethical in nature and frustrating to the primary team. In order for optimal care to proceed, ethical questions need to be acknowledged and addressed.

REFERENCES

Kontos, N., Freudenreich, O., & Querques, J. (2013). Beyond capacity: Identifying ethical dilemmas underlying capacity evaluation requests. *Psychosomatics, 54*, 103–110.
Kornfeld, D. S., Muskin, P. R., & Tahil, F. A. (2009). Psychiatric evaluation of mental capacity in the general hospital: A significant teaching opportunity. *Psychosomatics, 50*, 468–473.

8. Which of the following requires the greatest threshold for decision-making capacity?

A. A life-saving blood transfusion
B. Appointing a surrogate decision-maker
C. An oral antibiotic for a urinary tract infection
D. A lumbar puncture to evaluate for suspected meningitis
E. Consenting to participate in a drug trial for Alzheimer's disease

ANSWER: E

Decisions vary in the cognitive and emotional demands they place on patients. Therefore, impairment of decision-making capacity for one decision does not necessarily imply impairment for other decisions. A "sliding-scale" approach is often used in determining capacity, where clinicians have a low threshold for deeming the patient to have capacity to make decisions of low risk and high benefit, and a high threshold for deeming the patient to have capacity to make decisions of high risk and low benefit. An alternative approach maintains that the threshold for most medical decisions is fundamentally the same but that the complexity of the decision (including the number of options and their attendant risks/benefits) varies greatly, creating an illusion of a "sliding scale." Most patients who lack the capacity to make a particular medical decision are usually determined to *retain* the capacity to appoint a surrogate decision-maker, which can facilitate care delivery. Similarly, receiving a life-saving transfusion, a lumbar puncture, or an oral antibiotic are all interventions that can be life-saving, conferring low risk with clear benefit. Participating in research is associated with many unknown risks with potentially very little, if any, direct benefit. Therefore, the threshold is relatively "high" for allowing a patient to participate in research.

REFERENCES

Rosenstein, D. L., & Miller, F. G. (2011). Ethical issues. In J. L. Levenson (Ed.), *Textbook of psychosomatic medicine: Psychiatric care of the medically ill* (2nd ed., pp. 33–44). Washington, DC: American Psychiatric Publishing.

Sadock, B. J., & Sadock, V. A. Psychosomatic medicine. In *Kaplan and Sadock's synopsis of psychiatry* (11th ed., pp. 999–1081). Philadelphia, PA: Lippincott Williams and Wilkins.

QUESTIONS AND ANSWERS

This chapter has accompanying questions and answers which are available to subscribers as part of the Oxford eLearning platform. To access the questions, follow the link below, or go to http://oxford-elearning.oup.com/books.

http://oxford-elearning.oup.com/books/test/67/10.1093/med/9780190265557.003.0036

37.

CLINICAL VIGNETTE

DELIRIUM

Filza Hussain

A 70-year-old woman with Parkinson's disease underwent hip fracture repair surgery after falling at home. She was noted to be somnolent shortly after the surgery. Later that evening she was irritable and repeatedly tried to get up to go to the bathroom despite being reminded she had a urinary catheter in place. She was seen muttering to herself and picking at her clothes. Psychiatry was consulted after she flung a glass full of ice chips across the room at the nursing aide. Her family, who describe her as a "sweet little lady," were surprised and concerned by this behavior.

On examination with you, she is pleasant and cooperative. She has baseline mild cogwheel rigidity. She is unable to perform serial 7s and spell the word *world* backward. She is increasingly upset with you for "playing mind games" on her.

1. What is the most likely explanation for the patient's presentation?

A. Delirium
B. Postsurgical depression
C. Advancing Parkinson's disease
D. Major neurocognitive disorder
E. Adjustment disorder with behavioral disturbance

ANSWER: A

Delirium presents with an acute change in mental status accompanied by inattention, reduced awareness of surroundings, at least one additional cognitive deficit, and often a range of behavioral, emotional, and personality symptoms. It is frequently misdiagnosed as depression, other psychiatric disorders, or dementia. About 40% of psychiatry consults in the general hospital for depression end up being delirium. In delirium, a patient has difficulty focusing, sustaining, or shifting attention, which is thought to cause many of the other features of the condition. The sudden onset of cognitive and behavioral changes effectively rules out dementia, though, notably, episodes of confusion are common in neurocognitive disorder with Lewy bodies. Delirium is due to the direct neurophysiological effects of metabolic or inflammatory disturbances, as is illustrated in this case, whereas adjustment disorder is caused by psychological response to stress.

REFERENCES

van Meenen, L. C, van Meenen, D. M., de Rooij, S. E., & ter Riet, G. (2014). Risk prediction models for postoperative delirium: A systematic review and meta-analysis. *Journal of the American Geriatrics Society, 62*, 2383–2390.

Vardy, E. R., Teodorczuk, A., & Yarnall, A. J. (2015). Review of delirium in patients with Parkinson's disease. *Journal of Neurology, 262*, 2401–2410.

2. What is the value in early recognition of this patient's condition?

A. Prompts indicated medical workup
B. Prescription of an antidepressant
C. Transfer to a psychiatric unit
D. Transfer to a nursing home
E. No significant outcome

ANSWER: B

Delirium continues to be underrecognized in the general hospital. It is frequently misdiagnosed as depression or dementia. Nondetection is associated with poorer outcomes, including longer hospital stays, prolonged exposure to hospital pathogens, other causes of morbidity such as pulling out lines and increased mortality. Early detection prompts a medical workup and informs medical care with the goal of reducing morbidity in patients. Delirium is typically best managed in a medical setting where the underlying medical conditions can be treated; only rarely do the behavioral disturbances due to delirium or other neurocognitive disorders require admission to a geriatric psychiatric unit. Discharge to a nursing facility should be deferred until the patient is stable.

REFERENCES

Kat, M. G., de Jonghe, J. F., Vreeswijk, R., van der Ploeg, T., van Gool, W. A., Eikelenboom, P., & Kalisvaart, K. J. (2011). Mortality associated with delirium after hip-surgery: A 2-year follow-up study. *Age and Ageing*, *40*, 312–318.

Mittal, V., Muralee, S., Williamson, D., McEnerney, N., Thomas, J., Cash, M., & Tampi, R. R. (2011). Delirium in the elderly: A comprehensive review. *American Journal of Alzheimer's Disease and Other Dementias*, *26*, 97–109.

3. Which of the following are risk factors for the development of delirium? (Check all that apply.)

A. Age
B. Neurocognitive impairment
C. Polypharmacy
D. Functional impairment
E. Visual impairment
F. Elevated albumin
G. Elevated BUN

ANSWER: ALL BUT F

Advanced age, neurocognitive impairment, polypharmacy, functional impairment, visual impairment, *low* albumin, and elevated BUN have all been identified as risk factors for developing delirium.

REFERENCE

Oh, E. S., Li, M., Fafowora, T. M., Inouye, S. K., Chen, C. H., Rosman, L. M., ... Puhan, M. A. (2015). Preoperative risk factors for postoperative delirium following hip fracture repair: A systematic review. *International Journal of Geriatric Psychiatry*, *30*, 900–910.

4. Which of the following strategies are recommended as part of multicomponent interventions to prevent delirium? (Check all that apply.)

A. Frequent reorientation
B. Early mobilization
C. Promoting normal sleep–wake cycles
D. Correcting sensory deficits
E. Good hydration

ANSWER: ALL OF THE ABOVE

Nonpharmacological care bundles can prevent up to a third of delirium among at-risk patients. Common care bundles include Vanderbilt's ABCDE bundle and the CEDARTREE's Hospital Elder Life Program (HELP). Which of these interventions prevents delirium independently versus in combination with the others remains an area of active investigation.

REFERENCE

Kalish, V. B., Gillham, J. E., & Unwin, B. K. (2014). Delirium in older persons: Evaluation and management. *American Family Physician*, *90*, 150–158.

5. Which of the following may prolong or worsen the patient's condition?

A. Quetiapine
B. Lorazepam
C. Risperidone
D. Buspirone
E. Escitalopram

ANSWER: B

Benzodiazepines are deliriogenic and should be avoided in delirium with the exception of alcohol withdrawal delirium or when used in combination with a neuroleptic for acute tranquilization. Anticholinergics should also be avoided because they worsen delirium. Antipsychotics such as quetiapine and risperidone are commonly used to manage the behavioral and psychological feature of delirium, though it bears noting that no medication is approved by the FDA for delirium. In a patient with Parkinson's disease, quetiapine is typically preferred as a first-line agent. Buspirone does not have a role in acute management of delirium.

REFERENCE

Clegg, A., & Young, J. B. (2011). Which medications to avoid in people at risk of delirium: A systematic review. *Age and Ageing*, *40*, 23–29.

6. Which class of medications has been shown to prevent postoperative delirium?

A. Antidepressants
B. Mood stabilizers
C. Sedative–hypnotics
D. Opioids
E. Antipsychotics

ANSWER: E

Antipsychotics prevent delirium in a variety of postsurgical settings, particularly following orthopedic surgery.

REFERENCE

Fok, M. C., Sepehry, A. A., Frisch, L., Sztramko, R., Borger van der Burg, B. L. S., Vochteloo, A. J. H., & Chan, P. (2015). Do antipsychotics prevent postoperative delirium? A systematic review and meta-analysis. *International Journal of Geriatric Psychiatry, 30*, 333–344.

QUESTIONS AND ANSWERS

This chapter has accompanying questions and answers which are available to subscribers as part of the Oxford eLearning platform. To access the questions, follow the link below, or go to http://oxford-elearning.oup.com/books.

http://oxford-elearning.oup.com/books/test/67/10.1093/med/9780190265557.003.0037

38.

CLINICAL VIGNETTE

PSYCHOSOMATICS (HIV)

Mark Oldham

A 25-year-old Latino man with historical intravenous heroin use presents to your clinic with a chief complaint of panic attacks. After developing rapport with you, he confides that he has a history of recurrent sexual molestation from the ages of 6 to 9. He also shares a concern that he might have HIV because his partner, with whom he has been sexually active for 5 years, was recently hospitalized for confusion and ultimately diagnosed with AIDS. The patient routinely engages in unprotected receptive anal intercourse with his partner.

1. Which of the following factors place this patient at increased risk of contracting HIV? (Check all that apply.)

A. Substance use history
B. Trauma history
C. Sexual activity
D. Ethnicity
E. Gender
F. Age

ANSWER: ALL OF THE ABOVE

Each of these factors increases the patient's baseline risk of HIV. HIV rates remain higher among men who have sex with men (MSM), and anal intercourse (especially receptive) is associated with higher risk of contracting HIV than vaginal intercourse. Intravenous drug use is another well-established risk factor for HIV. Additionally, being young and Hispanic places the patient in a high-risk category for HIV positivity. Three of four people with HIV in the United States are men, and there is a growing recognition of the syndemic (*i.e.*, two epidemics that reinforce one another) of HIV and history of trauma. Historically, the four Hs for HIV risk were homosexuality, Haitian ethnicity, hemophilia (due to blood transfusions), and (IV) heroin use. The association between HIV and Hatian ethnicity has diminished, and transmission due to blood transfusion is effectively non-existent—at least in developed countries—now that blood donations are screened for HIV.

REFERENCES

Brezing, C., Ferrara, M., Freudenreich, O. (2015). The syndemic illness of HIV and trauma: Implications for a trauma-informed model of care. *Psychosomatics*, *56*, 107–118.

Scott, H. M., Vittinghoff, E., Irvin, R., Sachdev, D., Liu, A., Gurwith, M., Buchbinder, S. P. (2014). Age, race/ethnicity, and behavioral risk factors associated with per-contact risk of HIV infection among men who have sex with men in the United States. *Journal of Acquired Immune Deficiency Syndromes, 65*, 115–121.

Centers for Disease Control. HIV/AIDS: HIV by Group. Retrieved from http://www.cdc.gov/hiv/group/

2. You diagnose the patient with major depression and opioid use disorder and order several laboratory tests, including complete blood panel, comprehensive metabolic panel, serum thyroid stimulating hormone, immunoassay for HIV, and urine toxicology—the only notable result of which is the presence of HIV. You decide to start fluoxetine and titrate slowly to effect and refer him to a local HIV clinic. You speak with the infectious disease doctor, who recommends combination antiretroviral therapy (cART), and you confirm that the patient is on fluoxetine. Which of the following antiretrovirals should be avoided due to potential interaction with fluoxetine?

A. Zidovudine
B. Nevirapine
C. Indinavir
D. Efavirenz
E. Ritonavir

ANSWER: E

Ritonavir is a protease inhibitor commonly added as part of combination antiretroviral therapy (cART) regimens to "boost" CNS levels of other protease inhibitors (such as indinavir, darunavir, or fosamprenavir) by inhibition of p-glycoprotein. P-glycoprotein serves as an efflux pump, removing many xenobiotics from the brain. Ritonavir also has significant effects on the p450 system, inhibiting 2D6 and 3A4 while inducing 1A2. It increases CNS activity of fluoxetine via p-glycoprotein and p450 inhibition. In general, sertraline or paroxetine may be preferred in patients with HIV due to fewer potential interactions with HIV medications.

REFERENCE

University of Liverpool. Antidepressant treatment selector. (2016). Retrieved from www.hiv-druginteractions.org/

3. Which of the following antiretrovirals may worsen depression in this patient?

A. Zidovudine
B. Nevirapine
C. Indinavir
D. Efavirenz
E. Ritonavir

ANSWER: D

Both premarketing and postmarketing evidence suggest that efavirenz is associated with serious psychiatric adverse experiences, the most common being depression. In the premarketing study quoted in the package insert, intravenous drug use, depression history, and being on a psychotropic agent were all risk factors for developing depression on efavirenz.

REFERENCE

Sustiva (efavirenz) package insert. Retrieved from dailymed.nlm.nih.gov/

4. Which herb or supplement is best avoided in patients on combination antiretroviral therapy?

A. Ginseng
B. Melatonin
C. Milk thistle
D. St. John's wort
E. Omega-3 fatty acids

ANSWER: D

St. John's wort induces 3A4 and p-glycoprotein and should not be coadministered with a range of HIV medications. These metabolic effects may compromise efficacy of antiretroviral therapy. The other agents are not known to have significant interactions. Not listed here as options, ginkgo biloba induces 3A4, and garlic inhibits 2C9 and 3A4. The clinical relevance of these effects, though, remains unclear.

REFERENCES

Mills, E., Monori, V., Perri, D., Phillips, E., Koren, G. (2005). Natural health product–HIV drug interactions: A systematic review. *International Journal of STD and AIDS, 16*, 181–186.

University of Liverpool. Antidepressant treatment selector. (2016). Retrieved from www.hiv-druginteractions.org/

5. Which of the following best describes the relationship between HIV disease and trauma? (Check all that apply.)

A. Sexual trauma can transmit HIV.
B. HIV-positive men are more likely than HIV-negative men to have a history of trauma.
C. HIV-positive women report more intimate partner violence than HIV-negative women.
D. A trauma history may indirectly lead to HIV acquisition by way of intravenous drug use.

ANSWER: E

Each of the above statements is true. The high co-occurrence of HIV disease and trauma has been labeled a syndemic, defined as two epidemics that reinforce one another.

REFERENCE

Brezing, C., Ferrara, M., & Freudenreich, O. (2015). The syndemic illness of HIV and trauma: Implications for a trauma-informed model of care. *Psychosomatics, 56*, 107–118.

6. Which of the following sexual disorders is most likely to be found in this patient?

A. Coolidge effect
B. Erectile disorder
C. Delayed ejaculation
D. Premature ejaculation
E. Male hypoactive sexual desire disorder

ANSWER: B

Several factors increase the patient's risk of erectile disorder, not least of which is the high prevalence of hypogonadism found in HIV-positive men. Up to a quarter of young to middle-aged men with HIV have hypogonadism (colloquially "low T"). Specific HIV-related factors include poor clinical or nutritional status, co-morbid opioid use, and pituitary dysfunction. In addition, use of fluoxetine carries a risk of sexual side effects, including erectile disorder.

REFERENCE

Rochira, V., & Guaraldi, G. (2014). Hypogonadism in the HIV-infected man. *Endocrinology and Metabolism Clinics of North America, 43,* 709–730.

7. At your next visit the patient continues to have moderate symptoms of depression. He explains, "I can't tell if I'm coming or going. I keep forgetting things, and I'm clumsy." He is concerned that he will "lose his mind" like his partner did. Despite his complaints of memory impairment, he is fully oriented, recalls three objects after 5 minutes, and has an intact fist-edge-palm test. Urine toxicology screens have consistently been negative for any substances of abuse. Which of the following would be most appropriate at this time?

A. Evaluate for HIV-associated mild neurocognitive disorder.
B. Evaluate for HIV-1-associated minor cognitive/motor disorder.
C. Recommend lumbar puncture to rule out CNS infection.
D. Recommend brain MRI to evaluate for structural CNS disease.
E. Treat depression.

ANSWER: E

HIV-associated neurocognitive disorder (HAND) may occur in *nearly half of patients with HIV disease,* although thankfully in the era of combination antiretroviral therapy, HAND is now much more commonly either asymptomatic or mild rather than the devastating dementia prevalent through the early 1990s. The Frascati criteria published in 2007 represent the latest iteration of operationalized HAND diagnosis; these include HIV-associated asymptomatic neurocognitive impairment, mild neurocognitive disorder, and dementia. However, these *cannot be diagnosed during clinical depression or within a month of active substance use.* Management of depression takes precedence in this clinical situation. HIV-1-associated minor cognitive/motor disorder is an outdated term. Of note, whereas HAND is a more widely accepted diagnostic construct, *DSM-5* has adopted mild and major neurocognitive disorder due to HIV disease as new diagnostic categories.

REFERENCE

Antinori, A., Arendt, G., Becker, J. T., Brew, B. J., Byrd, D. A., Cherner, M., Clifford, D. B., Cinque, P., et al. (2007). Updated research nosology for HIV-associated neurocognitive disorders. *Neurology, 69,* 1789–1799.

8. Which of the following has been shown to prevent HIV-associated neurocognitive disorder?

A. Antiretroviral therapy with high CNS penetration
B. Selective serotonin reuptake inhibitors
C. NMDA receptor antagonists
D. Psychostimulants
E. None of the above

ANSWER: E

There is no question that combined antiretroviral therapy (cART; historically highly active antiretroviral therapy, or HAART) has transformed HIV from a death sentence to a chronic disease, and severe dementia due to HIV disease itself (likely an immune-mediated process) has given way to milder forms of neurocognitive impairment. In this way, cART has influenced the course and severity of HAND. It has not eliminated it though. Up to half of patients still have significant neurocognitive impairment. There is no clear evidence that cART regimens with high CNS penetration prevent HAND, though high-penetration regimens are generally recommended to lower HIV concentration in the cerebrospinal fluid. Psychostimulants may be used to treat symptoms of

HAND such as slowed processing speed but do not alter the disease course.

REFERENCE

Ellis, R. J., Letendre, S., Vaida, F., Haubrich, R., Heaton, RK, Sacktor, N., Clifford, D. B., Best, B. M., et al. (2014). Randomized trial of central nervous system-targeted antiretrovirals for HIV-associated neurocognitive disorder. *Clinical Infectious Diseases, 58*, 1015–1022.

QUESTIONS AND ANSWERS

This chapter has accompanying questions and answers which are available to subscribers as part of the Oxford eLearning platform. To access the questions, follow the link below, or go to http://oxford-elearning.oup.com/books.

http://oxford-elearning.oup.com/books/test/67/10.1093/med/9780190265557.003.0038

39.

CLINICAL VIGNETTE

MOOD DISORDERS (WITH SUICIDAL IDEATION)

Sarah Jillani

A 38-year-old man was brought to the emergency room by the police after his cousin called 911. He was found by his wife counting several pills that were laid out on the bed, which he planned to take to end his life. He appeared overwhelmed, restless, and perturbed. He stated, "I just want to give up my life." He endorsed severe depressive symptoms, feeling like he was a "loser" because he had lost his job as a teacher and believing he was a burden to his wife, saying she would be better off without him. He was unable to identify any reasons to live.

1. The next step in management of this patient should be:

A. Discharge to outpatient primary care with recommendations for management.
B. Discharge to outpatient psychiatric care.
C. Admit to the inpatient psychiatric unit for safety and stabilization.
D. Refer to group psychotherapy.
E. Refer to intensive outpatient treatment.

ANSWER: C

The severity of suicidal ideation, the frequency of the ideation, duration, reason for ideation, deterrents from committing suicide, or any action that the patient has taken toward suicide should all be assessed when evaluating suicide risk. This patient's interrupted suicide attempt, psychomotor activation, and anxiety are all risk factors for acute suicide completion and place him in a category of high risk for suicide. The inpatient psychiatric unit is the appropriate place for him to be evaluated, treated, and stabilized. Management in an outpatient setting would be inappropriate. Group psychotherapy alone would be inadequate treatment for the patient's severe depression and would provide insufficient monitoring of the patient's suicide risk. Intensive outpatient treatment would be an appropriate level of care following stabilization on an inpatient unit.

REFERENCE

Posner, K., Brown, G. K., Stanley, B. et al. (2011). The Columbia-Suicide Severity Rating Scale: Initial validity and internal consistency findings from three multisite studies with adolescents and adults. *American Journal of Psychiatry, 168*, 1266–1277.

2. Further history reveals that a few years ago the patient abruptly became "the life of the party," squandered his children's college fund on gambling, and was caught in an affair. He recalls how at the time it seemed "like I could do anything." During that time he was glad to feel rested after 3 hours of sleep and recalls looking into becoming a CEO. His friends told him that he needed to slow down. Two weeks after this very enjoyable period, his enthusiasm "crashed," leaving him depressed. He was treated with fluoxetine in the past, but it caused him to become restless, anxious, and irritable, so he stopped taking it. With this further information, the patient's most likely psychiatric diagnosis is:

A. Major depressive disorder
B. Bipolar I disorder, current episode depressed
C. Bipolar I disorder, current episode manic with mixed features
D. Cyclothymic disorder
E. Bipolar II disorder, current episode depressed

ANSWER: B

When a patient presents with a major depressive episode, it is necessary to inquire about previous manic or hypomanic symptoms because a major depressive episode may occur as part of bipolar disorder. Bipolar I disorder is a chronic, recurrent mood disorder characterized by the presence of at least one manic episode and usually recurrent major depressive episodes. A manic episode is a distinct period of abnormally and persistently elevated, expansive, or irritable mood lasting at least 1 week, or any duration if hospitalization is necessary. During the mood episode, symptoms such as grandiosity, inflated self-esteem, flight of ideas, goal-directed hyperactivity, pressured speech, excessive involvement in pleasurable activities, and marked impairment in occupational, social, and relationship functioning are prominent. Another key feature during a manic episode is the decrease need for sleep. Bipolar II disorder is also a chronic disorder that requires at least one hypomanic and one major depressive episode but is commonly marked by severe, recurrent, often psychotic depression. Cyclothymic disorder is characterized by a 2-year period during which there have been numerous periods of hypomanic symptoms that do not meet criteria for a hypomanic or manic episode and numerous periods of depressive symptoms that do not meet criteria for a major depressive episode. The current or most recent episode should be specified when diagnosing bipolar disorder.

REFERENCE

American Psychiatric Association. (2013). Depressive disorders. In *Diagnostic and statistical manual of mental disorders* (5th ed.). Washington, DC: American Psychiatric Publishing.

3. Which of the following may be appropriate for managing the patient's current depressive symptoms?

A. Quetiapine
B. Fluoxetine
C. Olanzapine
D. Valproic acid
E. Amitriptyline

ANSWER: A

Antidepressants are frequently used despite lack of evidence for efficacy for bipolar depression. A recent meta-analysis of antidepressants in bipolar depression demonstrated a pooled effect of antidepressants that were no different from placebo. Clinical trials have demonstrated the efficacy of lamotrigine, quetiapine, olanzapine-fluoxetine combination, and lurasidone in treatment of bipolar depression. Metabolic side effects are a serious concern with quetiapine and olanzapine-fluoxetine combination and should be carefully monitored. Valproic acid is not effective to treat bipolar depression.

REFERENCE

Geddes, J. R., & Miklowitz, D. J. (2013). Treatment of bipolar disorder. *Lancet, 381*, 1672–1682.

4. The patient expresses an interest in psychotherapy to recover from depression. Which of the following psychotherapeutic modalities is efficacious as an adjunctive intervention for bipolar depression?

A. Family-focused therapy
B. Interpersonal and social rhythm therapy
C. Cognitive behavioral therapy
D. All of the above

ANSWER: D

Psychotherapy is an underutilized intervention for treating bipolar depression. The STEP-BD study compared up to 30 sessions of family-focused therapy, interpersonal and social rhythm therapy, or cognitive behavioral therapy with a brief psychoeducational therapy for patients with bipolar depression who also received mood stabilizers. Patients in intensive psychotherapy recovered more rapidly and were more likely to be clinically well than those in brief treatment. No differences emerged among the three intensive psychotherapeutic modalities in symptoms or psychosocial functioning.

REFERENCE

Miklowitz, D. J., Otto, M. W., Frank, E., et al. (2007). Intensive psychosocial intervention enhances functioning in patients with bipolar depression: Results from a 9-month randomized controlled trial. *American Journal of Psychiatry, 164*, 1340–1347.

5. The patient is successfully treated for depression with quetiapine and referred to an outpatient clinic for maintenance treatment of bipolar disorder. Which agent has the strongest evidence for relapse prevention?

A. Lithium
B. Valproic acid
C. Lamotrigine
D. Carbamazepine
E. Oxcarbazepine

ANSWER: A

Lithium is a mood-stabilizing agent in the treatment of bipolar disorder. It is efficacious in depression, mania, and euthymic maintenance. It remains the most well-established medication for long-term treatment of bipolar disorder.

REFERENCE

Geddes, J. R., & Miklowitz, D. J. (2013). Treatment of bipolar disorder. *Lancet*, *381*, 1672–1682.

6. What is the greatest risk factor for suicide attempts in bipolar disorder?

A. Female gender
B. Prior suicide attempt
C. Acute mania
D. Recurrent hospitalizations
E. Increasing age

ANSWER: B

The most consistently demonstrated risk factor for suicide in bipolar disorder is prior suicide attempt. Suicide rates are high among patients with bipolar spectrum illness. The lifetime prevalence for suicide occurs in an estimated 10% to 15% of individuals with bipolar I disorder.

REFERENCE

Coryell, W., Kriener, A., Butcher, B. et al. (2015). Risk factors for suicide in bipolar I disorder in two prospectively studied cohorts. *Journal of Affective Disorders*, *190*, 1–5.

7. The most common psychiatric comorbidity in patients with bipolar disorder is:

A. Antisocial personality disorder
B. Alcohol use disorder
C. Autism spectrum disorder
D. Delusional disorder
E. Obsessive–compulsive personality disorder

ANSWER: B

Several psychiatric comorbidities are common with bipolar disorder. The most prevalent among them are substance use disorders such as alcohol, cocaine, and opioid use disorders, anxiety disorders such as generalized anxiety disorder, social phobia and panic disorders, attention deficit hyperactivity disorder, and borderline personality disorder. Up to 45% of patients with bipolar disorder also meet criteria for alcohol use disorder. Substance use disorder comorbidity is associated with poor symptom control in bipolar disorder. Addressing psychiatric comorbidity in bipolar disorder is essential to achieving euthymia and optimal functional outcome.

REFERENCE

Krishnan, K. R. (2005). Psychiatric and medical comorbidities of bipolar disorder. *Psychosomatic Medicine*, *67*, 1–8.

QUESTIONS AND ANSWERS

This chapter has accompanying questions and answers which are available to subscribers as part of the Oxford eLearning platform. To access the questions, follow the link below, or go to http://oxford-elearning.oup.com/books.

http://oxford-elearning.oup.com/books/test/67/10.1093/med/9780190265557.003.0039

40.

CLINICAL VIGNETTE

PERSONALITY DISORDERS

Sarah Jillani

A 40-year-old woman presents to your clinic feeling panicked and depressed. She has been having multiple arguments with her ex-fiancé and has become physically assaultive toward him. She reports a rapid fluctuation of mood in response to situational stressors accompanied by superficial cutting to cope with dysphoria and anxiety. She reports feeling empty. She says she becomes very close to people quickly, but her friendships are short-lived and frequently end when she feels as though she has been let down by others. She is taking lorazepam 2 mg for anxiety, prescribed by her primary care doctor.

1. The most likely personality disorder diagnosis is:

A. Borderline personality disorder
B. Narcissistic personality disorder
C. Histrionic personality disorder
D. Avoidant personality disorder
E. Obsessive–compulsive personality disorder

ANSWER: A

Personality disorders are pervasive, begin in early adulthood, and involve clinical presentations across several contexts. Borderline personality disorder is a heterogeneous diagnostic group characterized by a dysregulation of emotions and impulses, an unstable sense of self, and difficulties in interpersonal relationships, often accompanied by suicidal and self-injurious behavior often triggered by life (particularly interpersonal) stressors.

REFERENCES

American Psychiatric Association. (2013). Personality disorders. In *Diagnostic and statistical manual of mental disorders* (5th ed., pp. 645–684). Arlington, VA: American Psychiatric Publishing.

Leichsenring, F., Leibing, E., Kruse, J., New, A. S., & Leweke, F. (2011). Borderline personality disorder. *Lancet, 377,* 74–84.

2. The prevalence of borderline personality disorder in the outpatient psychiatric setting is:

A. 1%
B. 5%
C. 10%
D. 20%
E. 30%

ANSWER: C

Borderline personality disorder is the most common personality disorder. In the primary care setting, the prevalence of borderline personality disorder is estimated at 6%, with a prevalence of nearly 10% in the outpatient psychiatric setting. A large number of individuals with the disorder are undiagnosed and untreated.

REFERENCE

Gunderson, J. G. (2009). Borderline personality disorder: Ontogeny of a diagnosis. *American Journal of Psychiatry, 166,* 530–539.

3. Which of the following statements regarding the treatment of borderline personality disorder is TRUE?

A. Psychiatrist involvement should be limited to medication prescription to prevent conflict.
B. Pharmacotherapy is the mainstay of treatment of borderline personality disorder.

C. Dialectical behavior therapy reduces self-harm, parasuicidal behavior, and suicidal ideation.
D. Long-term psychodynamic psychotherapy is the preferred nonpharmacological treatment.
E. Benzodiazepines are the preferred pharmacological treatment.

ANSWER: C

Psychiatric management is led by the psychiatrist and includes monitoring safety, responding to crises, maintaining a therapeutic framework and alliance, educating the patient regarding the disorder, coordinating treatment with multiple clinicians, and assessing effectiveness of the treatment plan. Psychotherapy is the mainstay of treatment for borderline personality disorder, augmented in some cases by symptom-targeted pharmacotherapy. Dialectical behavior therapy has been shown to be effective for self-harm, parasuicidal behavior, and suicidal ideation. Pharmacotherapy is directed toward three clusters of symptoms: cognitive-perceptual symptoms (with low-dose antipsychotics), affective symptoms (with selective serotonin reuptake inhibitors), and impulsive-behavioral dyscontrol (with selective serotonin reuptake inhibitors and low-dose antipsychotics).

REFERENCES

American Psychiatric Association. (2001). Practice guideline for the treatment of patients with borderline personality disorder. *American Journal of Psychiatry, 158*(10 suppl.), 1–52.

Leichsenring, F., Leibing, E., Kruse, J., New, A. S., & Leweke, F. (2011). Borderline personality disorder. *Lancet, 377,* 74–84.

4. The patient reveals that when she is overwhelmed with distressing and painful feelings, she frequently burns herself with cigarettes and cuts herself superficially with a razor. Which of the following is most likely achieved by these actions?

A. Emotional regulation
B. Worsening dysphoria
C. Vindication for prior injury
D. Completed suicide
E. Improved ego strength

ANSWER: A

Self-injurious behavior in patients in borderline personality disorder is incompletely understood, and it may be associated with different motivations, meanings, or goals from one patient to another or at various times in the same patient. It may produce relief of dysphoria and may be accompanied by analgesia, suggesting the release of endogenous opiates during acute intensification of dysphoric states.

REFERENCE

Reitz, S., Kluetsch, R., Niedtfeld, I., Knorz, T., Lis, S., Paret, C., ... & Schmahl, C. (2015). Incision and stress regulation in borderline personality disorder: Neurobiological mechanisms of self-injurious behaviour. *British Journal of Psychiatry, 207,* 165–172.

5. Suicide completion occurs at what rate in borderline personality disorder?

A. 1% to 2%
B. 3% to 5%
C. 8% to 10%
D. 15% to 20%
E. 20% to 25%

ANSWER: C

Personality disorders are estimated to be present in more than 30% of individuals who die by suicide, about 40% of individuals who attempt suicide, and about 50% of psychiatric outpatients who die by suicide. In clinical populations, the rate of suicide of patients with borderline personality disorder is estimated to be between 8% and 10%, a rate far greater than that in the general population. However, since 60% to 70% of patients with borderline personality disorder make suicide attempts, suicide attempts that do not result in death are far more frequent than completed suicides in patients.

REFERENCE

Oldham, J. M. (2006). Borderline personality disorder and suicidality. *American Journal of Psychiatry, 163,* 20–26.

6. What is the most common psychiatric comorbidity in borderline personality disorder?

A. Autism spectrum disorder
B. Bipolar disorder
C. Schizophrenia
D. Major depressive disorder
E. Delusional disorder

ANSWER: D

Patients with borderline personality disorder often present with symptoms of depression. It can be difficult to distinguish between borderline personality disorder and major depressive disorder, especially when the two disorders co-occur. When major depressive disorder and borderline personality disorder co-occur, both conditions should be treated concurrently. Major depressive disorder co-occurring with borderline personality disorder does not respond as well to antidepressant medication as does major depressive disorder in the absence of borderline personality disorder. Major depressive disorder is not a significant predictor of outcome for borderline personality disorder, but borderline personality disorder is a significant predictor of outcome for major depressive disorder. Whereas borderline personality disorder and bipolar disorder can co-occur, the exact rates of comorbidity have not conclusively been characterized, and clinical diagnostic practice is often inaccurate in distinguishing the two conditions. The other options are much less likely to co-occur.

REFERENCE

Yoshimatsu, K., & Palmer, B. (2014). Depression in patients with borderline personality disorder. *Harvard Review of Psychiatry, 22*, 266–273.

QUESTIONS AND ANSWERS

This chapter has accompanying questions and answers which are available to subscribers as part of the Oxford eLearning platform. To access the questions, follow the link below, or go to http://oxford-elearning.oup.com/books.

http://oxford-elearning.oup.com/books/test/67/10.1093/med/9780190265557.003.0040

41.

CLINICAL VIGNETTE

PSYCHOPHARMACOLOGY (EXTRAPYRAMIDAL SYMPTOMS)

Filza Hussain

A 45-year-old man with schizophrenia comes to your clinic for an initial assessment at the request of his family members. They are concerned about the patient pacing excessively for the past 6 weeks. On interview, when you ask him to comment on the pacing and excessive walking, he notes, "I don't know, I just have to walk to feel better." On reviewing his history further, you discover that his psychiatrist recently added a second antipsychotic, ziprasidone, to control breakthrough symptoms. In addition, his medication regimen consists of a long-acting formulation of haloperidol and benztropine twice a day. On exam he demonstrates masked facies, cogwheel rigidity and rapid darting movements of his tongue.

1. What is the most likely explanation for this man's pacing?

A. Akathisia
B. Dystonia
C. Tardive dyskinesia
D. Medication nonadherence
E. Cocaine intoxication

ANSWER: A

Extrapyramidal side effects of antipsychotics include akathisia, tardive dyskinesia, parkinsonism, and dystonic reactions. Akathisia is a subjective sense of restlessness, accompanied by the urge to move, fidgeting while seated, rocking while standing, pacing, and crossing and uncrossing the legs while sitting.

REFERENCE

Miller, C. H., & Fleischhacker, W. W. (2000). Managing antipsychotic-induced acute and chronic akathisia. *Drug Safety, 22*, 73–81.

2. Which of the following pharmacological interventions would likely alleviate this patient's pacing?

A. Increasing the dose of ziprasidone
B. Adding lurasidone
C. Adding propranolol
D. Discontinuing benztropine
E. Watchful waiting

ANSWER: C

Akathisia is a dose-dependent adverse effect, and its optimal management involves prevention. Using the lowest effective dose and slow titration can prevent incidence of akathisia. Typical antipsychotics are more likely to cause akathisia, and among the typical agents the high-potency antipsychotics most commonly cause this effect. Akathisia is also common among the atypical aripiprazole; premarketing studies suggest that a third of patients on aripiprazole will develop akathisia. When akathisia emerges, the offending agent should be cross-titrated to another antipsychotic if clinically appropriate. Propranolol or other lipophilic beta-blockers are the most consistently effective treatment for acute akathisia. Addition of benzodiazepines would be a next choice. Adding a third antipsychotic such as lurasidone, discontinuing benztropine, or increasing the dose of ziprasidone would do little to alleviate the akathisia or could worsen the akathisia.

REFERENCE

Iqbal, N., Lambert, T., & Masand, P. (2007). Akathisia: Problem of history or concern of today. *CNS Spectrums, 12*(9 suppl. 14), 1–13.
Miller, C. H., & Fleischhacker, W. W. (2000). Managing antipsychotic-induced acute and chronic akathisia. *Drug Safety, 22*, 73–81.

3. Which of the following is most likely responsible for the cogwheel rigidity observed on exam?

A. Benztropine
B. Nonadherence to benztropine
C. Ziprasidone
D. Nonadherence to ziprasidone
E. Early Parkinson's disease

ANSWER: C

Cogwheel rigidity is a sign of parkinsonism and a well-established extrapyramidal side effect of antipsychotics. High-potency typical antipsychotics such as haloperidol and fluphenazine are associated with higher rates of EPS than low-potency and atypical antipsychotics. Among the currently available atypical antipsychotics, the risk from greatest to least is ziprasidone, aripiprazole, risperidone and paliperidone, asenapine and iloperidone, olanzapine, quetiapine, and clozapine. Benztropine is effective in treating antipsychotic-induced parkinsonism, but there is no evidence of nonadherence in the history. Parkinson's disease is on the differential diagnosis, but evidence of parkinsonism while using two antipsychotic agents at high risk of extrapyramidal symptoms makes primary Parkinson's disease less likely.

REFERENCE

Owen, J. (2011). Psychopharmacology. In J. Levenson (Ed.), *Textbook of psychosomatic medicine: Psychiatric care of the medically ill* (2nd ed.). Washington, DC: American Psychiatric Publishing.

4. Dopamine receptor blockade in which of the following pathways is mostly responsible for this patient's parkinsonism?

A. Mesolimbic pathway
B. Nigrostriatal pathway
C. Tuberoinfundibular pathway
D. Nucleus accumbens
E. Mesocortical pathway

ANSWER: B

The nigrostriatal pathway mediates movement, and when a substantial number of D_2 receptors are blocked here, this will produce various disorders of movement that can appear very much like those in Parkinson's disease; this is why these movements are sometimes called drug-induced parkinsonism. The positive symptoms of schizophrenia are treated by blockade of D_2 receptors specifically in the mesolimbic dopamine pathway. D_2 receptors in the mesolimbic dopamine system are also postulated to be the normal reward system of the brain, and the nucleus accumbens is widely considered to be the "pleasure center" of the brain. Antipsychotics also block D_2 receptors in the mesocortical dopamine pathway, where dopamine may already be deficient in schizophrenia. Blockade of the mesocortical dopamine pathway can cause or worsen negative and cognitive symptoms. Of historical note, the term *neuroleptic* (literally to "seize the nerve") was derived because patients would develop parkinsonian features; it was common practice to titrate typical neuroleptics to the "neuroleptic dose," or the dose at which parkinsonian features emerged, which at the time was thought to indicate sufficient central D_2 receptor blockade.

REFERENCE

Stahl, S. M. (2013). Antipsychotic agents. In *Essential psychopharmacology* (4th ed.). New York, NY: Cambridge University Press.

5. The patient's family reports that the darting tongue movements have been present for a number of years. Which of the following is the strongest risk factor for developing such movements in this patient?

A. Male gender
B. Race
C. Age
D. Dose of antipsychotic
E. Long-term exposure to antipsychotic

ANSWER: E

The darting tongue movements are characterized as tardive (or late-appearing, akin to the word *tardy*) dyskinesia. A recent study characterized the incidence of tardive dyskinesia as 5.5% for first-generation antipsychotics and 3.9% for second-generation antipsychotics. The greatest risk factor for developing tardive dyskinesia is prolonged exposure to antipsychotics. Other risk factors include older age, female gender, cocaine abuse, and presence of an affective disorder. Tardive dyskinesia can occur in 15% to 30% of patients with prolonged exposure to antipsychotics.

REFERENCE

Mehta, S. H., Morgan, J. C., & Sethi, K. D. (2015). Drug-induced movement disorders. *Neurologic Clinics, 33*, 153–174.

6. You consider switching from the combination of long-acting injectable haloperidol and oral ziprasidone to clozapine in order to have a more effective antipsychotic regimen. Which of the following are adverse effects associated with clozapine?

A. Renal insufficiency
B. Hypothyroidism
C. Metabolic syndrome
D. AV nodal conduction delay
E. Hyperparathyroidism

ANSWER: C

Clozapine outperforms other antipsychotics in the management of schizophrenia. Two failed trials of antipsychotics should prompt consideration of clozapine, and clozapine should be considered as a first- or second-line agent when there is a high risk for suicidality and aggression. There are a number of risks associated with clozapine, including myocarditis, agranulocytosis, seizures, risk of fatal cardiorespiratory suppression, increased risk of death in dementia-related psychosis, and metabolic syndrome. The first five of these represent black box warnings for clozapine, but the fifth one in particular (mortality risk in dementia-related psychosis) is generic to all antipsychotics. The metabolic syndrome is a collection of abnormal clinical and metabolic findings, including visceral adiposity, insulin resistance, increased blood pressure, elevated triglycerides and low HDL cholesterol levels. These are predictive of diabetes and cardiovascular disease.

REFERENCE

Warnez, S., & Alessi-Severini, S. (2014). Clozapine: A review of clinical practice guidelines and prescribing trends. *BMC Psychiatry, 14*, 102.

7. Which of the following statements regarding metabolic syndrome associated with atypical antipsychotics is TRUE?

A. The increased risk of diabetes, cardiovascular disease, and obesity in patients with schizophrenia is unrelated to the prescription of atypical antipsychotics.
B. Aripiprazole poses the greatest risk of metabolic syndrome among the atypical antipsychotics.
C. The psychiatrist should defer to the patient's primary care physician for monitoring of metabolic syndrome when atypical antipsychotics are used.
D. Metabolic parameters that should be monitored while one is on an atypical antipsychotic include weight, blood pressure, fasting plasma glucose, and lipids.
E. Ziprasidone poses the greatest risk of metabolic syndrome among the atypical antipsychotics.

ANSWER: D

Many studies indicate that the prevalence of diabetes, cardiovascular disease, and obesity is much higher in people with schizophrenia than in the general population, and some of the elevated disease risk has been attributed to the metabolic side effects of atypical antipsychotics. The pathophysiology of atypical antipsychotic-induced metabolic syndrome has not been fully elucidated. Increased food intake, weight gain, hyperglycemia, and lipid accumulation in adipose and liver tissue play a role in atypical antipsychotic-induced metabolic syndrome. Clozapine and olanzapine demonstrate the most severe metabolic risk profile; quetiapine and risperidone demonstrate moderate risk; and aripiprazole, ziprasidone, and lurasidone demonstrate relatively low risk. The recommended schedule for monitoring patients on second-generation antipsychotics is at baseline, at 12 weeks, and then annually. Parameters that should be monitored include weight, blood pressure, fasting plasma glucose, and fasting lipid profile. Additionally, weight should be monitored every 4 weeks during the first 12 weeks of treatment. There is moderate evidence to support the use of metformin as a prophylactic intervention against olanzapine-induced metabolic alterations.

REFERENCE

Mitchell, A. J., Vancampfort, D., Sweers, K., van Winkel, R., Yu, W., & De Hert, M. (2013). Prevalence of metabolic syndrome and metabolic abnormalities in schizophrenia and related disorders: A systematic review and meta-analysis. *Schizophrenia Bulletin, 39*, 306–318.

QUESTIONS AND ANSWERS

This chapter has accompanying questions and answers which are available to subscribers as part of the Oxford eLearning platform. To access the questions, follow the link below, or go to http://oxford-elearning.oup.com/books.

http://oxford-elearning.oup.com/books/test/67/10.1093/med/9780190265557.003.0041

42.

CLINICAL VIGNETTE

SCHIZOPHRENIA

Michael Maksimowski

You are consulted to see a guarded and suspicious 36-year-old woman who was found by the police on the street intoxicated on alcohol and cocaine. She is admitted to the medical floor to address dehydration and malnourishment. There are no family contacts listed in the patient's chart and no past psychiatric history within her medical records. The primary care team is concerned about the patient's verbal threats toward staff, especially when vitals are checked or medications are given. The patient confides in you that the nursing staff is attempting to poison her. She appears paranoid and is scanning the room while you interview her.

1. Which of the following matters should the psychiatric consultant attend to first?

A. The patient's poor hygiene
B. The patient's verbal threats
C. A chart review of the patient's medical course since admission
D. Screening for underlying depression
E. Staff's feelings about caring for a threatening patient.

ANSWER: B

Psychiatric consultants should determine whether a consult is urgent or nonurgent. Criteria for an urgent consult include a suicide attempt, active suicidal ideation with plan or intent, a patient with agitation or violent behavior, a patient with evidence of psychosis, or a patient demanding to leave against medical advice on whom the team would like a capacity assessment. The patient's verbal threats are likely due to underlying psychosis and warrant immediate evaluation and management because they constitute a danger to others. The other problems can be addressed after safety is established.

REFERENCE

Sadock, B. J., & Sadock, V. A. (2015). Psychosomatic medicine. *Synopsis of Psychiatry* (11th ed., pp. 813–838). Philadelphia, PA: Lippincott Williams and Wilkins.

2. After evaluating the patient and reviewing the labs, you suspect cocaine-induced psychosis. Which of the following clinical symptoms is a feature of cocaine intoxication?

A. Hypotension
B. Dyskinesias
C. Psychomotor slowing
D. Miosis
E. Bradycardia

ANSWER: B

Signs of cocaine intoxication include hypertension, tachycardia, tachypnea, mydriasis, diaphoresis, motor restlessness, dyskinesias, and tremor.

REFERENCE

Sadock, B. J., & Sadock, V. A. Cocaine-related disorders. *Synopsis of Psychiatry* (11th ed., pp. 421–428). Philadelphia, PA: Lippincott Williams and Wilkins.

3. The patient's paranoid beliefs persist even after the acute intoxication syndrome resolves. It is suspected that the patient has an underlying psychotic disorder. Which of the following objective findings in this patient is considered a positive symptom of schizophrenia?

A. Ambivalence to her current situation
B. Brief responses to questions
C. Lack of emotional expression
D. Belief that the nurses are poisoning her
E. Aloofness

ANSWER: D

Symptoms of schizophrenia are categorized into positive, negative, and cognitive symptoms. Positive symptoms of schizophrenia include delusions, hallucinations, disorganized thinking or speech, and disorganized or abnormal motor behavior that may sometimes manifest as catatonia. The negative symptoms of schizophrenia are diminished emotional expression, avolition (the inability to initiate and persist in goal-directed activities), alogia (diminished speech output), and asociality (lack of interest in social interactions). Cognitive deficits are common and are linked to vocational and functional impairment. Cognitive deficits include impairment in declarative and working memory, slower processing speed, abnormalities in sensory processing, reductions in attention, and social cognition deficits such as inaccuracy in inferring the intentions of other people.

REFERENCE

American Psychiatric Association. (2013). Schizophrenia spectrum and other psychotic disorders. In *Diagnostic and Statistical Manual of Mental Disorders* (5th ed., pp. 87–122). Arlington, VA: American Psychiatric Publishing.

4. The patient is admitted to the inpatient psychiatric unit, stabilized on paliperidone, and discharged to outpatient care. After 3 months, active psychotic symptoms are evident during an outpatient visit. The patient reported that she does not like to take a pill daily. The best management strategy to improve medication adherence is:

A. Initiate clozapine
B. Provide monetary reward for adherence
C. Increase the dose of paliperidone
D. Admit to the inpatient psychiatric unit
E. Administer a long-acting injectable

ANSWER: E

Medication adherence is a challenge in chronic illnesses such as schizophrenia. About two thirds of patients discontinue medications within 1 year of initiation of medication. Long-acting injectable antipsychotics confer a number of benefits such as eliminating daily pill ingestion and the abrupt loss of medication coverage. A long-acting injectable should be considered when a patient reports good clinical response to a medication but struggles to take the medication reliably. Currently risperidone, paliperidone, olanzapine, aripiprazole, haloperidol, and fluphenazine are available in long-acting injectable formulations. Clozapine should be considered following ineffectiveness of two antipsychotics and in some cases as first- or second-line agents when the patient is at high risk for suicide or aggression. Inpatient hospitalization may be indicated if the patient poses a danger to herself or others but it would not itself increase outpatient medication adherence. Monetary reward would not be a practical solution, but food vouchers or other rewards of limited value have been used effectively as part of contingency management programs to incentivize abstinence from stimulants. Increasing the dose of oral paliperidone would not improve medication adherence.

REFERENCE

Bera, R. B. (2014). Patient outcomes within schizophrenia treatment: A look at the role of long-acting injectable antipsychotics. *Journal of Clinical Psychiatry*, *75*(suppl. 2), 30–33.

5. The patient discovers that she is pregnant and chooses to remain on the long-acting injectable formulation of paliperidone during pregnancy given the benefit she has had from the medication. You are asked to perform a consultation on her shortly after she delivers. The postpartum management of this patient involves:

A. Immediate separation of mother from the infant
B. An automatic referral to the Department of Child and Family Services
C. An automatic admission to the inpatient psychiatric unit
D. A careful evaluation of the patient, including assessing for hallucinations and delusions, and for risk of harm to herself and to the infant.
E. Immediate discontinuation of paliperidone due to breastfeeding

ANSWER: D

The evaluation of patients with schizophrenia in the postpartum setting should be thorough, and particular attention should be paid to the safety of the patient and to that of the newborn infant. Many patients with schizophrenia are safely discharged with follow-up in outpatient care. Some may require inpatient admission especially if the patient is demonstrating rapid deterioration, command hallucinations, delusions involving the baby, suicidal ideation, aggression, or risk of harm to the infant. Many women with schizophrenia are able to parent, and a diagnosis alone does not warrant a social services referral. The presence of poorly controlled symptoms, concerns regarding the baby's safety, absence of a supportive partner or family, unstable housing status, and presence of mental health problems are predictors of social services supervision and possible custody loss. Paliperidone is excreted in breast milk. The risk of infant exposure to paliperidone is unknown, and monitoring for extrapyramidal side effects in the baby is recommended. However, this would not be an indication to abruptly discontinue the medication.

REFERENCE

Jones, I., Chandra, P. S., Dazzan, P., & Howard, L. M. (2014). Bipolar disorder, affective psychosis, and schizophrenia in pregnancy and the post-partum period. *Lancet, 384*, 1789–1799.

6. Which of the following confers an increased risk of schizophrenia?

A. Chromosome 22q11.2 deletion syndrome
B. Living in a rural environment
C. Young paternal age
D. Belonging to the ethnic majority group
E. Juvenile diabetes

ANSWER: A

Environmental risk factors for schizophrenia include birth in late winter, growing up in an urban environment, and belonging to certain ethnic minority groups. There is a strong contribution of genetic factors in determining risk for schizophrenia. A spectrum of risk alleles that are both common and rare contribute to the risk. The risk alleles are associated with other mental disorders such as autism spectrum disorder, intellectual impairment, and bipolar disorder. Chromosome 22q11.2 deletion syndrome is associated with high rates of schizophrenia and is one of the strongest risk factors for developing schizophrenia.

REFERENCE

Howes, O. D., & Murray, R. M. (2014). Schizophrenia: An integrated sociodevelopmental-cognitive model. *Lancet, 383*, 1677–1687.

7. Which of the following gender-related statements about schizophrenia is TRUE?

A. The incidence of schizophrenia is slightly higher in women than in men.
B. The age of onset is later in women, with a second, midlife peak.
C. Social functioning is poorly preserved in women.
D. Negative symptoms are common in women.
E. Thought disorganization is common in women.

ANSWER: B

A number of features distinguish the clinical expression of schizophrenia in women and in men. The incidence of the disorder is lower in women. The age of onset is later in women, and there is a second, midlife peak. Symptoms in women are more affect laden. Negative symptoms and thought disorganization are infrequent. Social functioning is better preserved.

REFERENCE

American Psychiatric Association. (2013). Schizophrenia spectrum and other psychotic disorders. In *Diagnostic and Statistical Manual of Mental Disorders* (5th ed., pp. 87–122). Arlington, VA: American Psychiatric Publishing.

QUESTIONS AND ANSWERS

This chapter has accompanying questions and answers which are available to subscribers as part of the Oxford eLearning platform. To access the questions, follow the link below, or go to http://oxford-elearning.oup.com/books.

http://oxford-elearning.oup.com/books/test/67/10.1093/med/9780190265557.003.0042

43.

CLINICAL VIGNETTE

SUBSTANCE USE DISORDERS (ALCOHOL)

Shirshendu Sinha

A 45-year-old corporate lawyer presents for treatment of problem drinking. He tried alcohol for the first time at age 17, drank occasionally through college, and began drinking heavily in law school. He reports having at least 6 beers daily and drinks up to 14 drinks in a day. He often wakes up with hangovers and arrives late at work. He states, "I have this intense urge to drink and keep thinking about alcohol all the time." He misses family events, has stopped playing tennis, and spends time at a local bar. His wife has threatened to move out with their children. He has been trying to cut down on his own but has not been able to do so. He denies any prior psychiatric diagnosis. Hee scored a 24 on the Alcohol Use Disorder Identification Test. He is eager to get help and has some insight into his problem with alcohol. He is interested in a treatment program.

1. Which of the following symptoms meet *DSM-5* criteria for alcohol use disorder? (Select all that apply)

A. Daily drinking
B. Failed attempts to quit
C. Legal consequences
D. Sacrifice activities due to use
E. Failure at role fulfillment due to use
F. Family history of alcohol use disorder
G. Craving with compulsion to use
H. Recent use of alcohol
I. Alcohol Use Disorder Identification Test score of 7
J. Use of alcohol in situations where it is hazardous

ANSWER: B, D, E, G, J

The symptoms (in parentheses) described here that meet the *DSM-5* diagnostic criteria of substance use disorders include unsuccessful attempts to cut down or control use (failed attempts to quit); important social, occupational, or recreational activities are given up or reduced because of use (sacrifice activities due to use); recurrent alcohol use resulting in a failure to fulfill major role obligations at work, school, or home (failure at role fulfillment due to use); a strong desire or urge to use (craving with compulsion to use); and recurrent alcohol use in situations in which it is physically hazardous (use of alcohol in situations where it is hazardous). *DSM-IV-TR* had separated use disorders into abuse and dependence, but these diagnostic criteria were combined in *DSM-5* with some exceptions. Because presence of legal problems, which was a diagnostic criterion option in substance abuse in *DSM-IV-TR*, does not correlate with substance abuse or dependence, it was abandoned in *DSM-5*. Craving, defined as a strong desire to use a substance, was added as a new diagnostic criterion for substance use disorders in *DSM-5*.

REFERENCE

American Psychiatric Association. (2013). Substance -related and Addictive Disorders. In *Diagnostic and statistical manual of mental disorders* (5th ed., pp 481–589). Arlington, VA: American Psychiatric Publishing.

2. Results from the National Epidemiologic Survey on Alcohol and Related Conditions, a large epidemiological study in the United States, which targeted clivilian adults 18 years and older in household and selected group quarters, indicatewhich of the following? (Select all that apply.)

A. Twelve-month prevalence of alcohol use disorder is about 14%.
B. Alcohol use disorder is significantly associated with anxiety disorders.

C. Lifetime prevalence of alcohol use disorder is about 30%.
D. Lower income has an inverse relationship with prevalence of alcohol use disorder.
E. Significant associations were found between 12-month and lifetime prevalence of alcohol use disorder and other substance use disorders, major depression, bipolar I disorders, and antisocial and borderline personality disorders.

ANSWER: A, C, E

A recent epidemiological study, known as the National Epidemiologic Survey on Alcohol and related Conditions-III (NESARC-III), aimed to identify the prevalence and correlates of *DSM*-5 substance use disorders. 36,309 in-person interviews were conducted on US civilians 18, years and older of households and selected group residential quarters. The 12-month and lifetime prevalence of alcohol use disorder was estimated at 13.9% and 29.1%, respectively. The 12-month and lifetime prevalences of severe alcohol use disorder was greatest among respondents with the lowest income level. Significant associations were found between 12-month and lifetime alcohol use disorder and other substance use disorders, major depressive and bipolar I disorders, and antisocial and borderline personality disorders. Associations between alcohol use disorder and panic disorder, specific phobia, and generalized anxiety disorder were modest.

REFERENCE

Grant, B. F., Saha, T. D., Ruan, W. J., Goldstein, R. B., Chou, S. P., Jung, J....Hasin D. S. (2016). Epidemiology of *DSM-5* drug use disorder: Results from the National Epidemiologic Survey on Alcohol and Related @ Conditions-III. *JAMA Psychiatry 73*, 39–47.

3. What is the most likely diagnosis that has been presented here?

A. Alcohol abuse
B. Alcohol use disorder, mild
C. Alcohol dependence
D. Alcohol use disorder, moderate
E. Alcohol use disorder, severe

ANSWER: E

For all substances including alcohol, the *DSM-IV* diagnoses of substance abuse and substance dependence have been replaced with a single diagnosis, substance use disorder. *DSM*-5 alcohol use disorder diagnosis required at least 2 of the 11 criteria in the 12 months preceding the interview. Per *DSM-5*, a mild alcohol use disorder is suggested by the presence of@ numerals? see apa explanation for consistency within sent or par/ 2-3 criteria, moderate by@ 4-5 criteria, and severe by @6 or more criteria. The patient described in this vignette meets the diagnostic criteria for alcohol use disorder, severe.

REFERENCE

American Psychiatric Association. (2013). Substance-related and addictive disorders. In *Diagnostic and statistical manual of mental disorders* (5th ed., pp 481–589). Arlington, VA: American Psychiatric Publishing.

4. The patient reports having significant urges to use alcohol. Which of the following scales has been used in research and clinical practice to measure urges?

A. Alcohol Use Disorders Identification Test (AUDIT)@are abbs ok in these answers? see full in par below for some/
B. Alcohol Time Line Follow Back (TLFB)
C. Audit Alcohol Consumption Questions (AUDIT-C)
D. CAGE - Adapted to Include Drugs (CAGE-AID)
E. Penn Alcohol Craving Scale (PACS)

ANSWER: E

PACS is a 5-item, self-administered, instrument for assessing craving. Current craving is often used as a treatment outcome measure because it is frequently a signal of impending relapse. The@full first or second? AUDIT @same name ear in chap? is a 10-item questionnaire that screens for hazardous or harmful alcohol consumption that is suitable in primary care settings and has been used in a variety of populations and cultures. The@ TLFB is a drinking assessment method that obtains estimates of daily drinking retrospectively over a specified period. It can be used to provide feedback to increase motivation for change. The AUDIT-C is a brief @3-item questionnaire about hazardous drinking. The CAGE-AID (an acronym for cut down, annoyed, guilty, eye-opener) AID is a commonly used,@ five-item tool used to screen for drug and alcohol use.

REFERENCE

Flannery, B. A., Volpicelli, J. R., & Pettinati, H. M. (1999). Psychometric properties of the Penn Alcohol Craving Scale. *Alcoholism: Clinical and Experimental Research, 23*, 1289–1295.

Schneekloth, T. D., Biernacka, J. M., Hall-Flavin, D. K., Karpyak, V M., Frye, M. A., Loukianova, L L.,... Mrazek D. A. (2012). Alcohol craving as a predictor of relapse. *American Journal on Addictions*, *21*(suppl. 1), S20–S26.

5. Which of the following medications have been approved by the United States Food and Drug Administrtion (FDA) for the treatment of alcohol use disorder? (Select all that apply.)

A. Fluoxetine
B. Naltrexone
C. Bupropion
D. Gabapentin
E. Acamprosate
F. Topiramate
G. Disulfiram

ANSWER: B, E, G

Naltrexone, acamprosate, and disulfiram have been approved by the @but abb usec in question and elsewhere/ FDA for the treatment of alcohol use disorder. Naltrexone, is effective in reducing alcohol craving and preventing alcohol-induced relapse. Mu opiate receptor antagonism of naltrexone and resultant blocking of centrally mediated reinforcing effects of alcohol are proposed explanations for naltrexone's effectiveness. It is available as a daily oral pill or as a monthly depot injection. Acamprosate is a small, flexible molecule that resembles GABA and decreases glutamatergic neurotransmission, by acting as an *N*-methyl-D-aspartate antagonist. It has been proposed that naltrexone helps sustain abstinence in detoxified alcohol-dependent individuals by reducing neuronal hyperexcitability during early recovery. Disulfiram inhibits the enzyme aldehyde dehydrogenase. When alcohol is ingested after disulfiram, toxic levels of acetaldehyde accumulate, leading to a host of unpleasant symptoms, which are deterrents to drinking alcohol.

ADDITIONAL READING :

Kleber, H. D., Weiss, R. D., Anton, R. F., Jr., George, T. P., Greenfield, S. F., Kosten, T. R.,...Connery H. S. (2006). Practice guidelines for the treatment of patients with substance use disorders. In *Amerian Psychiatric Association's practice guidelines for the treatment of psychiatric disorders* (2nd ed., pp 491–589). Washington, DC: American Psychiatric Press

6. In addition to psychosocial interventions, which of the following medications is most effective for the maintenance of complete abstinence of alcohol?)

A. Fluoxetine
B. Naltrexone
C. Bupropion
D. Gabapentin
E. Acamprosate
F. Topiramate
G. Disulfiram

ANSWER: E

Acamprosate was approved by the FDA in 2004 to treat alcohol dependence through preventing relapse and promoting abstinence. The best evidence for a pharmacotherapeutic agent in patients seeking to remain abstinent as opposed to reducing their drinking levels is for acamprosate. Length of abstinence following treatment with acamprosate has also been demonstrated to be associated with genetic variants in GRIN2B, the gene that encodes the GluN2Bsubunit of NMDA receptors.

REFERENCE

Helton, S. G., & Lohoff, F. W. (2015). Pharmacogenetics of alcohol use disorders and comorbid psychiatric disorders. *Psychiatry Research,230*, 121–129.
Kleber, H. D., Weiss, R. D., Anton, R. F., Jr., George, T. P., Greenfield, S. F., Kosten, T. R., Connery H. S. (2006). Practice guidelines for the treatment of patients with substance use disorders. In *American Psychiatric Association's practice guidelines for the treatment of psychiatric disorders* (2nd ed.). Washington, DC: American Psychiatric Publishing.

7. Which of the following FDA-approved medications used for treatment of alcohol use disorders is more effective if administered after a period of sobriety?

A. Fluoxetine
B. Naltrexone
C. Bupropion
D. Gabapentin
E. Acamprosate
F. Topiramate
G. Disulfiram

ANSWER: E

Acamprosate was approved by the FDA in 2004 to treat alcohol dependence through preventing relapse and promoting abstinence. Data suggest that acamprosate presumably works best in controlling the desire to drink after a period of abstinence.

REFERENCE

Helton, S. G., & Lohoff, F. W. (2015). Pharmacogenetics of alcohol use disorders and comorbid psychiatric disorders. *Psychiatry Research, 230*, 121–129.

Kleber, H. D., Weiss, R. D., Anton, R. F., Jr., George, T. P., Greenfield, S. F., Kosten, T. R., Connery H. S. (2006). Practice guidelines for the treatment of patients with substance use disorders. In *American Psychiatric Association's practice guidelines for the treatment of psychiatric disorders* (2nd ed., pp. 481–589). Washington, DC: American Psychiatric Publishing.

8. Which of the following is available as a depot injection for alcohol use disorder?

A. Naltrexone
B. Gabapentin
C. Acamprosate
D. Topiramate
E. Disulfiram

ANSWER: A

Naltrexone, a mu receptor antagonist, is available as a monthly depot injection under the trade name Vivitrol® and is approved for the management of alcohol use disorder and opioid use disorder.

REFERENCE

https://www.vivitrol.com/Content/pdf/prescribing_info.pdf

9. Which of the following medications is effective in treatment for alcohol use disorder and relapse@ hy? -related symptoms of insomnia, dysphoria, and cravings?)

A. Valproic acid
B. Fluoxetine
C. Pregabalin
D. Gabapentin
E. Clozapine

ANSWER: D

Beneficial effects of gabapentin for the treatment of alcohol use disorder were found over the 12-week course of treatment on (A) the rates of complete abstinence and on rates of eliminating heavy drinking; (B) the number of heavy drinking days and the number of drinks consumed per week; and (C) severity of craving, insomnia, and dysphoria. Results followed a linear dose effect, with greatest efficacy achieved at the 1,800-mg dose. Laboratory measures of GGT provided validation of gabapentin's effects on self-reported drinking outcomes. Significant effects were found to persist after treatment in study completers who participated in the follow-up assessment that was conducted 24 weeks after initial administration. Gabapentin was well tolerated, with no deaths and no drug-related adverse effects. Gabapentin has not been approved by the FDA for the treatment of alcohol use disorders.

REFERENCE

Mason, B. J., Quello, S., Goodell, V., Shadan, F., Kyle, M., & Begovic, A. (2014). Gabapentin treatment for alcohol dependence: A randomized clinical trial. *JAMA Internal Medicine, 174*, 70–77.

10. During treatment in the residential facility, the patient agrees to take acamprosate to support abstinence. Which of the following laboratory tests should be obtained to determine the starting dose of acamprosate?

A. Complete blood count
B. Aspartate aminotransferase
C. EKG
D. Creatinine clearance
E. Serum electrolytes

ANSWER: D

Acamprosate is generally well tolerated; diarrhea is the most common side effect. Because acamprosate is exclusively excreted by the kidneys, creatinine clearance should be monitored, and caution must be taken with patients who have renal impairment.

REFERENCE

Saivin, S., Hulot, T., Chabac, S., Potgieter, A., Durbin, P., & Houin, G. (1998). Clinical pharmacokinetics of acamprosate. *Clinical Pharmacokinetics, 35*, 331–345.

11. The overactivity of which of the neurotransmitters produces symptoms of acute alcohol withdrawal?

A. Serotonin
B. Dopamine

C. Glutamate
D. GABA
E. Norepinephrine

ANSWER: C

When alcohol is removed from the body of chronic heavy regular alcohol drinkers, a "hyperglutamatergic" state develops, which in combination with reduced GABA function produces excessive excitatory signaling, contributing to the potentially life-threatening alcohol withdrawal syndrome.

REFERENCE

Holmes, A., Spanagel, R., & Krystal, J. H. (2013). Glutamatergic targets for new alcohol medications. *Psychopharmacology, 229*, 539–554.

QUESTIONS AND ANSWERS

This chapter has accompanying questions and answers which are available to subscribers as part of the Oxford eLearning platform. To access the questions, follow the link below, or go to http://oxford-elearning.oup.com/books.

http://oxford-elearning.oup.com/books/test/67/10.1093/med/9780190265557.003.0043

INDEX